PHLEBOTO...

H A N D B O O K

fourth edition

RB
45.15
. G37
1996

Diana Garza, EdD, MT (ASCP), CLS
Associate Professor
Department of Health Care Administration
College of Health Sciences
Texas Woman's University-Houston Center
Houston, Texas

Adjunct Associate Professor
Division of Laboratory Medicine
University of Texas M.D. Anderson Cancer Center

Kathleen Becan-McBride, EdD, MT (ASCP), CLS (NCA)
Professor, Department of Clinical Laboratory Sciences
Programs in Medical Technology and Clinical Cytogenetics
School of Allied Health Sciences

Professor, Department of Pathology and Laboratory Medicine
Medical School

Texas–Mexico Border Coordinator for Health Services Projects
The University of Texas–Houston Health Science Center
Texas Medical Center
Houston, Texas

Assistant Director, Greater Houston Area Health Education Center

Contributing Author: **Marilyn Wolfe-Kirk, RN**
Infection Control Coordinator
Shriners Hospital for Crippled Children
Houston, Texas

Appleton & Lange
Stamford, Connecticut

Prentice Hall International (UK) Limited, *London*
Prentice Hall of Australia Pty. Limited, *Sydney*
Prentice Hall Canada, Inc., *Toronto*
Prentice Hall Hispanoamericana, S.A., *Mexico*
Prentice Hall of India Private Limited, *New Delhi*
Prentice Hall of Japan, Inc., *Tokyo*
Simon and Schuster Asia Pte. Ltd., *Singapore*
Editora Prentice Hall do Brasil Ltda., *Rio de Janeiro*
Prentice Hall, *Upper Saddle River, New Jersey*

Library of Congress Cataloging-in-Publication Data

Garza, Diana.
    Phlebotomy handbook / Diana Garza, Kathleen Becan-McBride. — 4th ed.
        p.   cm.
    Includes bibliographical references and index.
    ISBN 0–8385–8086–6 (pbk. : alk. paper)
    1. Phlebotomy—Handbooks, manuals, etc.   I. Becan-McBride, Kathleen, 1949—   II. Title.
    [DNLM: 1. Blood Specimen Collection--handbooks.   2. Bloodletting--handbooks.   QY 39 G245p 1996]
    RB45. 15. G37   1996
    616.07′561—dc20
    DNLM/DLC   95–42358
    for Library of Congress   CIP

ISBN 0-8385-8086-6

9 780838 580868   90000

Acquisitions Editor: Cheryl L. Mehalik
Production Editor: Elizabeth Ryan
Production Service: Spectrum Publisher Services, Inc.
Designer: Libby Schmitz

PRINTED IN THE UNITED STATES OF AMERICA

To my husband, Peter McLaughlin; my children, Lauren, Kaitlin, and Kevin; and my parents for their affection, patience, and constant support.

Diana Garza

To my husband, Mark; my sons, Patrick and Jonathan; my parents; my sister; and my parents-in-law for their support and devotion.

Kathleen Becan-McBride

CONTENTS

APPENDICES

PREFACE

The overall goal of *Phlebotomy Handbook,* fourth edition, is to link the phlebotomist (i.e., the health care provider in the blood collection role—such as the nurse, phlebotomist, medical laboratory technician, and others) to the latest information, techniques, skills, and equipment for the provision of safe and effective collection procedures, for the improvement of diagnostic and therapeutic laboratory testing, for enhancement of customer satisfaction, and, ultimately, for the promotion of better health outcomes.

Currently, the entire health care industry is undergoing change, including empowering patients with more information and education, implementing major cost-containment efforts, and emphasizing improvement of the quality of care. Thus, the practice of phlebotomy is dramatically affected by these trends. The role of the phlebotomist is expanding to encompass additional patient care duties and responsibilities, a more patient-sensitive role, and better communication with patients, family members, and other members of the health care team. For example, the title *phlebotomist* has changed in many health care facilities to *clinical assistant, medical assistant, patient associate,* or *patient care technician.* Cross-training has encompassed blood collection as well as other procedures such as electrocardiograms. Many nurses have expanded their responsibilities to include blood collection for laboratory testing. The tasks of health care providers are becoming blended as health care teams work for high-quality, cost-effective, patient care.

With this in mind, the *Phlebotomy Handbook,* fourth edition, has been enhanced and revised with:

- Five new chapters—Chapter 3, "The Circulatory System;" Chapter 7, "Complications in Blood Collection;" Chapter 8, "Pediatric Phlebotomy;" Chapter 10, "Home, Hospital Bedside, and Nursing Home Collections;" Chapter 11, "Urinalysis and Body Fluid Collections"
- Updated information throughout, including blood collection equipment and techniques; legal issues and professional liability; and interpersonal communication skills
- Chapters divided into five sections that conclude with a case study relating to each chapter's content

- Key terms, objectives, and study questions with each chapter
- Color atlas including heart, veins, and artery overviews
- Second color that enhances text information

Phlebotomy Handbook has additional companion resources that are cross-referenced to the text. If sitting for certification, consider the *Phlebotomy Examination Review,* which is keyed to the *Handbook* and will aid in preparation. An *Instructor's Manual* that contains a test bank of questions, as well as other instructional material, is also available.

ACKNOWLEDGMENTS

We are indebted to many contributions from individuals, companies, and health care organizations for assistance in preparing the first, second, and third editions of this textbook. They have served as a framework from which we redesigned the fourth edition.

We are grateful to Becton-Dickinson Vacutainer System, the College of American Pathologists, the University of Texas M.D. Anderson Cancer Center, Texas Woman's University, and the University of Texas–Houston Health Science Center for their support and permission to work on this project. We particularly wish to thank our contributing author Marilyn Wolfe-Kirk, RN, for her expertise in pediatrics, Estella Woodard, MT(ASCP) and Peter McLaughlin, MD for their assistance with the venipuncture photography, Jim Lemoine for his photography services, Charlene E. Nix for assistance with graphics, and Martha Garza for her assistance in manuscript preparation. These individuals worked diligently often under short time constraints.

We are grateful to our families for tolerating the many hours we spent writing the four editions of this textbook.

OVERVIEW

I

*T*he practice of phlebotomy, like any other health professional skill, has certain characteristics that balance knowledge and theory with practical expertise. These characteristics include a recognizable definition or identity, a means of assigning tasks and responsibilities, and an established network for communication with other members of the health care team. Moreover, essential basic functions of the human body must be well understood before technical skill and expertise can be acquired. Over the years, the practice of phlebotomy has developed these characteristics in sophisticated and elaborate ways. Part I, comprising the first three chapters of this book, defines phlebotomy practice in the current environment and creates a foundation of essential knowledge of the human body. In addition, the color atlas in Part I provides illustrations pertaining to the anatomy and physiology sections.

Chapter 1, Phlebotomy and Health Care Settings, describes a working framework for the phlebotomist (e.g., nurse, patient care technician, clinical assistant) in a health care environment that is rapidly changing. Emphasis is on roles and responsibilities, on communication, and on the vital link that the phlebotomist plays in providing quality health care services.

Chapter 2, Basic Anatomy and Physiology of Body Systems, provides an overview of the structure and function of each body system. Particular emphasis is on identifying the anatomic regions of the body, the structural levels of the body, the role of homeostasis, and the relation of body functions to testing for diagnostic, therapeutic, and monitoring purposes.

Chapter 3, The Circulatory System, highlights the structures and functions of the circulatory system, as well as the specific role of the heart, vessels, and blood are described. Emphasis is on the arterial and venous system, blood flow and oxygen transport, identification of veins that are used for venipuncture, the cellular and noncellular components of blood, the phases of hemostasis, and blood pressure.

one

1

PHLEBOTOMY AND HEALTH CARE SETTINGS

Chapter Outline

Chapter Objectives
The Health Care Team and
Health Care Facilities
Organizational Structures within
Health Care Facilities
Radiology/Medical Imaging
Nuclear Medicine
Radiation Therapy
Occupational Therapy
Physical Therapy
Encephalography and
Electrocardiography
Pharmacy

Support Services
Total Quality Management
Department of Clinical
Laboratory Medicine
Clinical Laboratory Personnel
Clinical Laboratory Sections
Interdepartmental Relationships
The Laboratory in the
Physician's Office
Self Study
Key Terms
Study Questions

Chapter Objectives

Upon completion of Chapter 1, the learner is responsible for the following:

1. Identify the various types of health care facilities.

2. Describe the departments in a health care facility.

3. Identify the health care providers in the health care facilities who generally perform phlebotomy procedures.

4. Outline the role of each clinical laboratory worker and the educational level and work experience required for each position.

5. Describe the departments and sections of the clinical laboratory and the laboratory tests conducted in each area.

6. Describe the various organizational structures of clinical laboratories as they relate to the health facility's personnel, departments, and sections.

The development of new diagnostic techniques, clinical laboratory technology, and automated instruments has greatly increased the volume of laboratory testing. As a result, various health care workers (e.g., phlebotomists, laboratorians, nurses, patient care technicians, clinical assistants, health care assistants, medical assistants) are taking greater roles in phlebotomy and other specimen collection processes. The major functions of phlebotomy are to obtain patients' blood specimens by venipuncture and microcollection techniques and to facilitate collection and transportation of other clinical laboratory specimens.

Traditionally, training in blood collection techniques has usually occurred on a one-to-one basis as part of on-the-job training. However, because of the increase in the number of laboratory assays and the need for quality assurance not only of laboratory assays, but also of laboratory test results, many colleges, universities, and health care institutions have implemented blood collection courses and curricula to prepare individuals to assume the responsibilities and tasks of phlebotomy.

THE HEALTH CARE TEAM AND HEALTH CARE FACILITIES

In the past, health care was provided in physicians' offices, clinics, and hospitals. In addition, health care services were provided by numerous specialized health care workers (e.g., nurse, respiratory therapist, phlebotomist, perfusionist, nutritionist). Now, as technological advances and pressures to lower health care costs drive the health care facilities to become more patient centered, health care workers are working as a team to find the balance between quality and cost-effectiveness. As a result, the tasks of health care workers are becoming blended; for example, more nurses are taking blood samples for laboratory testing, whereas many phlebotomists have become **clinical assistants** (or **patient care technicians**) as they help with patient care duties, which include collecting patients' blood for laboratory assays.[1] Furthermore, health care and laboratory testing have expanded into numerous types of facilities. Hence, health care delivery has evolved into different levels of care that are referred to as *primary, secondary,* and *tertiary care.*[2]

Primary care is care given to maintain and monitor normal health ✔ and to prevent diseases by means of laboratory screenings and immunizations. Blood cholesterol screening, blood glucose screening, and other laboratory screening tests are examples of this level of care. Other examples include treatment of minor injuries, diagnosis and treatment of minor disorders such as a cold or a sore throat, regular checkups for infants, immunizations, prenatal care during a normal pregnancy, and treatment of chronic illnesses and diseases such as diabetes mellitus.

A primary health care physician is usually called a *family practitioner,* or a *general internist.* Other primary health care workers include nurse practitioners, nurse midwives, nurse specialists, and physician assistants (PAs). A major task of these primary health care workers is to refer patients to the correct specialist if the patient needs a higher level of care.

Secondary care is specialized care involving a physician who is an ✔ expert on a particular group of diseases, a group of organ systems, or an organ. For example, an ophthalmologist is a specialist who diagnoses and treats eye disorders exclusively.

Tertiary care is highly specialized and oriented toward unusual and ✔ complex diagnoses and therapies. Sophisticated instrumentation and technology, such as computed tomography (CT) scanners, are used in the treatment and diagnosis of patients in an acute-care hospital environment. Acute care hospitals are characterized by hospital stays of less than 30 days.

Ambulatory care is personal health care provided to an individual ✔ who is not a bed-ridden patient in a health care institution. It involves all primary care health services, including laboratory testing services, provided to noninstitutionalized patients. Once the almost exclusive domain of physicians, nurses, and dentists, ambulatory care now includes PAs, laboratory technologists, phlebotomists, optometrists, health assistants, nurse practitioners, nurse midwives, and other personnel working in a multidisciplinary team effort. Increasingly, health care in the United States is shifting from inpatient care in hospitals to ambulatory care facilities. Thus, blood and other patient specimens are being collected at a higher rate in ambulatory care facilities than in hospitals.

Ambulatory care is divided into two major categories: care provided by private physicians or group practice and care provided in an organized setting that is independent from a private practitioner or a group of practicing physicians. This latter form includes (1) hospitals that provide emergency services and outpatient clinic care; (2) emergicenters that have the same 24-hour, 7-day-a-week access that hospital emergency services provide; (3) freestanding "surgicenters"; (4) health department clinics; (5) community health centers (CHCs); (6) rural health clinics; (7) health maintenance organizations (HMOs); (8) community mental health centers; (9) school-based clinics; (10) prison health clinics; (11) multiphasic screening centers; and (12) organized home health care.

✔ A **health maintenance organization (HMO)** is a comprehensive group practice center financed by prepayment or regular monthly accounts. Facilities are usually integrated with the hospital, screening center, clinic, and physicians' offices located in one central area.

✔ **Multiphasic screening centers** provide laboratory, radiological, and electrocardiographic screening examinations for preventive medicine and

✔ early detection of disease. **Community health centers (CHCs)** offer services to the community and are supported mainly by federal funds. Almost all CHCs are primary care centers located in low-income areas, and members of the community are usually diagnosed and treated at these centers on an ambulatory basis.[3]

Many of these health care settings have on-site laboratory services. However, in some ambulatory care settings, blood and other patient specimens are sent by courier to a large independent laboratory. Thus, each member of the health care team involved in blood collection must know the proper phlebotomy techniques and procedures, as well as the protocols for transporting blood specimens to reference laboratories.

In the past, clinical laboratories with a high level of technological and organizational complexity have existed in secondary and tertiary care hospitals. However, health care reform is organizationally merging and shifting these highly technological clinical laboratories to independent sites not fixed in one hospital environment. These laboratories are receiving the patients' blood and other specimens by courier service from ambulatory and hospital settings, and subsequent test results are sent to the health care facilities through computer networks. Such changes in the health care delivery system are a result of cost-containment efforts. More health care services outside the domain of secondary and tertiary hospitals will continue to develop in order to decrease the health care costs of these highly sophisticated and technological facilities.

As a result of shifts in care to ambulatory sites and an overabundance of hospital beds, acute-care hospitals are decreasing in numbers. However, their types and functions will continue to play a role in health care delivery. Within hospitals, increased analyte testing at the bedside will continue to expand blood collection responsibilities into the realm

✔ of **patient-focused laboratory testing.** Thus, each member of the health care team involved in blood collection must learn the test procedure, quality control parameters, and preventive maintenance protocols required for patient-focused laboratory testing (see Chapter 10).

Hospitals are classified in many ways. For example, one type of classification, referred to as *clinical,* is based on the type of patients treated. Clinical hospitals include general hospitals that serve patients with various illnesses, and special-care hospitals that serve only patients with a few types of illnesses. Included in the special-care classification are pediatric, geriatric, cancer, maternity, and psychiatric hospitals.

Another type of classification for hospitals pertains to the type of ownership or control (i.e., governmental v. nongovernmental). Within the governmental classification are federal hospitals such as Veterans Administration (VA) hospitals, military hospitals, and US Public Health Service hospitals, as well as state, county, and city facilities. Governmental hospitals have a public tax base for support of health care facilities.

State hospitals usually provide long-term psychiatric and chronic (long-term) care. Also, some state hospitals are affiliated with state medical universities and thus serve as teaching facilities that provide general, acute (short-term) care. Teaching hospitals usually provide highly specialized (tertiary) services, such as organ transplantations and cardiac bypasses.[4] These hospitals are generally committed to the threefold mission of education, research, and patient care. In addition, teaching hospitals provide a disproportionate number of charity patient services.

Nongovernmental hospitals differ in ownership and thus in control. For example, the largest group of nongovernmental hospitals are referred to as *community hospitals* because they are owned by the community. The governing board includes representatives from the community and relates the needs of the community to the hospital. Other types of nongovernmental hospitals include church hospitals and privately owned hospitals.

Hospital size is commonly designated by the number of patients seen per day and the number of beds in the hospital. This bed number may be recorded as the number of adult beds, the number of pediatric beds, or both.

A new type of hospital has an institution for medical treatment and surgical needs adjacent to a hotel, or adjoining a hotel, to accommodate the patient's recovery period. The hotel provides comfortable living arrangements for the patient and his or her family, while the hospital is located nearby for follow-up medical treatment. Another new type of hospital is referred to as a p*ostoperative recovery center,* or a **long-term rehabilitation center.** Such facilities accommodate long-term recovery care for patients and are less costly because they do not have the highly technological surgical rooms and intensive-care units (ICUs) needed for acute care.

Because of the emergence of these new types of hospitals, many traditional acute-care hospitals are organizing specialty activities that focus on diagnosing and treating specific diseases such as heart disease or cancer. These services are offered on either an inpatient or an outpatient basis.

✔ Besides hospitals, a growing number of **birth centers** are providing prenatal and postpartum care for women who have normal pregnancies. Routine laboratory tests are usually performed on site; thus, phlebotomy techniques are a must in these facilities.

✔ **Home health care services** are medical services that are provided in a patient's home under a physician's direction. These services are becoming more popular because when patients are recovering from a disease, an illness, or an injury, caring for the patients at home is less costly than caring for them in a hospital. Phlebotomists, nurses, home health care assistants, and other health care workers are now being employed by companies and hospitals offering home health care services. These health care workers travel to homes throughout the community, collecting blood from patients and then transporting the blood to the clinical laboratory for testing. Various patient-focused laboratory testing is also performed in the home by these health care providers.

✔ **Medical group practices** usually consist of physicians, nurses, and other health care professionals who offer medical care to individuals in need of diagnosis and treatment. The services may be general or specific, depending on the practice group. The number of medical group and physician's office laboratories is increasing because (1) new developments in laboratory technology have produced complex laboratory analyzers that are now simple to operate and relatively inexpensive, (2) the laboratory results can be obtained while the patient is in the office, and (3) the amount of money generated by these laboratories is providing an additional incentive for physicians.

ORGANIZATIONAL STRUCTURES WITHIN HEALTH CARE FACILITIES

Health care settings are organizationally designed into departments, functional activities, or both. Traditionally, hospitals and other health care facilities have been separated by departments, which can be listed according to medical specialties, as shown in Table 1–1. More subspecialized medical departments are usually organized around organs and organ systems, as shown in Table 1–2. Alternatively, health care settings may be categorized according to the therapy or services provided to the patient (e.g., occupational or physical therapy, pharmacy).

TABLE 1–1. DEPARTMENTS FOUND IN MOST LARGE HEALTH CARE FACILITIES

Department	Brief Description
Internal medicine	General diagnosis and treatment of patients for problems of one or more internal organs
Pediatrics	General diagnosis and therapy for children
Surgery	Diagnosis and treatment in which the physician physically alters a part of the patient's body
Anesthesiology	Preparing the patient for specialized treatment and/or surgery
Pathology and laboratory medicine	Diagnosis, both before and after treatment, using anatomic and/or clinical laboratory test results
Obstetrics/gynecology	Diagnosis and treatment relating to the sexual reproductive system of females, using both surgical and nonsurgical procedures
Psychiatry/neurology	Diagnosis and treatment for people of all ages with mental, emotional, and nervous system problems, using primarily nonsurgical procedures
Radiology/medical imaging	Diagnosis and treatment, primarily through the use of x-ray, ultrasonography, and other internal imaging procedures
Allergy	Diagnosis and treatment of persons who have allergies or "reactions" to irritating agents
Geriatrics	Diagnosis and treatment of the elderly population
Oncology	Diagnosis and treatment of malignant (life-threatening) tumors
Proctology	Diagnosis and treatment of diseases of the anus and rectum
Rheumatology	Diagnosis and treatment of joint and tissue diseases, including arthritis
Family medicine/general practice	Care of medical problems of all family members so that a different physician is not necessary for each family member by age level or sex
Neonatal–perinatal	Study, support, and treatment of newborn and prematurely born babies and their mothers
Physical medicine	Diagnosis and treatment of disorders and disabilities of the neuromuscular system
Plastic surgery	Correction of the loss or deformity of tissues, including skin

As managed health care systems develop throughout the United States, the traditional departments within health care settings are restructuring by cross-training personnel to perform tasks in multiple departments. For example, a clinical laboratorian acquires responsibilities in **radiology/medical imaging** and in laboratory testing. The following sections describe major departments within health care facilities. Because patient blood collection may be required before, during, or after patient health care is provided in any one of these departments, health care workers should become familiar with all the departments.

TABLE 1–2. MEDICAL DEPARTMENTS LISTED BY ORGANS AND ORGAN SYSTEMS

Department	Organs and Organ Systems
Orthopedics	Bones and joints
Ophthalmology	Eyes
Otolaryngology	Ears, nose, and throat
Urology	Sexual and reproductive system for males and renal system for females and males
Cardiology	Heart
Dermatology	Skin
Neurology	Nervous system
Hematology	Blood system
Immunology	Immune system
Gastroenterology	Esophagus, stomach, and intestines
Nephrology	Kidneys
Endocrinology	Organs and tissues that produce hormones (e.g., estrogens, testosterone, cortisol)
Cardiovascular	Heart and blood circulation
Pulmonary	Lungs

Radiology/Medical Imaging

The radiology department uses ionizing radiation for treating disease, fluoroscopic and radiographic x-ray instrumentation and imaging methods for diagnosing disease, and radioactive isotopes for both diagnosing and treating disease (Fig. 1–1). These procedures involve fluoroscopic, tomographic, and radiographic analysis of the chest, abdomen, heart, bones, and other parts of the body with manual, automated, stationary, or mobile equipment.

Almost every patient admitted to a hospital (inpatient or outpatient), or to another health care facility, becomes a patient in the radiology department at some time during his or her stay. In radiology, patients and employees must be protected against exposure to unnecessary irradiation from radiological instrumentation. On occasion, the health care worker may need to go to the radiology department to obtain blood laboratory specimens from a patient. Thus, the phlebotomist should become acquainted with the location and the safety requirements of this department.

Radiology studies sometimes require that the patient be injected with dye. If the phlebotomist finds that the patient has received radiology dyes prior to blood collection, he or she should communicate the patient's name and possible dye interference to the clinical laboratory

Figure 1–1. X-ray equipment.

supervisor who receives the blood specimens. The supervisor can then communicate with the laboratory director, the clinical pathologist, and the attending physician to determine whether the dye will interfere in the requested laboratory assays.

Nuclear Medicine

The **nuclear medicine** department uses radioactive materials in the diagnosis and treatment of patients and in the study of the disease process. This department is primarily involved in diagnosis and in procedures requiring the introduction of a radioactive tracer into the patient, usually by intravenous injection. The resulting emitted rays are detected by sensitive crystals on the complex instrumentation, which provides sequential imaging and a graphic representation of the radioactivity. The nuclear medicine procedures differ from the radiology procedures predominantly in that the latter use rays transmitted through the patient, whereas the former use rays emitted from the patient; the result is images that provide more anatomic than functional information. As with the radiology department, the health care workers collecting blood should acquaint themselves with the location and safety requirements of the nuclear medicine department.

The radioisotopes that are introduced into a patient for nuclear medicine studies may interfere with laboratory assays. Thus, the blood collector who finds that the patient from whom he or she must collect blood is not in the hospital room, but rather in the nuclear medicine department, should ask employees in nuclear medicine if the patient has already had a radioisotopic injection. If so, the health care worker should report this information to the specimen control supervisor, who will then follow up to determine whether the injection will interfere with laboratory assays.

Radiation Therapy

✔ The department of **radiation therapy** applies high-energy x-rays, cobalt, elution, and other types of radiation in the treatment of disease, particularly cancer (Fig. 1–2). The instrumentation used in radiation therapy presents a problem of irradiation greater than that of the radiology department. Thus, safety precautions against unnecessary irradiation are extremely important for patients and employees.

Occupational Therapy

✔ The department of **occupational therapy** helps the patient to become as independently active as feasible within the limitations of his or her mental or physical disability. The occupational therapist collaborates with other health care professionals (e.g., social worker, nursing staff, at-

Figure 1–2. Radiation therapy equipment.

tending physician, physical therapist) to plan a therapeutic program of rehabilitative activities for the patient. Because the patient may spend a considerable amount of time in the occupational therapy department, health care workers who collect blood should become aware of this department's location if they must collect blood from patients who have been taken to this department to undergo therapy.

Physical Therapy

The role of the **physical therapy** department is to eliminate the patient's disability or to restore, as completely as possible, his or her mental or physical abilities that have been impaired by illness or injury. Rehabilitation within this department requires the use of heat and/or cold, water therapy, ultrasound or electricity, and other physical techniques to restore useful activity. Because patient rehabilitative services are usually extensive and time consuming, the health care worker may, on occasion, need to collect specimens in the physical therapy department.

Encephalography and Electrocardiography

Another department that the health care worker should be aware of is the **encephalography** department. The electroencephalograph (EEG) is an instrument that records brain waves. It is a sensitive instrument; therefore, the patient must be taken to a special shielded area that is protected against outside electrical or static interference.

The purpose of the department of electrocardiography is to provide a diagnostic service for the patient. The **electrocardiograph (ECG or EKG)** records the electric current produced by the contractions of the heart muscle and is used to assist in the diagnosis of heart disease or to indicate progress in recovery from heart disease.

Pharmacy

Almost everyone knows that a pharmacist dispenses medications ordered by a physician. In addition, however, the pharmacist is involved with members of the health care team as a primary consultant on drug therapy. On many occasions, the pharmacist must inform clinical laboratory personnel of a patient's blood level of a certain drug when the patient is involved in drug therapy. So that therapeutic drug levels can be monitored, blood specimens must be drawn at certain time intervals. A health care worker may be responsible for collecting the blood specimens for therapeutic drug monitoring and may need to communicate with the pharmacy department regarding the time intervals of the blood collections.

Support Services

In addition to the aforementioned departments, most hospitals and many other types of health care facilities have support services departments. These support services include the following: dietary, housekeeping, physical plant, grounds, security, information system management, purchasing, personnel, and laundry. These service departments are indirectly involved with patient care; thus, the phlebotomist will usually not be directly involved with the activities of these departments. However, health care workers involved in blood collection should be aware of these departments in their work settings.

Total Quality Management

✔ Managers of health care institutions must have some means of identifying whether quality health care is being provided to the patients. The **total quality management (TQM)** department in a health care facility usually has a total quality improvement model focused on continuous improvement in the health care facility. The improvement is to provide better quality care for the patient through better quality techniques of the health care providers.[5] The fundamental goal of TQM is to identify and take advantage of opportunities for improvement in care.

All health care workers are directly affected by TQM. Thus, it is important to become knowledgeable of the TQM department and its overall responsibilities and tasks. (These functions are discussed in greater depth in Chapter 15.)

DEPARTMENT OF CLINICAL LABORATORY MEDICINE

The rapid advances in clinical laboratory automation, procedures, and computer technology are reflected in the fact that the clinical laboratory has grown faster than most other areas in health care delivery. Sophisticated technology and automation have provided new dimensions in the diagnosis and treatment of disease.

The clinical laboratory department comprises two major areas: clinical pathology and anatomic pathology. In the clinical pathology area, blood and other types of body fluids and tissues [e.g., urine, cerebrospinal fluid (CSF), biopsy specimens, gastric secretions] are analyzed (Fig. 1–3). In the area of anatomic pathology, autopsies, cytological procedures, and surgical pathological procedures are performed. The primary purpose of the clinical laboratory is to provide patient services, but this laboratory also is usually involved in research and development and teaching so that the patient is ensured high-quality laboratory services.

Figure 1–3. Clinical laboratory areas.

Clinical Laboratory Personnel

Laboratory Directors. The laboratory personnel are frequently directed by a pathologist or a clinical laboratory scientist with a doctorate degree (Fig. 1–4). The organizational structure of the clinical laboratory is constantly being revised (Fig. 1–5); within this structure, the personnel are directed by a complementary relationship between the pathologist and the administrative technologist.

The pathologist is a physician who usually has extensive education in *pathology*—the study and diagnosis of diseases through the use of laboratory test results. He or she directs the physician–patient services of the clinical laboratory. The pathologist also has the following responsibilities: assists in establishing policies and test protocols; provides consultation services concerning laboratory results to medical-dental

Figure 1–4. Organizational structure of a typical clinical laboratory.

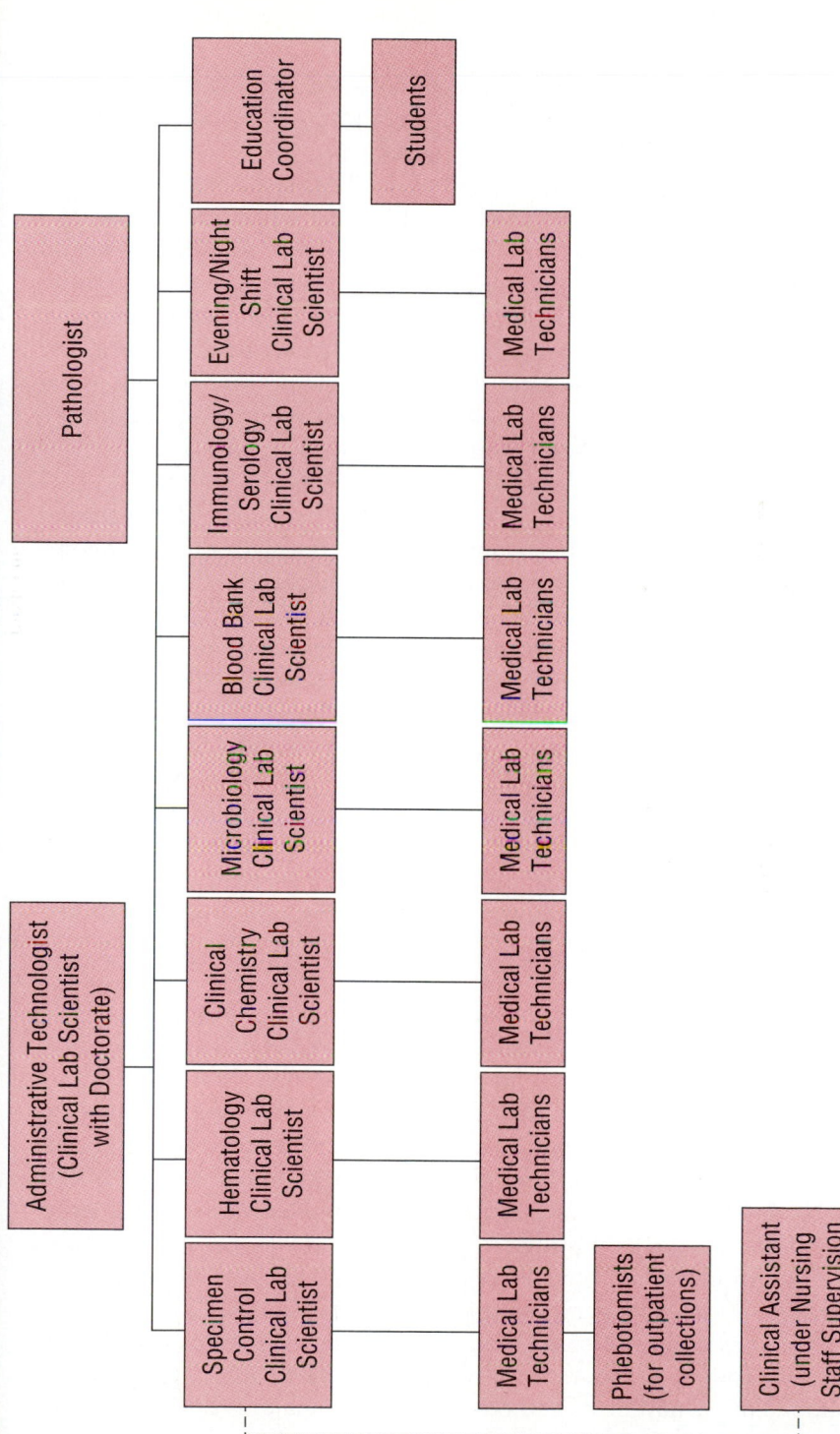

Figure 1–5. Organizational structure becoming increasingly common in clinical laboratories.

staff; teaches continuing education programs for laboratory personnel; and provides consultation on and interpretation of surgical and autopsy tissue, cytological, and bone marrow specimens.

The administrative technologist is a medical technologist (or clinical laboratory scientist) who has had additional education in management and administration. He or she is the director of administrative and technical services. The administrative technologist also has the following responsibilities: sets up laboratory procedures and policies; employs laboratory personnel; performs budgetary functions of the laboratory; and provides for orientation and training of new personnel, continuing education of technical and supervisory staff, and assignment of duties to personnel commensurate with their qualifications.

Technical Supervisors of Clinical Laboratory Sections. The technical supervisor in each of the clinical laboratory sections is a clinical laboratory scientist with additional experience and education in his or her section, such as specimen control, hematology, microbiology, or clinical chemistry. He or she assumes the following responsibilities: prepares daily work schedules to provide adequate coverage and effective use of personnel; maintains levels of supplies and reagents commensurate with the workload; ensures that clinical laboratory personnel follow policies and procedures; provides technical instructions and training of personnel in his or her section; supervises personnel in his or her section; maintains a current procedural manual; assists the administrative technologist in budget preparation; and recommends to the administrative technologist the selection, transfer, discipline, and discharge of personnel.

✔ *Clinical Laboratory Scientist (Medical Technologist).* The **clinical laboratory scientist (CLS),** who is also referred to as a *medical technologist (MT),* has a bachelor's degree in a biological science, which includes 1 year or more of study in a CLS program. Some states have licensing examinations for CLSs. Many CLSs become certified by passing national certification examinations. With this educational background, the CLS may become a technical supervisor once he or she acquires work experience in the clinical laboratory.

The duties and responsibilities of the CLS include the following: performs various chemical, microscopic, microbiological, or immunologic tests pertaining to patient care and diagnosis; records and reports test results following laboratory procedures; participates in research and development of new test methods; assumes a major responsibility for preventive maintenance, troubleshooting, and quality control of instruments and safety conditions in the clinical laboratory; participates in continuing education and in-service programs; and assists in teaching pathology residents and medical technology and medical laboratory technician students.

Medical Laboratory Technician. The **medical laboratory technician (MLT),** who is also referred to as a *clinical laboratory technician (CLT),* is a graduate of a 2-year certificate or associate degree MLT program. Some states require licensing of the MLT and have a licensing examination for this category. Many MLTs become certified by passing MLT or CLT national certification examinations.

Under supervision by a CLS and/or a technical supervisor, the MLT performs routine tests and procedures in any assigned laboratory department. He or she records and reports results, following laboratory procedures, and notifies the supervisor about any abnormal results. Other duties and responsibilities include the following: prepares specimens for reference laboratories, prepares reagents as needed, draws blood as required, observes safety procedures and maintains the laboratory area and equipment, and participates in continuing education and in-service programs.

Phlebotomist. Usually, the **phlebotomist** must have a high school diploma or its equivalent to enter phlebotomy training. The training varies from one health care center to another and may require a few weeks to months, depending on the institution. The phlebotomist may become certified by passing a national certification examination.

Under the supervision of the specimen control technical supervisor, the phlebotomist has the following typical duties and responsibilities:

1. Collects adequate and correct blood specimens by venipuncture or microtechnique on adults, children, and infants
2. Follows departmental policies to correctly identify the patient before any blood specimen is drawn and to correctly label all specimens drawn
3. At all times shows concern for and understanding of the patient and promotes the comfort and well-being of the patient as much as possible while performing collection duties (patience and persistence are needed when the phlebotomist is dealing with patients from whom blood specimens are difficult to obtain)
4. Starts glucose tolerance procedures and collects remaining specimens at required times; draws other timed specimens as indicated
5. Picks up a variety of clinical specimens other than blood and delivers them to the laboratory

6. Sorts and processes specimens received in the central specimen receipt area of the department; is responsible for orderly and timely flow of specimens to the technical areas
7. Maintains accurate and orderly log records and worksheets, where required, according to established departmental and hospital protocol
8. Projects an image of professionalism in appearance and conduct at all times

Clinical Assistant. The clinical assistant usually must have a high school diploma or its equivalent. He or she is a phlebotomist who works on a particular hospital floor or in a specific section and who has interdisciplinary health care team responsibilities. In addition to obtaining and transporting patients' blood specimens for laboratory testing, he or she is responsible, under the supervision of the nursing staff director, for direct patient care (e.g., transporting meals to patients, transporting patients in wheelchairs to physical therapy).

Clinical Laboratory Sections

✔ *Clinical Chemistry.* The **clinical chemistry** section is one of the largest areas in the clinical laboratory. In this section, the laboratory procedures that are conducted (Table 1–3) include the quantitative measurement of serum proteins, blood glucose, serum lipids (triglycerides, cholesterol), serum iron and iron-binding levels, serum electrolytes (sodium, potassium, bicarbonate, chloride), blood gases [partial pressure of oxygen (P_{O_2}), partial pressure of carbon dioxide (P_{CO_2}), pH, serum creatinine, blood urea nitrogen (BUN), vitamins (ascorbic acid, vitamin B_{12}, folic acid), and enzymes lactate dehydrogenase (LD), alanine aminotransferase (ALT), creatine phosphokinase (CPK)]. Also, the clinical chemistry section usually has a toxicology area for drug analysis and an area for hormone analysis. Other procedures generally included in clinical chemistry are bilirubin and liver function analysis, and CSF and gastric fluid analysis.

The clinical chemistry section has become highly automated; thus, most of the chemical procedures use less patient's blood for each analysis than was used originally. Automation has greatly increased the efficiency and quality assurance within the clinical chemistry section (Fig. 1–6, page 25).

✔ *Hematology.* In the **hematology** section, laboratory assays are used to identify diseases of blood-forming tissues. In addition, other processes can be evaluated through changes in the blood. Coagulation tests, clinical microscopy, and urinalysis are frequently performed in the hema-

Plate 1. Superficial anatomy of the heart. Anterior (sternocostal) view of the heart showing major anatomic features. (Coronary arteries are shown in red, coronary veins in blue.) *(From Martini FH:* Fundamentals of Anatomy and Physiology, *3rd ed. Englewood Cliffs, NJ, Prentice Hall, 1995, p 685, with permission.)*

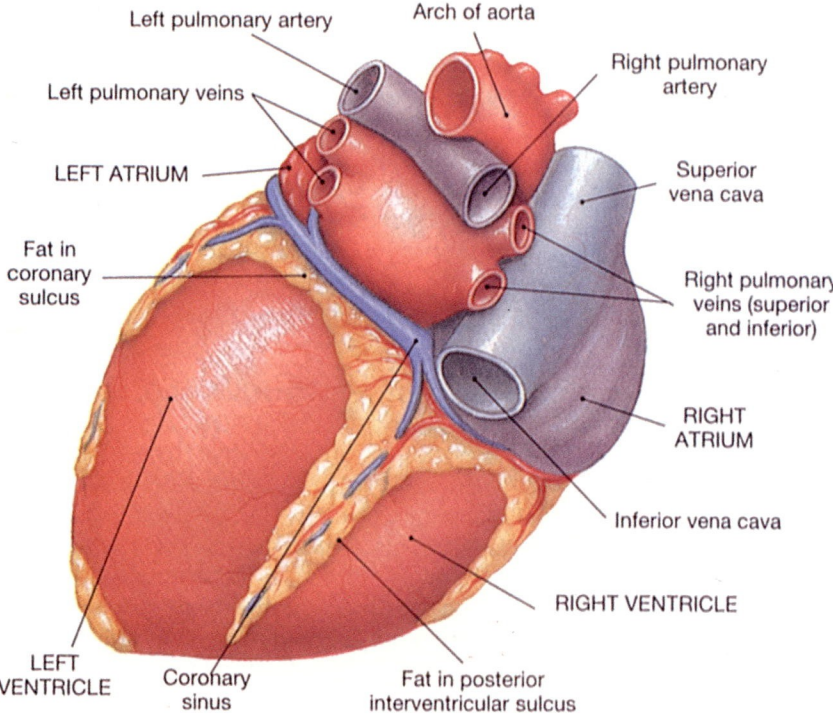

Left pulmonary artery

Arch of aorta

Right pulmonary artery

Left pulmonary veins

LEFT ATRIUM

Superior vena cava

Fat in coronary sulcus

Right pulmonary veins (superior and inferior)

RIGHT ATRIUM

Inferior vena cava

RIGHT VENTRICLE

LEFT VENTRICLE

Coronary sinus

Fat in posterior interventricular sulcus

Plate 2. Superficial anatomy of the heart. The posterior (diaphragmatic) surface of the heart. (Coronary arteries are shown in red, coronary veins in blue.) *(From Martini FH:* Fundamentals of Anatomy and Physiology, *3rd ed. Englewood Cliffs, NJ, Prentice Hall, 1995, p 685, with permission.)*

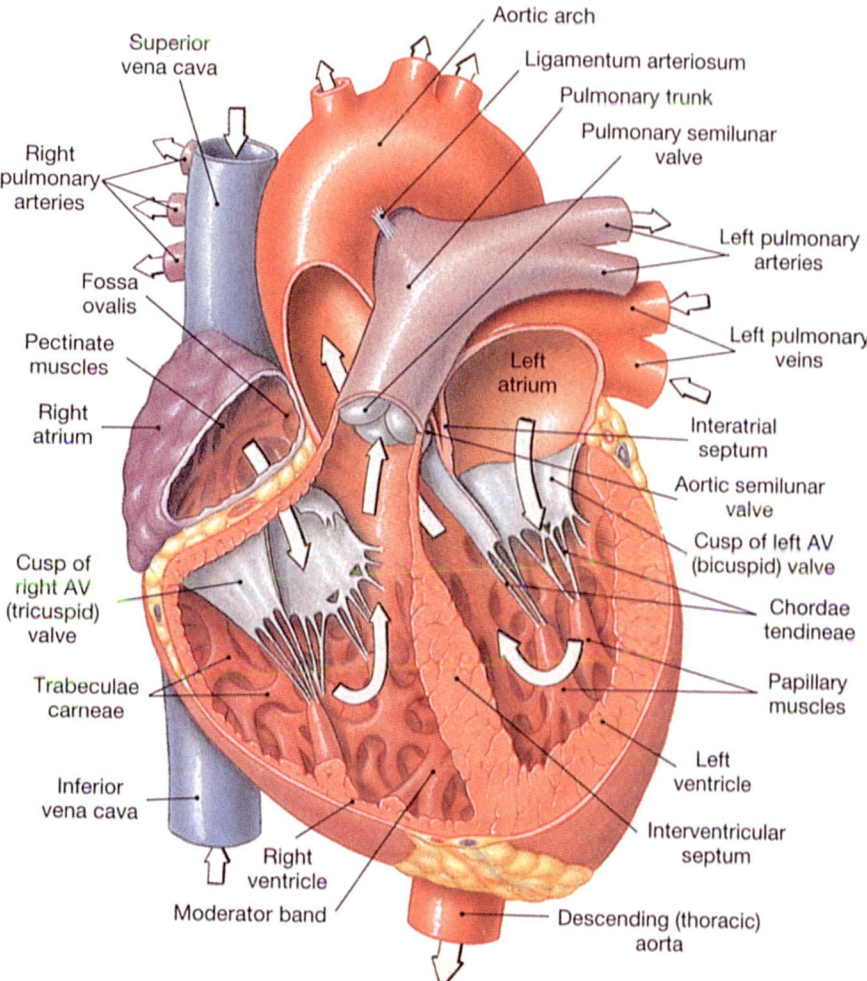

Plate 3. Sectional anatomy of the heart. A diagrammatic frontal section through the heart showing major landmarks and the path of blood flow through the atria and ventricles. *(From Martini FH:* Fundamentals of Anatomy and Physiology, *3rd ed. Englewood Cliffs, NJ, Prentice Hall, 1995, p 686, with permission.)*

Plate 4. The pulmonary circuit. *(From Martini FH: Fundamentals of Anatomy and Physiology, 3rd ed. Englewood Cliffs, NJ, Prentice Hall, 1995, p 750, with permission.)*

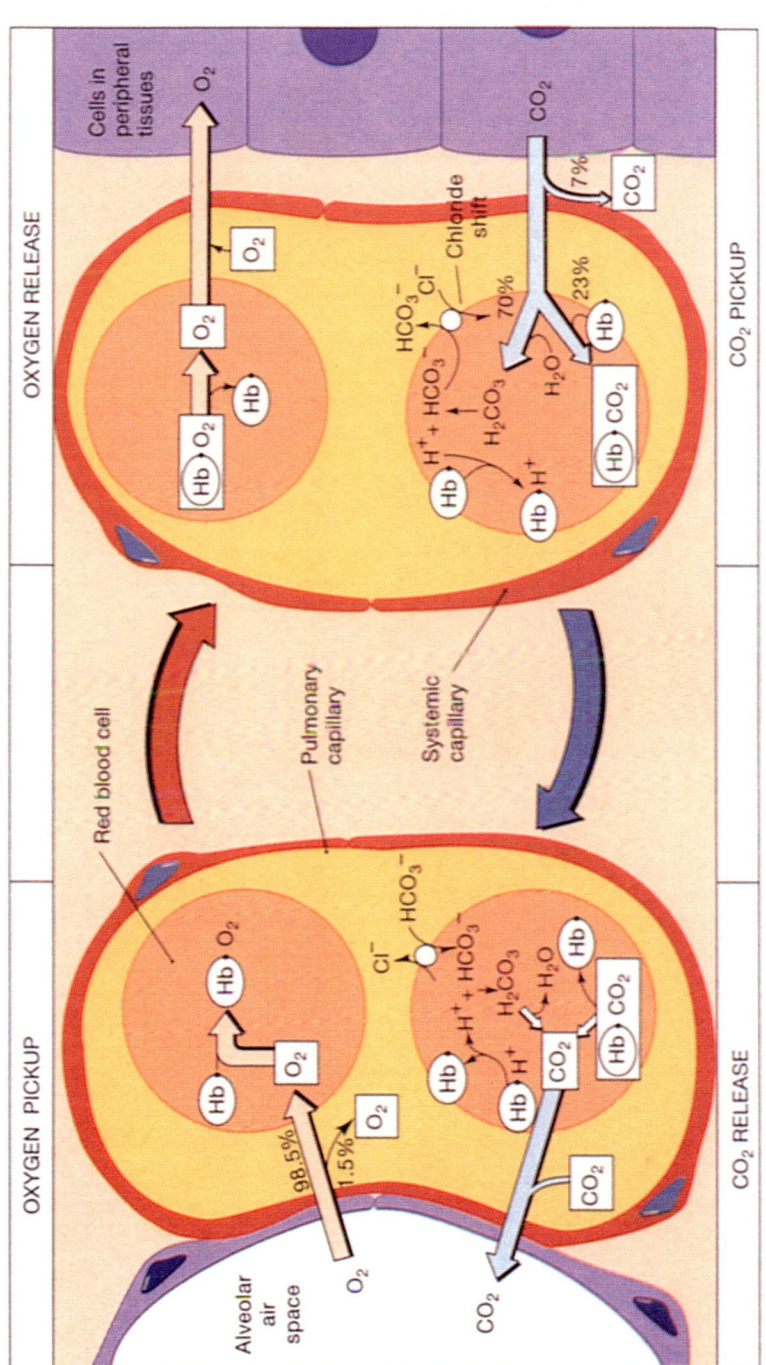

Plate 5. A summary of the primary gas transport mechanisms. *(From Martini FH: Fundamentals of Anatomy and Physiology, 3rd ed. Englewood Cliffs, NJ, Prentice Hall, 1995, p 862, with permission.)*

Plate 6. An overview of the arterial system. *(From Martini FH:* Fundamentals of Anatomy and Physiology, *3rd ed. Englewood Cliffs, NJ, Prentice Hall, 1995, p 751, with permission.)*

Plate 7. An overview of the venous system. *(From Martini FH:* Fundamentals of Anatomy and Physiology, *3rd ed. Englewood Cliffs, NJ, Prentice Hall, 1995, p 761, with permission.)*

Plate 8. Venous drainage of the abdomen and chest. *(From Martini FH:* Fundamentals of Anatomy and Physiology, *3rd ed. Englewood Cliffs, NJ, Prentice Hall, 1995, p 763, with permission.)*

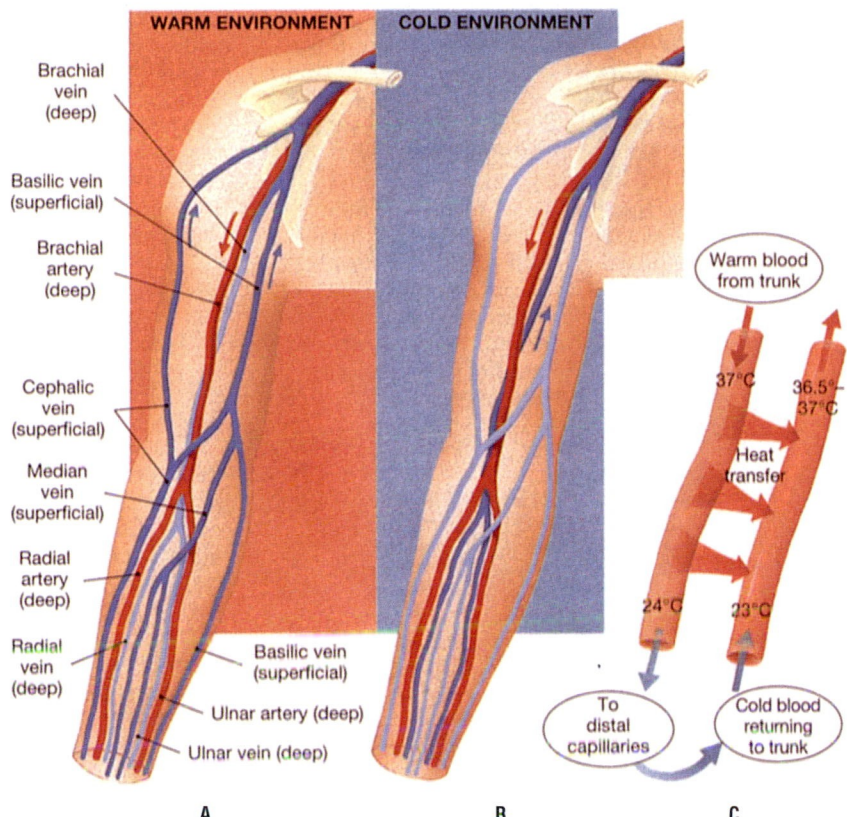

Plate 9. Circulation through vessels of the forearm in warm and cold environments. **A.** Circulation through the blood vessels of the forearm in a warm environment. Blood enters the limb in a deep artery and returns to the trunk in a network of superficial veins. These veins radiate heat into the environment through the overlying skin. **B.** Circulation through the blood vessels of the forearm in a cold environment. Blood now returns to the trunk via a network of deep veins that flow around the artery. The amount of heat loss is reduced, as is indicated in **C.** **C.** Countercurrent heat exchange occurs as heat radiates from the warm arterial blood to the cooler venous blood flowing in the opposite direction. By the time the arterial blood reaches distal capillaries, where most of the heat loss to the environment occurs, it is already 13°C cooler than it was when it left the trunk. This mechanism reduces the rate of heat loss while conserving body heat. In effect, the countercurrent exchange traps heat near the trunk. *(From Martini FH:* Fundamentals of Anatomy and Physiology, *3rd ed. Englewood Cliffs, NJ, Prentice Hall, 1995, p 971, with permission.)*

	Additive	Laboratory Use
Purple/ Lavender:	*Dry EDTA (K$_2$) (Potassium) *Dry EDTA (Na$_2$) (Sodium) *Liquid EDTA (K$_3$) (Potassium)	Whole blood or plasma hematology procedures. Tube inversion must occur for proper mixing.
Light Blue:	*3.8% Na (Sodium) citrate *3.2% Na (Sodium) citrate	Whole blood for routine coagulation procedures. Tube inversion must occur for proper mixing.
Red:	*None	Serum for chemistry, serology/immunology, and blood banking procedures.
Gray:	*Potassium Oxalate/ sodium fluoride *Sodium fluoride *Potassium oxalate *Lithium iodoacetate *Lithium iodoacetate/ lithium heparin	Whole blood or plasma required for glucose determinations. Glycolytic inhibition of specimen occurs to stabilize glucose results for up to 24 hours at R.T. for lithium iodoacetate and up to 3 days with sodium fluoride. Tube inversion should occur for proper mixing.

Plate 10. Color-coded blood collection tubes.

	Additive	Laboratory Use

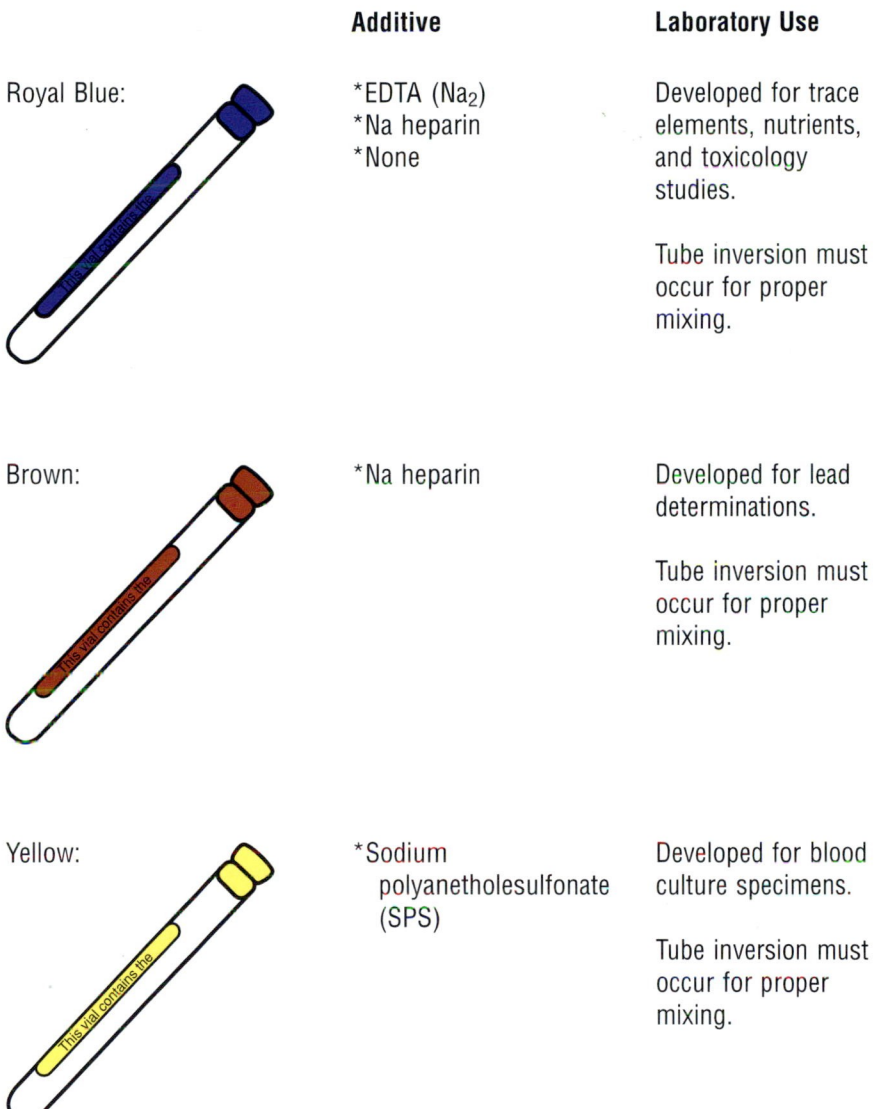

Royal Blue:

*EDTA (Na$_2$)
*Na heparin
*None

Developed for trace elements, nutrients, and toxicology studies.

Tube inversion must occur for proper mixing.

Brown:

*Na heparin

Developed for lead determinations.

Tube inversion must occur for proper mixing.

Yellow:

*Sodium polyanetholesulfonate (SPS)

Developed for blood culture specimens.

Tube inversion must occur for proper mixing.

Plate 10. Color-coded blood collection tubes (*continued*).

	Additive	**Laboratory Use**
Green:	*Li (Lithium) heparin *NH$_2$ (Ammonium) heparin *Na (sodium) heparin	Plasma required in chemistry and cytogenetics. Tube inversion must occur for proper mixing.
Black:	*3.8% Buffered Na (Sodium) Citrate	Whole blood for the hematology procedure— Westergren Sedimentation Rate
Yellow/Black Red/Green Red/Yellow Green/Black:	*Mottled tubes have gel barriers	Dependent upon manufacturer, the mottled tube colors indicate gel barrier with or without anticoagulants.

Plate 10. Color-coded blood collection tubes (*continued*).

TABLE 1–3. SUMMARY OF MAJOR TESTS PERFORMED IN THE CLINICAL LABORATORY SECTIONS

Clinical Chemistry Procedures

Total proteins

Glucose and glucose tolerance

Glycated hemoglobin

Triglycerides

Total cholesterol

HDL cholesterol

Iron

Total iron-binding capacity (IBC or TIBC)

Electrolytes [sodium (Na^+), potassium (K^+), chloride (Cl^-), bicarbonate (HCO^-)]

Magnesium

Blood gases [pH, partial pressure of carbon dioxide (P_{CO_2}), partial pressure of oxygen (P_{O_2})]

Creatinine

Uric acid

Blood urea nitrogen (BUN)

Enzymes [e.g., lactate dehydrogenase (LD), alanine aminotransferase (ALT), creatine phosphokinase (CPK)]

Drug analysis (e.g., gentamicin, tobramycin, primidone, phenytoin, digoxin, quinidine, salicylates, blood alcohol, barbiturates)

Bilirubin

Hormones [e.g., thyroxine (T_4), insulin, testosterone, luteinizing hormone, parathyroid hormone, prolactin, cortisol]

Clinical Microbiology Procedures

Acid-fast bacilli (AFB) smear	Fungus direct smear	Ova and parasites
Anaerobic culture	GC culture	Pinworm preparation
Culture and sensitivity (C&S)	Gram staining	Stool culture
AFB culture	Occult blood	Strep screening
Fungus culture	Nose/throat culture	Urine culture
Blood culture		

Hematology and Coagulation Procedures

CSF cell count	Hemoglobin	RBC count
Differential	Hemoprofile	Reticulocyte count
Eosinophil count	LE cell preparation	Sedimentation rate
Fecal leukocyte count	Nasal eosinophil count	Sickle-cell preparation
Hematocrit	Platelet count	WBC count
CBC	Partial thromboplastin time (PTT)	Thrombin time
Fibrin split product	Prothrombin time (PT)	
Fibrinogen		

TABLE 1–3. SUMMARY OF MAJOR TESTS PERFORMED IN THE CLINICAL LABORATORY SECTIONS (*continued*)

Clinical Microscopy and Urinalysis Procedures		
Hemosiderin	**Routine UA**	Synovial fluid analysis
Pregnancy test		Seminal fluid analysis

pH	Bilirubin	
Specific gravity	Nitrites	
Protein	Urobilinogen	
Sugar	Ascorbic acid	
Ketones	Occult blood	
	Leukocytes	

Immunohematology Procedures (Transfusion Medicine)		
ABO and Rh$_O$ (D) typing	Antibody screen indirect	Rh phenotyping and
ABO grouping	Coombs' test	genotyping
Antibody identification	Antibody titer	Rh$_O$ (D) typing
Hepatitis B core antigen and antibody	Direct Coombs' test	
Hepatitis B surface antigen (HB$_S$Ag) and antibody		
HIV-1 testing		

Clinical Immunology/Serology Procedures		
Amebiasis screening	Cold agglutinins	Rheumatoid factor
Antinuclear antibody (ANA)	CSF/VDRL	RPR
ASO screening	Syphilis antibody (FTA-ABS)	RPR quantitative
ASO titer	Infectious mononucleosis	*Salmonella* agglutinins
Brucella antibody	MHA-TP	Q fever
C-reactive protein	*Proteus* OX antibodies	
Borrelia burgdorferi (Lyme disease) antibody	Rubella HIA	
Francisella tularensis antibody		
Legionnaires' disease antibody		

Abbreviations: ASO, anti-streptolysin O; CBC, complete blood count; CSF, cerebrospinal fluid; FTA-ABS, fluorescent treponemal antibody absorption; GC, gonococcus; HDL, high-density lipoprotein; HIA, hemagglutination-inhibition antibody; HIV-1, human immunodeficiency virus—type 1; LE, lupus erythematosus; MHA-TP, microhemagglutination–*Treponema pallidum;* RBC, red blood cell; RPR, rapid plasma reagin; UA, urinalysis; VDRL, Venereal Disease Research Laboratory; WBC, white blood cell.

tology section. Hematologic results are extremely valuable diagnostic tools and are an integral part of a patient's examination. Most health care facilities require that the hematologic assay referred to as the *complete blood count (CBC)* be run on every individual admitted as a patient to the health care facility. The five components of the CBC count are as follows:

Figure 1–6. Johnson & Johnson clinical diagnostic E9501RC analyzer. *(Courtesy of Johnson & Johnson Co., Rochester, NY.)*

1. Red blood cell (RBC) count
2. White blood cell (WBC) count
3. Hemoglobin (Hgb or Hb)
4. Hematocrit (Hct or Crit)
5. Differential white count (Diff)—manual or automated

Other assays evaluated in the hematology section include the reticulocyte count, the erythrocyte sedimentation rate (ESR), and the erythrocyte indices [mean corpuscular volume (MCV), mean corpuscular hemoglobin (MCH), and mean corpuscular hemoglobin concentration (MCHC)]. Many of these assays are automated, and a blood specimen can be tested simultaneously for various hematologic parameters (Fig. 1–7).

Coagulation tests, usually performed in the hematology section, are conducted to determine the clotting ability of the blood. The two most common coagulation assays are prothrombin time (PT) and partial thromboplastin time (PTT). Screening tests and confirmatory assays for classic hemophilia are performed in the coagulation area. Also, other procedures, such as platelet counts and fibrinogen assays, help to detect coagulation problems such as disseminated intravascular coagulation (DIC) disease.

The clinical microscopy and urinalysis area uses microscopic and chemical procedures to screen urine specimens for abnormalities. Generally, each patient admitted to a health care facility must have a uri-

Figure 1–7. Coulter Counter systems. *(Courtesy of Coulter Electronics, Inc., Hialeah, FL.)*

nalysis performed on his or her random sample. (See Chapter 11 for urine collection information.) Assays performed on a urine specimen include the determination of pH, specific gravity, protein, sugar, ketones, bilirubin, nitrites, urobilinogen, ascorbic acid, and occult blood levels. Also, a microscopic examination may be performed to identify the presence or absence of crystals, casts, WBCs, and RBCs.

✔ *Clinical Microbiology.* Personnel in the section of **clinical microbiology** have the principal task of culturing and identifying bacterial pathogens and their toxins. In addition, personnel in this section evaluate bacterial sensitivity to a particular antibiotic; thus, when a microbiological specimen is collected, the physician usually requests a culture and sensitivity (C&S) test. (*Sensitivity* refers to the inhibition of bacterial growth by an antibiotic.)

The bacterial pathogens are classified according to (1) how they appear after Gram staining; (2) the shape of the microorganisms—rod-shaped (bacilli), circular-shaped (cocci), or spiral-shaped (spirochetes); and (3) the microorganisms' requirements for oxygen (aerobic) or lack of oxygen (anaerobic). Major methods for analysis in this section include determining (1) how these microorganisms grow in culture, (2) their biochemical properties, and (3) the sensitivity of the microorganisms to antibiotics.

In addition to analyzing bacterial pathogens, personnel in the clinical microbiology section identify pathogenic parasites, fungi, and viruses, and often they perform the occult (hidden) blood test (guaiac test). This procedure tests for blood in feces (stool), urine, and other patient secretions.

The specimens for microbiological analysis may be highly infectious and thus are considered biohazardous. Extreme caution and care must be taken in collecting and processing these specimens.

Clinical Immunology/Serology. The **clinical immunology/serology** section has the major tasks of running procedures to determine antigen–antibody reactions and identifying diseases having antigen–antibody pathogenesis. Common serological tests run in the clinical immunology/serology section include the Venereal Disease Research Laboratory (VDRL), rapid plasma reagin (RPR), fluorescent treponemal antibody absorption (FTA-ABS), cold agglutinins, febrile agglutinins, rubella, anti-streptolysin O (ASO) titer, anti–DNase B, fungus antibody, and Monospot (Ortho Diagnostics, Raritan, NJ) tests. As an example of diseases that are identified in this section, the VDRL and RPR tests are used to identify syphilis. The FTA-ABS test is a procedure used to confirm a syphilitic infection with spirochetes. The cold aggutinins test is mainly for primary atypical pneumonia. The febrile agglutinins procedure is used to test for typhoid fever, paratyphoid, brucellosis, and tularemia. The ASO titer is used to test for a streptococci infection, and Monospot tests are for infectious mononucleosis.

Blood Banking (Immunohematology)—Transfusion Medicine. The blood bank, sometimes referred to as **immunohematology,** or *transfusion medicine,* has the major task of providing blood products to patients. These blood products, collected from volunteer donors and given to the patients (recipients), include whole blood, packed RBCs, platelets, and fresh frozen plasma. Before blood may be given to patients, the donor and the recipient must have their blood grouped and typed. In addition, other procedures run in the blood bank include the antibody screening test, the Rh antibody titer test, the direct antiglobulin (Coombs') test, the human immunodeficiency virus (HIV) procedure, and the hepatitis B surface antigen (HB_SAg) test.

✔ *Cytology.* In the **cytology** section of the laboratory, body fluids and other tissue specimens are processed for detection and diagnostic interpretation of cell changes that might indicate cancer. The cytology section also usually screens Pap smears for early diagnosis of malignant diseases of the female genital tract.

Histology. The preparation and processing of tissue samples removed during surgery, autopsy, or other medical procedures are the primary
✔ tasks of personnel in the **histology** section. Following preparation of the tissue, the anatomic pathologist microscopically examines and evaluates the patient's tissue sample.

✔ *Cytogenetics.* In the **cytogenetics** section, detailed study of individual chromosomes (Fig. 1–8) that detect relationships to clinical disease, both congenital and acquired, is undertaken. The cytogenetic tasks re-

Figure 1–8. Photograph of karyotype. *(Courtesy of University of Texas, M.D. Anderson Hospital, Division of Laboratory Medicine, Houston, TX).*

quire competence in preparing specimens of peripheral blood, bone marrow, solid tissue, and amniotic fluid through cell cultures and chromosomal analysis. On occasion, the phlebotomist may draw blood specimens for chromosomal analysis.

Deoxyribonucleic Acid Probe Analysis. The **deoxyribonucleic acid** ✔
(DNA) probe analysis section is a fairly new section in the clinical laboratory. Depending on the type of health care facility, personnel in this section may run tests for genetic disorders, malignant disorders, infectious pathogens, or DNA fingerprinting in forensic medicine. The genetic disorders that have been diagnosed with DNA probes include sickle-cell anemia, Duchenne muscular dystrophy, and cystic fibrosis.[6] Some leukemias and lymphomas can be identified and classified with the use of DNA probes; for example, HIV is an infectious pathogen that can be detected with such analysis. Because DNA probe technology is expected to grow rapidly in the next few years, most likely the nurse, the phlebotomist, the clinical assistant, or another health care provider will collect many blood specimens for this section of the clinical laboratory.

Education and Research. The large clinical laboratory usually conducts ongoing research in the development of new procedures recently described in the medical literature, as well as basic research contributing to the clinical laboratory sciences. This work is performed by the pathologists, medical technologists, and other doctorate staff.

In addition to research, the large clinical laboratory department generally provides, or is affiliated with, a university for teaching programs. The educational programs include (1) a pathology residency program to teach physicians the subspecialty of pathology; (2) a medical technology program to teach qualified college seniors or graduates the concepts, theories, and techniques of clinical laboratory sciences; (3) a medical laboratory technician program to train college freshmen and sophomores the basic techniques and concepts in clinical laboratory sciences; and (4) a phlebotomy program to train individuals to collect blood.

The department of **clinical laboratory medicine,** with its various ✔
sections, may be a department within a health care facility or may be a consolidated laboratory of various health care facilities that serves many institutions and facilities by using courier services and computer technology (Fig. 1–9).[7] Also, some departments of clinical laboratory medicine are converting into specialized laboratories to enhance technological advances and to provide cost-effectiveness for patients. Thus, phlebotomists collecting blood specimens may be involved in transporting the specimens to various specialized laboratory facilities (Fig. 1–10).

Figure 1–9. Consolidated laboratory.

INTERDEPARTMENTAL RELATIONSHIPS

Clinical laboratory test results provide important data to the physician for diagnosing and monitoring patients and depend on smooth interrelationships with all other hospital departments. For example, a physician requests laboratory tests to be performed on a patient. The laboratory tests are performed upon admission of the patient to the hospital. When the patient's specimens and the requisition slips specifying the clinical laboratory procedures to be performed arrive at the clinical laboratory, they are sent to the appropriate section(s) for analysis. The test results are recorded in the clinical laboratory and returned to the patient's medical chart to be reviewed by the attending physician. This information must be as timely as possible, and coordination between the clinical laboratory and the nursing staff is important. The appropriate charges for the laboratory tests are directed to the patient's account at the business office.

Information resulting from the laboratory test requires that clinical laboratories coordinate activities with other hospital departments such as nursing, pharmacy, and dietary. Because the effects of diet and medication(s) on laboratory test results have been well documented, coordination and cooperation among the laboratory, medical staff, nursing staff, dietary department, and pharmacy are required to prevent false test results. This team of health care providers must be aware of the total patient care plan in relation to the clinical laboratory collection and test procedures so that laboratory test results can be efficiently used for the best possible patient care.

THE LABORATORY IN THE PHYSICIAN'S OFFICE

As discussed earlier, physician's office and medical group laboratories are increasing in numbers throughout the United States. Each group practice of physicians has unique office laboratory needs owing to its subspecialty. For example, a medical group of internists specializing in

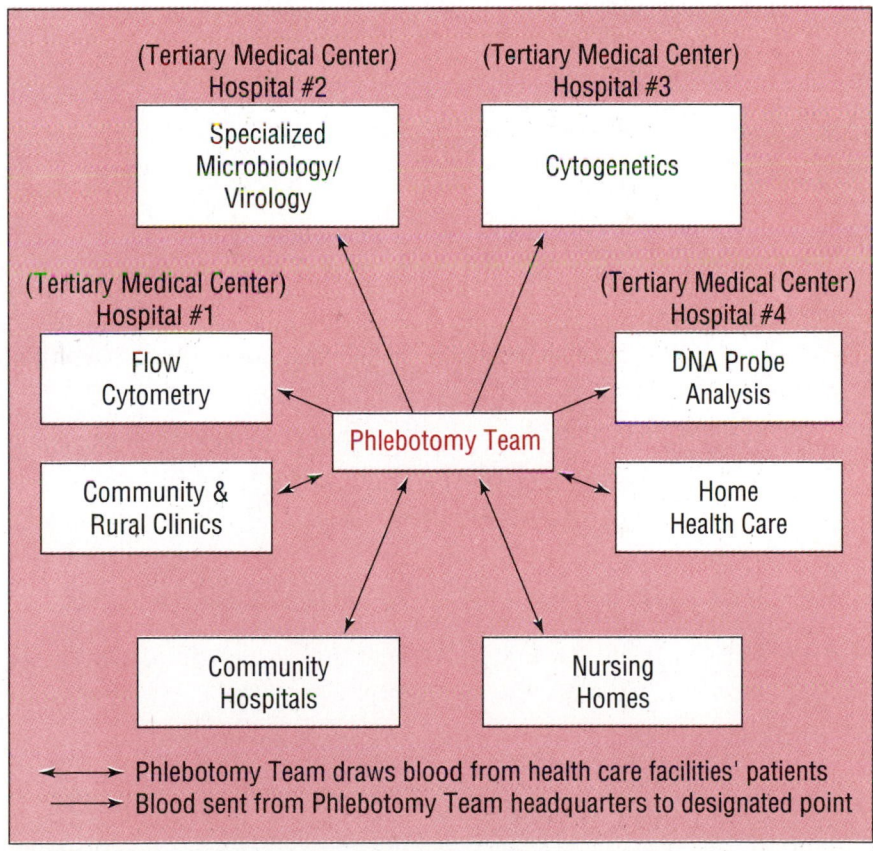

Figure 1–10. Specialized laboratory testing.

medical care of the diabetic patient needs laboratory tests for glucose monitoring, whereas obstetric group practices need laboratory assays related to pregnancy testing. In addition, because the laboratory services are provided only for the office patients, the office laboratories are usually small and have all the clinical laboratory areas (e.g., clinical chemistry, hematology, clinical microbiology) located in one room. The blood collector working in a medical group or physician's office laboratory will frequently need to acquire multidisciplinary laboratory skills to assist in all phases and areas of laboratory testing.

✔ Key Terms

Ambulatory Care

Birth Centers

Clinical Assistants

Clinical Chemistry

Clinical Immunology/Serology

Clinical Laboratory Medicine

Clinical Laboratory Scientist (CLS)

Clinical Microbiology

Community Health Centers (CHCs)

Cytogenetics

Cytology

Deoxyribonucleic Acid (DNA) Probe Analysis

Electrocardiograph (ECG or EKG)

Encephalography

Health Maintenance Organization (HMO)

Hematology

Histology

Home Health Care Services

Immunohematology

Long-Term Rehabilitation Center

Medical Group Practices

Medical Laboratory Technician (MLT)

Multiphasic Screening Centers

Nuclear Medicine

Occupational Therapy

Patient Care Technicians

Patient–Focused Laboratory Testing

Phlebotomist

Physical Therapy

Primary Care

Radiation Therapy

Radiology/Medical Imaging

Secondary Care

Tertiary Care

Total Quality Management (TQM)

Study Questions

1. In which of the following hospital departments is ionizing radiation used for treating diseases and fluoroscopic and radiographic x-ray instrumentation used for diagnosing diseases?
   a. radiology
   b. radiation therapy
   c. nuclear medicine
   d. occupational therapy

2. The electroencephalograph (EEG) is an instrument that records
   a. the electric current produced by contraction of the heart muscle
   b. brain waves
   c. signals from the skeletal muscles

3. Which of the following clinical laboratory sections performs the VDRL test?
   a. clinical chemistry
   b. hematology
   c. clinical immunology
   d. clinical microbiology

4. Blood glucose determinations are usually performed in which of the following laboratory sections?
   a. clinical chemistry
   b. hematology
   c. clinical immunology
   d. clinical microbiology

5. Of the following personnel, which individual is sometimes referred to as a *clinical laboratory scientist?*
   a. medical laboratory technician
   b. medical technologist
   c. phlebotomist

6. Which of the following is/are primary health care provider(s)?
   a. nurse
   b. nurse midwife
   c. cardiologist
   d. internist

7. Which of the following refer(s) to primary care?
   a. computed tomography
   b. blood glucose screening
   c. immunizations
   d. prenatal checkup

8. ICU is an abbreviation for
   a. interactive computer unit
   b. intravascular cardiac unit
   c. intensive-care unit
   d. interaxial computerized unit

9. ALT is performed in which clinical laboratory section?
   a. clinical microbiology
   b. hematology
   c. clinical chemistry
   d. urinalysis

10. The Diff is classified as what type of procedure?

    a. urinalysis   c. clinical immunology

    b. hematology   d. immunohematology

REFERENCES

1. Parsons ML, Murdaugh CL: *Patient-Centered Care: A Model for Restructuring*. Gaithersburg, MD, Aspen Publishers, 1994.
2. Rakich JS, Longest BB, Darr K: *Managing Health Services Organizations*. Baltimore, Health Professions Press, 1992.
3. Himmelstein DU, Woolhander S: A national health program for the United States. *N Engl J Med* 320:102, 1989.
4. Kovner A: *Health Care Delivery in the United States*. New York, Springer-Verlag, 1990.
5. Gaucher EJ, Coffey RJ: *Total Quality in Healthcare: From Theory to Practice*. San Francisco, Jossey-Bass, 1993.
6. Beyler SA: Diagnosis of genetic diseases in the preimplantation embryo. *Lab Med* 24:643–647, 1993.
7. Steiner J, Root J, Burk E: Lab regionalization: Structural options for the age of managed competition. *Med Lab Observ* July:48–51, 1994.

two

BASIC ANATOMY AND PHYSIOLOGY OF BODY SYSTEMS

Chapter Outline

Chapter Objectives

Upon completion of Chapter 2, the learner is responsible for the following:

1. Describe the anatomic surface regions and cavities of the body.

2. Identify the eight structural levels of the human body.

3. Describe the role of homeostasis in normal body functioning.

4. Describe the purpose, function, and structural components of the 11 body systems.

5. Recognize examples of disorders associated with each body system and the common diagnostic tests associated with each system.

ANATOMIC REGIONS

The human body has distinctive characteristics; that is, a backbone, bisymmetry, body cavities, and 11 major organ systems: integumentary, skeletal, muscular, nervous, respiratory, digestive, urinary, reproductive, endocrine, lymphatic, and cardiovascular. This chapter highlights the basic **anatomy** (structural components of the body) and **physiology** (functional components) of each system except the cardiovascular system, which is covered in Chapter 3.

Body regions can be categorized in various ways. One way is to begin at the top and to work down. In this manner, the body can be described as having the following regions:[1]

- Head and neck
- Upper torso
- Lower torso (female and male)
- Back
- Arms
- Legs
- Hands and feet

The body can also be described by surface regions, body planes, and body cavities. The front, **anterior,** or **ventral** surface of the body is separated into thoracic, abdominal, and pelvic cavities. The back, **posterior,** or **dorsal** surface is divided into cranial and spinal cavities. Each of these cavities houses one or more organs. Areas and directions of the body can be described by their distance from or proximity to one of the **body planes** (Fig. 2–1 and Table 2–1). The **sagittal plane** runs lengthwise from front to back, dividing the body into right and left halves. The **frontal plane** runs lengthwise from side to side, dividing the body into anterior and posterior sections. The **transverse plane** runs crosswise, or horizontally, dividing the body into upper and lower sections. **Medial** means toward the midline, and **lateral** means toward the sides of the body. *Normal anatomic position* refers to an erect standing position with arms at rest and palms forward.

STRUCTURAL ORGANIZATION

The design of the human body is elaborate and sophisticated. A human body can be divided into eight structural levels (Fig. 2–2): atoms; molecules (chemical constituents); small structures within cells, or organelles; cells (the basic living units of all plants and animals); tissues (groups of similar cells); organs (two or more tissues); organ systems (groups of organs); and the organism (the human body) itself. Trillions of cells make

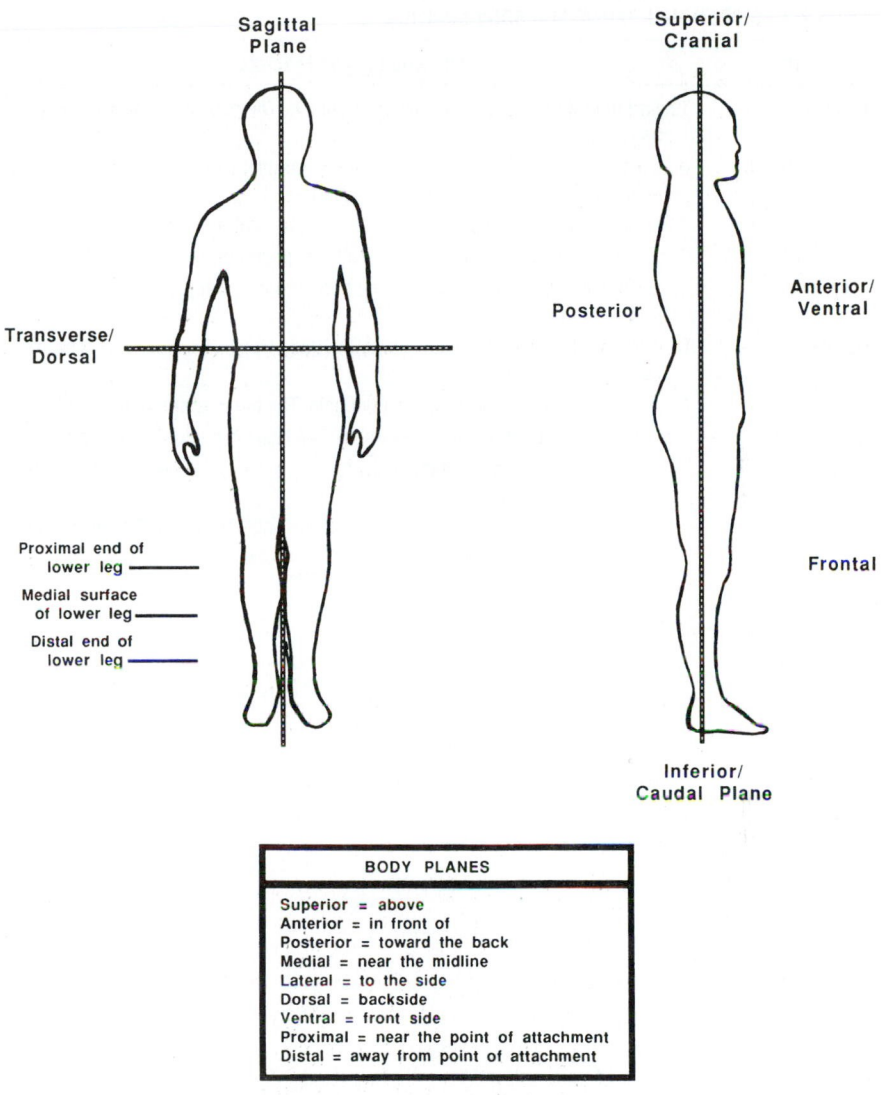

Figure 2–1. Body planes.

up each individual. Similar groups of cells are combined into tissues such as muscles or nerves, and tissues are combined into systems such as the circulatory or reproductive system. These organ systems work simultaneously to serve the needs of the body. No one system works independently of the others.

TABLE 2–1. DIRECTIONAL TERMS FOR BODY POSITION

Term	Description and Example
Right/Left	Toward the right/left side of the body. (Example: The patient has scar tissue on the right arm.)
Inferior/Superior	A structure or organ below/above another. (Example: The forehead is superior to the nose. The nose is inferior to the eyes.)
Anterior (ventral)	Front of the body. (Example: Toes are anterior, or ventral, to the heel.)
Posterior (dorsal)	Back of the body. (Example: The spinal cord is posterior, or dorsal, to the heart.)
Proximal	Closer to the point of attachment to the body trunk. (Example: The knee is proximal to the ankle.)
Distal	Farther from the point of attachment to the body trunk. (Example: The toes are distal to the ankle.)
Lateral	Away from the midline of the body. (Example: The hip is lateral to the navel.)
Medial	Toward the midline of the body. (Example: The heart is medial to the arms.)
Superficial	Closer to the outer surface of the body. (Example: Skin is superficial to muscles or bone.)
Deep	Internal or farther from the outer surface of the body. (Example: The heart and lungs are deep organs.)

Eight Levels of Organization

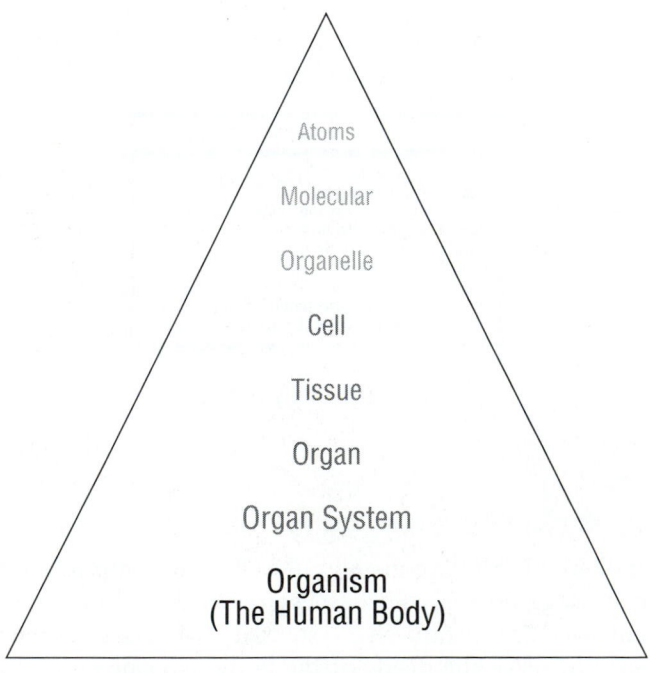

Figure 2–2. Eight levels of organization.

Before the major organ systems and their functions are discussed, a basic understanding of the human cell is necessary. Figures 2–3 and 2–4 illustrate a basic cell and its structures and some examples of specific cell morphologies. The size and shape of a cell depend on its function. Some cells fight disease-causing viruses and bacteria; some transport gases such as oxygen (O_2) and carbon dioxide (CO_2); some produce movement, store nutrients, or manufacture proteins, chemicals, or liquids; and others, such as the egg and the sperm, can create a new life. At the same time, other cells contribute to thoughts and emotions. Despite such diverse functions, several cells have basic structural elements in common. The cell membrane encloses the contents of the cell. This membrane serves as a protective barrier that selectively allows certain substances to move in or out. Nutrients and O_2 are taken in through the membrane only when needed, and wastes are eliminated as they build up. Most cells also have a **nucleus,** which is enclosed inside a nuclear membrane. The nucleus (*nuclei* for two or more) is commonly thought of as the control mechanism of the cell that governs the functions of the individual cell (i.e., growth, repair, reproduction, and metabolism). Inside the nucleus is a **nucleolus** and threadlike chromatin, which also aide in cell metabolism and reproduction. The nucleus contains a blueprint of itself in the genetic material so that it can reproduce itself when

Endoplasmic reticulum
Vacuole
Nucleolus
Mitochondria
Centriole
Nucleus
Lysosome
Vacuole
Cytoplasm
Golgi apparatus
Cell membrane

Figure 2–3. Basic cellular structure and components.

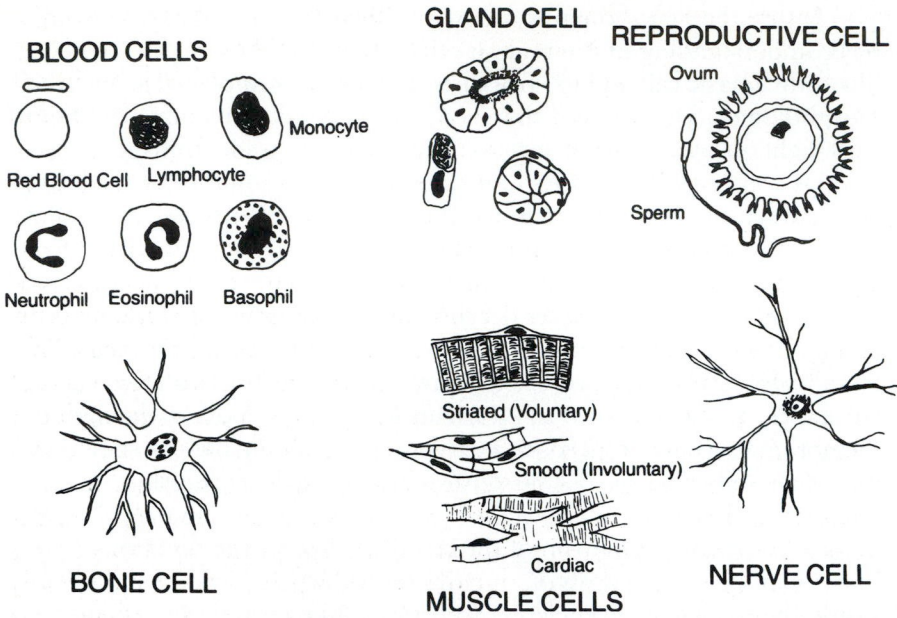

Figure 2–4. Various cell structures.

necessary. If the nucleus of a cell is damaged or destroyed, in most cases the cell will die. However, even though red blood cells (RBCs) lose their nuclei when they mature, the cells continue to live and carry O_2 for several months. Another component of the cell, the **cytoplasm,** contains mostly water with dissolved nutrients and fills up the rest of the cell membrane. Within the cytoplasm are smaller structures called *organelles*. The names and functions of these organelles are as follows:

- **Mitochondria.** Produce energy for the cell.
- **Ribosomes.** Assemble amino acids into proteins.
- **Endoplasmic reticulum.** Acts as transport channel between the cell membrane and the nuclear membrane.
- **Lysosomes.** Release digestive enzymes into vacuoles, or small pouches, for digestion of food particles.
- **Golgi apparatus.** Stores proteins.
- **Centriole.** Plays a role in cell division.

Cells communicate with each other in sophisticated reactions using electrical impulses (such as from one nerve cell to another) or in chemical reactions that result in the release of hormones or other enzymes and proteins to stimulate a particular function. The study of cellular structures and processes has captivated clinical laboratory scientists for years. With technologies such as flow cytometry, amplification of genetic material, and specific probing, the ways of seeking information about cellular functions continue to expand.

Deoxyribonucleic acid (DNA) is a long molecule commonly described as a *double helix* or *twisted ladder*. The molecule contains thousands of genes, which carry the code for an individual's genetic makeup, such as eye color, sex, and height. An individual's DNA contains the *DNA-coded blueprint* that was inherited from that person's parents. Genes also instruct the body to make the proteins needed to sustain life. Although each nucleus has a complete set of genes (except the egg and the sperm, each of which contains half a set), only certain genes are used in each cell to perform the cell's specific functions. DNA also duplicates exact copies of itself. An individual's DNA directs the development, growth, and functioning of all body systems and makes each individual's body unique, except in the case of identical twins.

Survival is the primary function of the human body, and many complex processes work independently and together to achieve this function. In human physiology, the body strives for a steady state, or homeostasis. Literally, *homeostasis* means "remaining the same." It is a condition in which a healthy body, although constantly changing and functioning, remains in a normal, healthy condition. Homeostasis, or a steady-state condition, allows the normal body to stay in balance by compensating with changes. For example, if the body is taking in too much water, it responds to this imbalance by excreting water from the kidneys (urine), skin (perspiration), intestines (feces), and lungs (water in expiration) (Fig. 2–5). A healthy body maintains constancy of its chemical components and processes in order to survive. Each organ system and body structure plays a part in maintaining homeostasis.

Another important function of the human body is metabolism. This process involves making necessary substances or breaking down chemical substances in order to use energy. Catabolism is a series of chemical reactions produced in cells to change complex substances into simpler ones while simultaneously releasing energy. This process provides energy for all body functions, whether for moving a chair or for allowing a heart to beat. Conversely, anabolism is a process by which cells use energy to make complex compounds from simpler ones. It allows synthesis of body fluids such as sweat, tears, saliva, and chemical constituents (enzymes, hormones, and antibodies). Both phases are required to maintain metabolic functions in a healthy individual.

Figure 2–5. Homeostasis.

As mentioned previously in a normal, healthy body, structural and functional aspects work together. Organization of all the body structures, such as cells, tissues, organs, and systems, together with proper functioning, such as digestion, respiration, circulation, nerve sensitivity, movement, and secretion, provide for a healthy individual. Systems working together can keep a body metabolizing properly and in homeostasis, which is the basis of survival.

Laboratory testing can provide a wealth of information about the individual organ systems and the integrated processes. Specimens, such as blood, bone marrow, urine, cerebrospinal fluid (CSF), pleural fluid, biopsy tissue, seminal fluid, and others, can be microscopically analyzed, assayed, and cultured to determine pathogenesis.[1,2]

MAJOR BODY SYSTEMS

This section summarizes the functions of the organ systems (Fig. 2–6). For each body system, a corresponding figure provides a brief summary of the structure, function, disorders, and diagnostic tests for that system.

Integumentary System

The **integumentary system** consists of the skin, hair, sweat and oil glands, teeth, and fingernails (Fig. 2–7). It is primarily involved in protective and regulatory functions. Intact skin protects the deeper tissues by providing a barrier to entering microorganisms and foreign bodies and by protecting such tissues from heat, cold, and other hazardous exposures. The skin also prevents water loss or allows for perspiration as needed by the body during exercise, fever, or weather conditions. Sebaceous glands in the skin produce oils for hair and skin protection, and sweat glands produce perspiration, which helps cool the body as needed and eliminates some waste. **Melanin** in the skin provides skin color and protects underlying tissues from absorbing ultraviolet rays. Ultraviolet light stimulates production of inactive vitamin D in the skin. The liver and kidneys then activate vitamin D so that it is beneficial to the body. Other functions of the skin are to store fat in the layers next to the underlying tissues and to allow an individual to experience sensations such as touch, temperature, pain, and pressure. Hair on the head provides protection by acting as a heat insulator, eyebrows keep perspiration out of the eyes, eyelashes protect eyes from foreign objects, and hairs in the nasal passages filter out dust and harmful microorganisms.

BODY FUNCTIONS				
Protection, Support, and Movement	Control and Regulation	Fluids and Transport	Environmental Exchange	Birth
BODY SYSTEMS				
Integumentary Skeletal Muscular	Nervous Endocrine	Cardiovascular Lymphatic	Respiratory Digestive Urinary	Reproductive

Figure 2–6. Body functions and systems.

Components:
- Skin, sweat and oil glands
- Hair
- Fingernails
- Teeth

Functions:
- Protects underlying tissues
- Regulates body temperature
- Eliminates some wastes
- Receives sensory stimuli such as touch, pressure, temperature, pain
- Prevents water loss

Disorders:
- Acne
- Burns
- Carcinoma and other skin cancers
- Fungal infections
- Herpes
- Impetigo
- Keloid
- Pediculosis
- Pruritus
- Psoriasis

Diagnostic Tests:
- Biopsies
- KOH preparations for skin scrapings
- Tissue cultures
- Microbiological cultures

Figure 2–7. Integumentary system.

Likewise, fingernails protect the tips of the hands. Teeth aide in breaking up food to begin the digestive process.

Integumentary system disorders include bacterial infections such as acne, impetigo (caused by *Staphylococcus aureus*), and decubitis ulcers; viral infections such as fever blisters or cold sores, rubeola, rubella, chickenpox, and herpes zoster (shingles); fungal infections such as ringworm and athlete's foot; allergic reactions such as dermatitis and eczema; psoriasis; and skin cancers such as malignant melanoma.

Diagnostic tests for many of these conditions involve skin scrapings; bacteriologic, viral, or fungal tissue cultures; potassium hydroxide (KOH) preparations; or biopsy staining procedures.

Skeletal System

The skeletal system refers to all bones and joints of the body. This system comprises primarily two types of tissue: bone and cartilage. Bone is composed of cells surrounded by calcified intercellular substances that allow for a rigid structure. Cartilage is composed of similar cells, but these cells are surrounded by a gelatinous material, instead of calcified substances, that allows for more flexibility. Likewise, tendons and ligaments provide flexibility and leverage. The skeletal system serves the body in five major ways: support, protection for softer tissues (brain and lungs), movement and leverage, hematopoiesis (blood cell formation) in the bone marrow, and mineral storage (Fig. 2–8).

More than 200 bones are contained in the human body, and they are classified into four groups on the basis of their shapes. Long bones include leg bones (e.g., femur, tibia, fibula) and arm and hand bones (e.g., humerus, radius, ulna, phalanges). Short bones include carpals and tarsals, or wrist and ankle bones, respectively. Among flat bones are several cranial bones, the ribs, and the scapulae (or shoulder blades). Finally, irregular bones include cranial bones (e.g., sphenoid, ethmoid) and bones of the vertebral column (e.g., vertebrae, sacrum, coccyx).

Bones are connected to each other by a variety of joints that permit flexion, extension, abduction (away from median), adduction (toward median), rotation, and combinations of these movements (Fig. 2–9). Bone structure differs between male and female skeletons. Besides being somewhat larger and heavier, the male has a pelvis that is deeper with a narrow pubic arch. In contrast, the female pelvis is shallow and broad and has a wider pubic arch to facilitate childbirth.

In general, bones consist of several layers covered by a membrane, the periosteum. The periosteum contains blood vessels that bring blood from inside to the outer layer. The outer layer, compact bone, is more rigid and heavier than the inner layer, which is like a honeycomb. This inner layer is called *spongy bone* but is just as strong as compact bone. In the center of a bone is the marrow, which produces most blood cells. Approximately 5 billion RBCs are produced daily by about ½ lb (227 g) of bone marrow. Marrow is located in all the bones of an infant, but in adults it is in the skull, sternum (or breastbone), vertebrae, hipbones, and ends of the long bones.[1]

Components:
- Bones
- Cartilage
- Tendons
- Ligaments
- Joints

Functions:
- Provides support
- Protects organs
- Allows leverage and movement
- Produces blood cells
- Stores minerals

Disorders:
- Arthritis
- Bursitis
- Gout
- Osteomyelitis
- Osteoporosis
- Rickets
- Tumors

Diagnostic Tests:
- Alkaline phosphatase (ALP)
- Calcium
- Complete blood cell (CBC) count
- Erythrocyte sedimentation rate (ESR)
- Phosphorus
- Synovial fluid analysis
- Uric acid
- Vitamin D

Figure 2–8. Skeletal system.

Minerals stored in bones include calcium and phosphorus. When these minerals are needed in other parts of the body, they are released from bone through the bloodstream.

Skeletal system disorders include inflammatory conditions such as arthritis and bursitis; gout; bacterial infections such as osteomyelitis; porous bone conditions such as osteoporosis; developmental conditions such as gigantism, dwarfism, and rickets; and bone tumors. Laboratory assessment of skeletal system disorders can include serum calcium and phosphate levels, serum alkaline phosphatase (ALP) levels, uric acid, vitamin D, erythrocyte sedimentation rate (ESR), complete blood cell (CBC) counts, microscopic analysis, and microbial cultures of the bone marrow and synovial fluid (fluid between joints and bones).

Muscular System

The **muscular system** refers to all muscles of the body, including those ✔ attached to bones and those along walls of internal structures such as the heart. On the basis of location, microscopic structure, and neural

Figure 2–9. Skeleton. *(From Guy JF: Learing Human Anatomy: A Laboratory Text and Workbook. Norwalk, CT, Appleton & Lange, 1992, p 15, with permission.)*

✔
✔
✔ control, muscles are classified as follows: (1) skeletal (striated voluntary) muscles—attached to bones; (2) visceral (nonstriated (smooth) involuntary) muscles—line the walls of internal structures such as veins and arteries; and (3) cardiac (striated involuntary) muscles—make up the wall of the heart (Fig. 2–10). Muscles provide movement, maintain posture, and produce heat. Movement takes place not only during locomotion, but also during body movements, changes in the size of openings, and propulsion of substances (e.g., propulsion of blood through veins or passage of food through intestines). Posture is maintained during sitting and standing by continued partial contraction of specific muscles. Muscle cells that provide mechanical energy for movement also release energy in the form of heat. All three muscle types work by extending, contracting, conducting, and being easily stimulated.

Skeletal muscles (more than 400 in humans) compose approximately 40 percent of a man's body. In contrast, women have less muscle and more fat than that in men. Muscles are strongest at about age

Components:
- Skeletal muscle
- Cardiac muscle (heart)
- Smooth muscle (walls of hollow organs)

Functions:
- Permits movement
- Produces heat
- Maintains posture

Disorders:
- Atrophy
- Muscular dystrophy (MD)
- Myalgia
- Tendinitis

Diagnostic Tests:
- Autoimmune antibodies
- Creatine phosphokinase (CPK)
- CK isoenzymes
- Lactic acid
- Lactate dehydrogenase (LDH or LD)
- Myoglobin

Figure 2–10. Muscular system.

25, but with proper nutrition and exercise, they can remain strong throughout life. Without sufficient exercise, muscles become smaller and weaker. Glycogen is the form of stored glucose in muscles. Without stores of glycogen, muscles must wait for glucose, which is transported through the bloodstream. Exercise increases the amount of glycogen available for muscles, which in turn allows them to function more easily.

Muscular system disorders include muscular dystrophy (MD), conditions that disrupt nerve stimulation (as in severe accidents or myasthenia gravis), muscle cramps and tendinitis, and viral infections such as multiple sclerosis (MS) and polio.

Laboratory testing of muscular system disorders often involves clinical assays of specific muscle enzymes such as creatine phosphokinase (CK) and lactate dehydrogenase (LDH), analysis of autoimmune antibodies, microscopic examination, or culturing of biopsy tissue.

Nervous System

The nervous system provides communication in the body, sensations, thoughts, emotions, and memories. Nerve impulses and chemical substances regulate, control, integrate, and organize body functions. The nervous system is composed of specialized nerve cells (neurons), the brain, the spinal cord, brain and cord coverings, fluid, and the nerve impulse itself. An estimated 10 billion neurons or more reside in the human body, most of which are in the brain. Sensory neurons transmit nerve impulses to the spinal cord or the brain from muscle tissues. Motor neurons transmit impulses to muscles from the spinal cord or the brain. Both the brain and the spinal cord are covered by protective membranes (meninges). Between these protective membrane layers are CSF-filled spaces that provide a cushion for the brain and the spinal cord. The brain has many vitally important areas. Along with the cranial nerves, its functions include all mental processes and many essential motor, sensory, and visceral responses. The spinal cord and the spinal nerves control sensory (touch), motor (voluntary movement), and reflex (knee-jerk) functions. Reflexes are responses to stimuli that do not require communication with the brain. A simple reflex, such as moving a finger from something hot, occurs even before the brain realizes the pain. Specific cranial and spinal nerves control all complex or simple action processes in the body. In summary, the nervous system is the primary communication and regulatory system in the body (Fig. 2–11).

Nervous system disorders include infectious conditions such as encephalitis, meningitis, tetanus, herpes, and poliomyelitis, and conditions such as amyotrophic lateral sclerosis (ALS), MS, Parkinson's disease,

Components:
- Brain
- Spinal cord
- Nerves
- Sense organs: eyes, ears, tongue, and sensory receptor in the skin

Functions:
- Allows communication throughout the body and regulates body functions
- Detects sensations
- Controls movements and physiological functions
- Controls intellectual processes

Disorders:
- Amyotrophic lateral sclerosis (ALS)
- Encephalitis
- Epilepsy
- Hydrocephaly
- Meningitis
- Multiple sclerosis (MS)
- Neuralgia
- Parkinson's disease
- Shingles

Diagnostic Tests:
- Acetylcholine receptor antibody
- Cerebrospinal fluid (CSF) analysis
- Cholinesterase
- Drug levels

Figure 2–11. Nervous system.

cerebral palsy (CP), tumors, epilepsy hydrocephaly, neuralgia, and headaches. Laboratory diagnosis of nervous system disorders is not very specific. Chemical assays can reveal drug interactions, as well as hormonal, protein, and enzyme alterations. Infections can be detected by bacterial, viral, or fungal cultures or by the presence of specific antibodies in the CSF.

Respiratory System

Respiration allows for the exchange of gases between blood and air. Once gases enter the blood, the circulatory system transports them between lungs and tissues. Together, the respiratory and circulatory systems carry O_2 to the cells and remove CO_2 from tissue cells. Oxygen allows the body to burn its fuel from the nutrients eaten; it makes up about one fifth of the air around us. The average person inhales and exhales about 15 times per minute, or approximately 20,000 times per day. As a person breathes in, the O_2 travels through air passages to the lungs. In the lungs, the exchange of gases occurs. Oxygen is exchanged for CO_2, which is then breathed out as the person exhales.

The main components of the **respiratory system** are in the head, the neck, and the thoracic cavity and include the nose, the pharynx, the larynx, the trachea, the bronchi, and the lungs (Fig. 2–12).

Receptors in the nose provide the sense of smell and allow for changes in voice. The nose also functions as the primary filter for air entering the body. It catches impurities and chemical substances that may irritate the respiratory system. In the nose, the throat, and the bronchial tree, mucus is continuously produced to trap unwanted particles and to prevent them from entering the lungs or vocal cords. Tiny hairlike cilia line the passageways and sweep the mucus to the nose and mouth so that it can be coughed up, sneezed, or swallowed. The pharynx is a

Components:
- Nasal cavity
- Pharynx
- Larynx
- Trachea
- Bronchi
- Lungs

Functions:
- Filters air, exchanges gases
- Supplies oxygen and removes carbon dioxide
- Helps regulate blood pH
- Protects vocal cords

Disorders:
- Respiratory tract infections
- Tonsillitis
- Asthma
- Bronchitis
- Cystic fibrosis
- Emphysema
- Pleurisy
- Pneumonia
- Tuberculosis
- Respiratory distress syndrome
- Respiratory syncytial virus
- Rhinitis

Diagnostic Tests:
- Alkaline phosphatase (ALP)
- Arterial blood gases
- Complete blood cell (CBC) count
- Bronchial washings
- Drug levels
- Electrolytes
- Microbiological cultures
- Pleuracentesis
- Sputum cultures
- Tuberculin skin test

Figure 2–12. Respiratory system.

tubelike passageway for both food and air. Along with the larynx (voice box), it determines the quality of voice. The trachea and the bronchial passages provide openings for outside air to reach the lungs. Within the bronchi are grapelike **alveolar sacs** that are enveloped by capillaries and allow diffusion between air and blood. The lungs are structured into millions of branches of alveoli with surrounding capillaries and therefore can quickly take in large amounts of O_2 and release large amounts of CO_2 if they are functioning properly. The lungs are soft and spongy and reach from just above the collarbone down to the diaphragm. They have no muscles; consequently, the diaphragm and other surrounding muscles help enlarge and contract the chest cavity as respiration occurs. Humans have two lungs; the right lung has three lobes, and the left lung has only two, to allow room for the heart. An adult's lungs hold 3 to 4 qt (approximately 3 to 4 L) of air, depending on how vigorously the person is moving or exercising. In patients with pneumonia, the alveolar sacs become inflamed, and fluid or waste products block the minute air spaces, thus normal O_2 and CO_2 exchange is difficult.

Red blood cells transport O_2 and CO_2 as part of a molecule called *hemoglobin*. After O_2 crosses the respiratory membranes (in the lung) into the blood, about 97 percent of the O_2 combines with the iron-containing heme portion of hemoglobin. The remaining 3 percent dissolves in plasma. Hemoglobin carries O_2 from the alveolar capillaries through the blood vessels to the tissue capillaries. Oxygen and CO_2 rapidly combine with hemoglobin to form oxyhemoglobin and carbaminohemoglobin, respectively (Fig. 2–13).

Association (chemical combination) and dissociation (chemical release) with hemoglobin depends on the gaseous pressure. In lung capillaries, O_2 pressure [partial pressure of oxygen (PO_2)] increases and

Hb = hemoglobin
PO_2 = pressure of O_2
PCO_2 = pressure of CO_2

Figure 2–13. Oxygen (O_2) and carbon dioxide (CO_2) transport by hemoglobin.

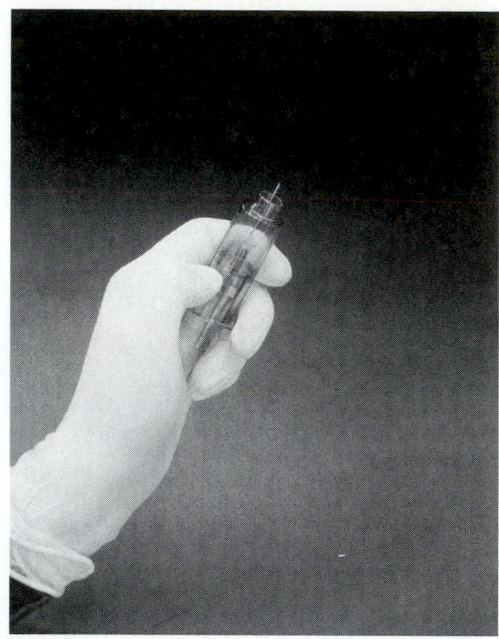

clot retracts to bring torn edges closer together. In phase five **(fibrinoly-** ✔
sis), final repair and regeneration of the injured vessel occurs, and the
clot slowly begins to dissolve as other cells carry out further repair.

The coagulation process (phase three) is a result of numerous coagulation factors. For simplicity, it is divided into two systems: intrinsic

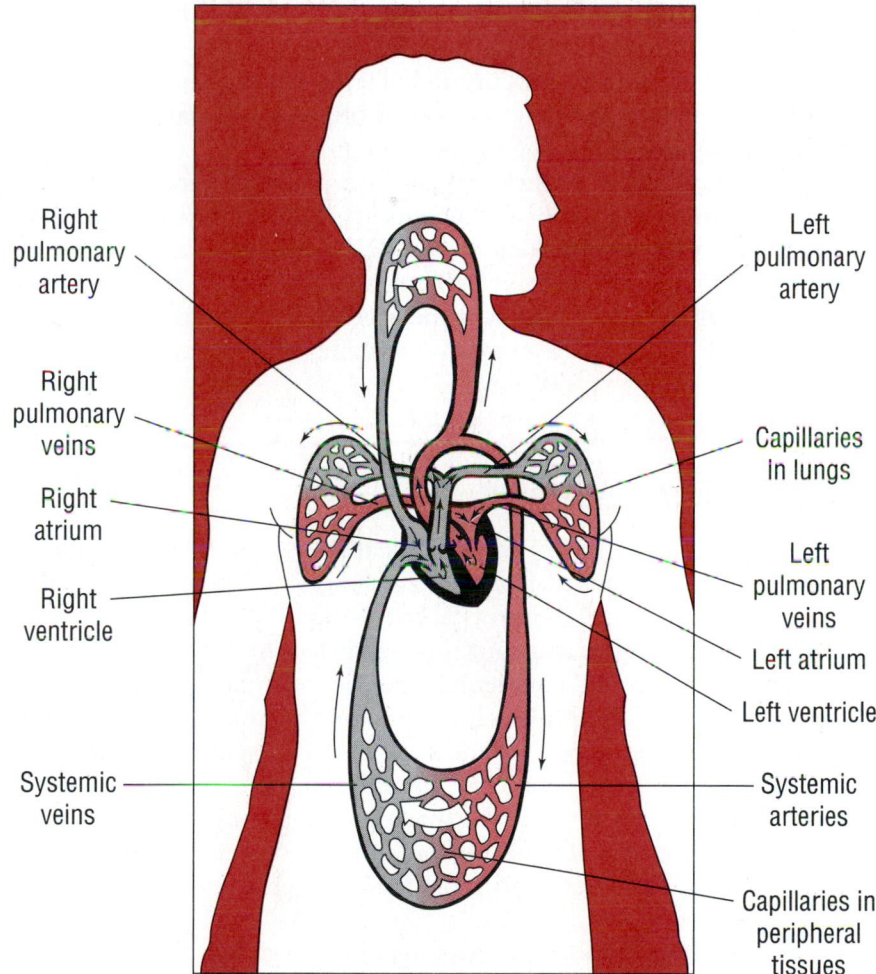

Figure 3–10. Overview of the pattern of circulation. Venous blood flow is on the left
side of the diagram, and arterial flow is on the right side. RA, right atrium; RV, right
ventricle; LA, left atrium; LV, left ventricle. *(From Martini F: Fundamentals of
Anatomy and Physiology, 2nd ed. Englewood Cliffs, NJ, Prentice Hall, 1992, p 673,
with permission.)*

and extrinsic. All coagulation factors required for the **intrinsic system** are contained in the blood, whereas the **extrinsic factors** are stimulated when tissue damage occurs. For example, blood vessels are lined with a single layer of flat endothelial cells and are supported by subendothelial cells and collagen fibers. Normally, endothelial cells do not react or attract platelets; however, they do produce and store some clotting factors. When the clotting sequence is initiated by vessel injury, endothelial cells react with degranulated platelets in forming the fibrin plug (Fig. 3–11).[2]

Large- or medium-sized veins and arteries require rapid surgical intervention to prevent bleeding. However, bleeding of small arteries and veins can be controlled by the hemostatic process.

Disorders of the hemostatic process are serious. Overactive clotting can cause clots within the body, such as an embolus or a thrombus, or disseminated intravascular coagulation (DIC) disease. Drugs such as heparin and Coumadin (warfarin), which suppress clotting factors, can be used to prevent such problems. On the other hand, if clotting factors are not produced by the body, excessive bleeding may occur, as in hemophilia.

DIAGNOSTIC ASSESSMENT

The number of RBCs, their morphological traits, and their hemoglobin content can be determined from an anticoagulated blood specimen in the clinical hematology laboratory. Platelets and WBCs can be assessed on the basis of number and morphological features. The results of a WBC differential count enumerate specific cell lines in percentages. Platelet function, as well as each coagulation factor, can be measured from anticoagulated blood specimens in the coagulation section of the clinical hematology laboratory. In addition, bone marrow, which is removed by a physician from the iliac crest of the hip, can be stained and studied microscopically in the hematology laboratory for the detection of abnormal numbers and morphological characteristics of blood cells.

Tests for blood types and cross-matches for donor blood are done in an immunohematology, a transfusion, or a blood banking laboratory. Serum and plasma constituents, including nutrients, metabolic wastes, respiratory gases, regulatory substances, and protective substances, can all be evaluated in the clinical chemistry laboratory.

Blood pressure and **pulse rate** measurements are performed as part of routine physical assessments (Figs. 3–4 to 3–6). High blood pressure can cause a stroke when a vessel ruptures in the brain. Having slightly

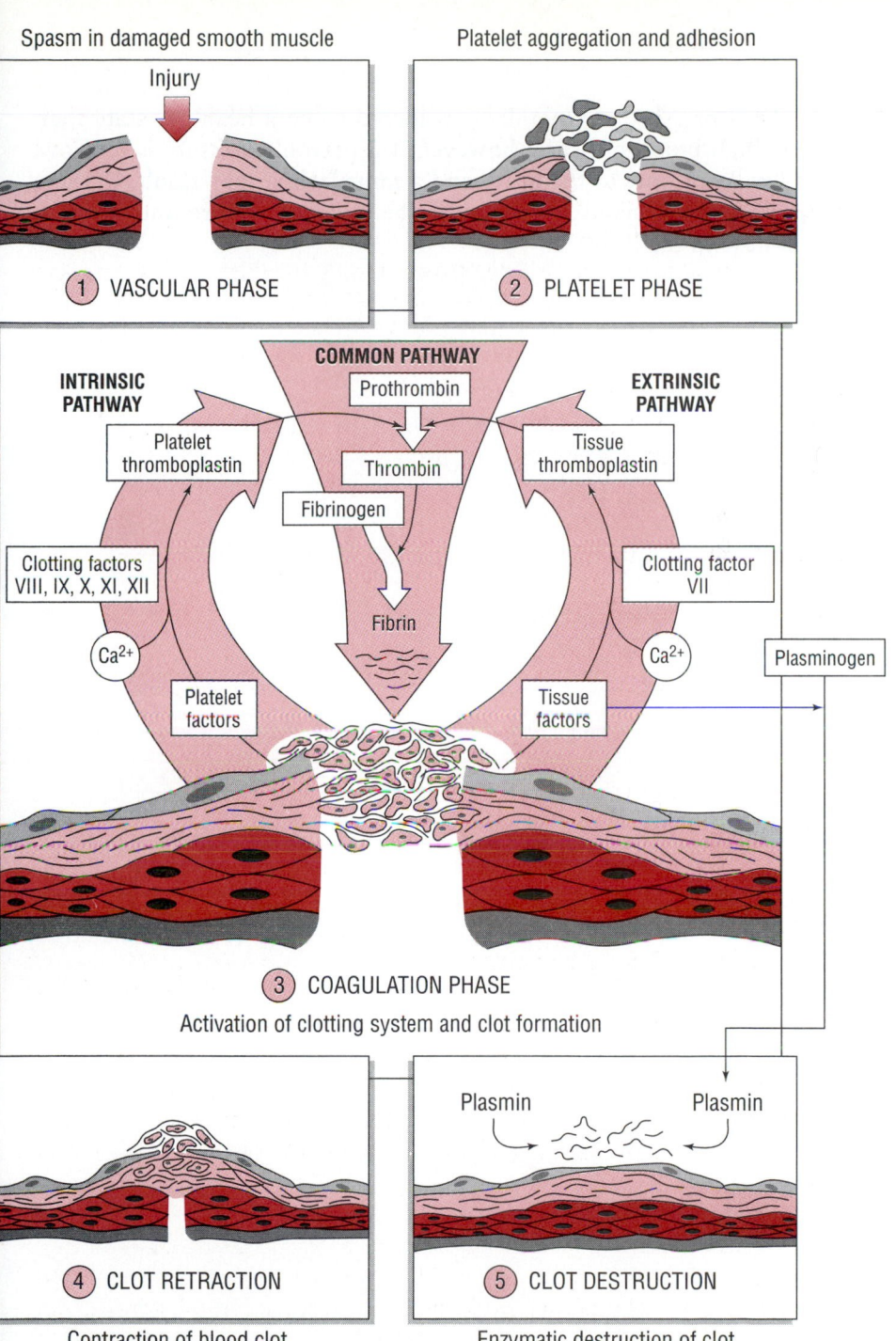

Figure 3–11. Clotting response. *(From Martini F: Fundamentals of Anatomy and Physiology, 2nd ed. Englewood Cliffs, NJ, Prentice Hall, 1992, p 625, with permission.)*

low blood pressure is generally considered to be a healthier state than having high blood pressure; however, if a person's pressure is too low, blood will not flow to the head, and a faint feeling may result. In these cases, the best response is to lower the head to restore and increase blood flow to the head.

✔ Key Terms

ABO BLOOD GROUP SYSTEM

ANTICOAGULANT

AORTA

ARTERIES

ARTERIOLES

ATRIA

BASILIC VEIN

BLOOD

BLOOD PRESSURE

BLOOD VESSELS

BUFFY COAT

CAPILLARIES

CARDIOVASCULAR SYSTEM

CEPHALIC VEIN

CIRCULATORY SYSTEM

COAGULATION

CROSS-MATCH TESTING

DIASTOLIC PRESSURE

DIFFERENTIAL

EXTRINSIC FACTORS

FIBRIN

FIBRINOLYSIS

GRANULOCYTES (BASOPHILS, NEUTROPHILS, EOSINOPHILS)

HEART

HEMATOPOIETIC

HEMOSTASIS

INFERIOR VENA CAVA

INTRINSIC SYSTEM

LYMPHOCYTES

MEDIAN CUBITAL VEIN

MEGAKARYOCYTES

MONOCYTES

PLASMA

PLATELETS (THROMBOCYTES)

PULMONARY CIRCUIT

PULSE RATE

RED BLOOD CELLS (RBCs, OR ERYTHROCYTES)

RH FACTOR

SERUM

SUPERIOR VENA CAVA

SYSTEMIC CIRCUIT

SYSTOLIC PRESSURE

VASOCONSTRICTION

VEINS

VENAE CAVAE

VENTRICLES

VENULES

WHITE BLOOD CELLS (WBCs OR LEUKOCYTES)

Study Questions

1. Whole blood consists of which of the following?
   - a. water
   - b. solutes
   - c. cells
   - d. tissue

2. Which type of blood cell is most numerous in the circulating blood?
   - a. red blood cell
   - b. white blood cell
   - c. platelet
   - d. macrophage

3. Identify the four chambers of the heart.
   - a. right atrium, right ventricle
   - b. superior vena cava, inferior vena cava
   - c. left atrium, left ventricle
   - d. ascending aorta, descending aorta

4. The liquid portion of an anticoagulated blood specimen is called
   - a. plasma
   - b. serum
   - c. cellular components
   - d. oxygenated blood

5. Which of the following veins are most commonly used for venipuncture procedures?
   - a. popliteal
   - b. brachial
   - c. median cubital
   - d. cephalic
   - e. basilic

6. Functions of the blood include which of the following?
   - a. transportation of gases, enzymes, and hormones
   - b. regulation of pH and electrolytes
   - c. regulation of body temperature
   - d. transportation of waste products

7. Blood pressure is reported in which of the following ways?
   - a. diastolic pressure only
   - b. diastolic pressure/systolic pressure
   - c. systolic pressure/diastolic pressure
   - d. systolic pressure only

8. Which of the listed circulating blood cells have no nuclei?
   - a. neutrophils
   - b. erythrocytes
   - c. basophils
   - d. eosinophils

9. The most common blood type is

    a. A   c. AB
    b. B   d. O

10. The coagulation process occurs in phases that include the

    a. vascular phase   c. coagulation phase
    b. platelet phase   d. clot-retraction phase

REFERENCES

1. Guy JF: *Learning Human Anatomy: A Laboratory Text and Workbook.* Norwalk, CT, Appleton & Lange, 1992.
2. Martini F: *Fundamentals of Anatomy and Physiology,* 2nd ed. Englewood Cliffs, NJ, Prentice Hall, 1992.

Phlebotomy Case Study

DORSAL HAND COLLECTION

Mr. Whitefield, a phlebotomist who recently completed his training program at Amber Community College, acquired a position at Oakhaven Hospital on the early morning shift. One morning, he was informed by the nurse on the orthopedic floor that any blood collections from Patient Davis should be taken while Mr. Davis is in the supine position and that all collections should be taken from the left dorsal hand.

Questions:

1. Is the dorsal area the same as the proximal area? Explain.

2. Should Mr. Davis sit up or lie down during the blood collection?

3. *Orthopedic* refers to what type of specialty?

EQUIPMENT AND PROCEDURES

II

*P*hlebotomy practice is best described by what phlebotomists do. Part II answers the following technical questions:

- What tools (supplies and equipment) do I need?
- How do I prepare myself and the patient?
- How do I do a venipuncture?
- How do I perform a finger stick?
- What can go wrong and how can I prevent it from happening?

Building on the knowledge from the first three chapters, Part II highlights technical skills. It is divided into four chapters that describe the supplies, equipment, techniques, and complications associated with phlebotomy practice.

Chapter 4, Blood Collection Equipment, describes and illustrates the latest supplies and equipment necessary for the collection of blood. Emphasis is on anticoagulated and nonadditive blood collection tubes, the importance of color coding, and the use of gloves, syringes, needles, microcollection equipment, specimen collection chairs and trays, and other supplies needed for a safe and effective collection procedure. Safe handling of blood specimens is highlighted.

Chapter 5, Venipuncture Procedures, provides a comprehensive description and illustrations of each step of the blood collection process. It includes a discussion of patient identification, as well as the venipuncture procedure itself. Emphasis is on proper preparation, technique, and collection.

Chapter 6, Skin Puncture Procedures, provides a detailed description and illustrations of each step of the skin puncture procedure. Emphasis is on site selection, finger sticks, and blood smear preparation.

Chapter 7, Complications in Blood Collection, describes the complications that occur during the blood collection process and the reasons for their occurrence. Emphasis is on recognition and prevention of these complications, the effects of the patient's physical disposition on the integrity of the specimen, and the interfering effects of drugs and other substances in the blood. Guidelines for specimen rejection are also presented.

four

4

BLOOD COLLECTION EQUIPMENT

Chapter Objectives

Upon completion of Chapter 4, the learner is responsible for the following:

1. List the various types of anticoagulants used in blood collection, their mechanisms for preventing blood from clotting, and the vacuum collection tube color codes for these anticoagulants.

2. Describe the latest phlebotomy safety supplies and equipment, and evaluate their effectiveness in blood collection.

3. Identify the various supplies that should be carried on a specimen collection tray when a skin puncture specimen must be collected.

4. Identify the types of equipment needed to collect blood by venipuncture.

5. Describe the special precautions that should be taken and the techniques that should be used when various types of specimens must be transported to the clinical laboratory.

Traditionally, in most clinical laboratories, serum, plasma, or whole blood has been used to perform various assays. More recently, though, heparinized whole blood has become the specimen of choice for the latest clinical laboratory instruments used in stat (immediate) situations. Using whole blood as a specimen decreases the time involved in acquiring the test result because centrifugation is not required prior to laboratory testing.

Each assay may require a different type of anticoagulant. These anticoagulants are discussed in detail later in this chapter.

Figure 4–1. Vacuum tube (VACUTAINER). *(Courtesy of Becton-Dickinson VACU-TAINER Systems, Franklin Lakes, NJ.)*

Venipuncture with a **vacuum (evacuated) tube** [VACUTAINER ✔ (Becton-Dickinson VACUTAINER Systems, Franklin Lakes, NJ)], as shown in Figure 4–1 is the most direct and efficient method for obtaining a blood specimen. The evacuated tube system requires three components: the evacuated sample tube, the double-pointed needle, and a special plastic **holder (adapter).** One end of the double-pointed needle ✔ enters the vein, the other end pierces the top of the tube, and the vacuum aspirates the blood (Fig. 4–2). Vacuum tubes may contain silicon to decrease the possibility of hemolysis and to prevent the clot from adhering to the wall of the tube. This convenient system eliminates the need for syringes and consists of disposable needles and tubes. The tubes are available in different sizes (Fig. 4–3) and can be purchased in glass or unbreakable plastic. The external tube diameter and length plus the maximum amount of specimen to be drawn into the vacuum tube are the two criteria used to describe vacuum tube size (Table 4–1). The smaller sizes (e.g., 2 mL) are useful for pediatric and geriatric collections and can be purchased with different types of anticoagulants as well as chemically clean or sterile glassware. Each vacuum tube is color coded according to the anticoagulant contained within the tube (Table 4–2).

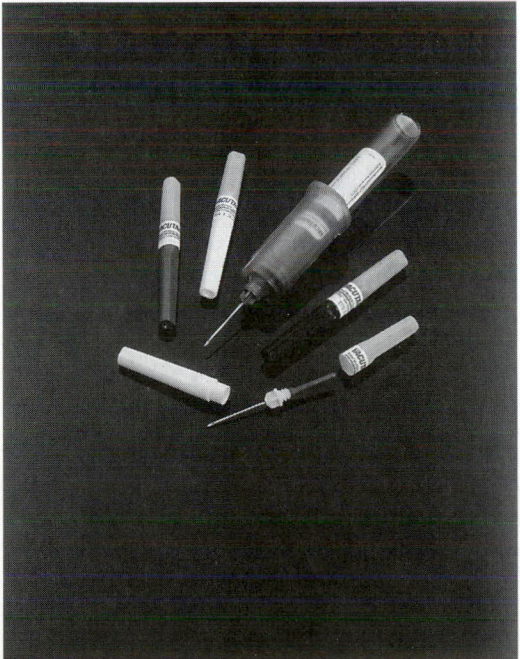

Figure 4–2. Holder-needle combination with inserted VACUTAINER. *(Courtesy of Becton-Dickinson VACUTAINER Systems, Franklin Lakes, NJ.)*

Figure 4–3. Venoject II tubes. *(Courtesy of Terumo Medical Corporation, Somerset, NJ.)*

Many tubes are specifically designed to be used directly with chemistry, hematology, or microbiology instrumentation. In these cases, the tube of blood is identified by its bar code and is pierced by the instrument probe, and some sample is aspirated into the instrument for analyses. Use of these *closed systems* minimizes laboratory personnel's risk of exposure to blood. In addition, some tubes have plastic tops or screw-on enclosures around the rubber stopper to minimize exposure to blood left on the top of the cap or blood splatters that can occur during cap removal.

Evacuated tubes are also used for transferring blood from a syringe into the tubes. The syringe needle is simply pushed through the top of the tube, and blood is automatically pulled into the tube because of the vacuum. The plunger must not be pushed down if the tubes are being filled from the syringe because it is extremely hazardous. Also, pushing the plunger may damage cellular components because of the forceful expulsion of blood. Specialized tubes and bottles that may fit the adapter are also available for blood culture collection.

TABLE 4–1. TYPICAL SIZES OF BLOOD COLLECTION VACUUM TUBES

External Diameter × Length (mm)	Draw Volumes (mL)
10.25 × 50	2.0
10.25 × 64	3.0
10.25 × 82	4.0
13 × 75	2.0
13 × 75	4.0
13 × 75	5.0
13 × 100	4.2
13 × 100	6.0
13 × 100	7.0
13 × 100	15.0
16 × 75	7.0
16 × 100	10.0

The expiration dates of tubes should be monitored continuously. Such monitoring is most easily accomplished with a computerized inventory system; however, routine rotation of stocked supplies and careful checking of phlebotomy trays and carts should also be the responsibility of each phlebotomist.

TABLE 4–2. SPECIMEN TYPE AND COLLECTION VACUUM TUBES

Specimen Type	Collection Tubes (Stopper Color / Type)	Additive
Clotted blood/serum	Gray and red	Polymer barrier
	Yellow and red	Polymer barrier
	Gold	Polymer barrier
	Red	None
Whole blood/plasma	Green and gray	Polymer barrier and lithium heparin
	Green and red	Polymer barrier and lithium heparin
	Light blue	Trisodium citrate
	Lavender (purple)	EDTA (K_3) or EDTA (K_2) or EDTA (Na_2)
	Gray	Sodium fluoride and potassium oxalate
	Green	Lithium heparin
	Green	Sodium heparin
Clotted blood/serum	Royal blue	No additive; but sterile tube for trace elements
	Brown	No additive or sodium heparin, but lead-free glass and sterile for lead determinations
Whole blood	Lavender (purple)	EDTA (K_3) or EDTA (K_2) or EDTA (Na_2)
	Green	Lithium heparin, sodium heparin, or ammonium heparin
	Yellow	Sodium polyanetholesulfonate (SPS)

The holder of the evacuated tube system has a large opening for the blood vacuum tube and a small opening at the other end for needle insertion. Various manufacturers have modified the adapter to reduce the risk of accidental needle sticks. For instance, Becton-Dickinson VACUTAINER Systems (Franklin Lakes, NJ) developed the Safety-Lok Needle Holder (Fig. 4–4), which has a protective shield so that the blood collector can slide the protective shield over the needle and lock it in place after the needle is withdrawn from the puncture site. This single-use adapter is fairly large and requires a large biohazardous sharps container for disposal. However, it provides effective, immediate containment of a used needle.

Another protective holder that provides effective, immediate containment of a used needle is the Saf-T Clik holder (Ryan Medical, a division of Winfield Industries, San Diego, CA) (Fig. 4–5). It reduces the risk of cross-contamination and fits any standard blood collection needle.

Figure 4–4. Safety-Lok Needle Holder. *(Courtesy of Becton-Dickinson VACU-TAINER Systems, Franklin Lakes, NJ.)*

Figure 4–5. Saf-T Clik shielded blood needle adapter. *(Courtesy of Ryan Medical, a division of Winfield Industries, San Diego, CA.)*

The Safety-Gard Phlebotomy System has been developed as a safety device for blood collection (Fig. 4–6). The blood collector can single-handedly retract a used blood collection needle and then safely recover the needle while it is enclosed and locked inside the holder. This holder system provides safe disposal of the needle because it remains locked within the Safety-Gard Needle Holder. A companion biohazardous container (Fig. 4–7), for use with the Safety-Gard Needle Holder, is also available. This system provides protection from needle sticks by removing used needles from the holder without user contact with the needles.

Another vacuum tube assembly developed to prevent needle sticks is the Pro-Ject Safety needle holder (Pro-tec Containers, Inc., Irvine,

Figure 4–6. Safety-Gard Phlebotomy System. *(Courtesy of Becton-Dickinson VACUTAINER Systems, Franklin Lakes, NJ.)*

CA). This safety needle holder for blood collection is reusable and has a needle-release mechanism that allows the phlebotomist to eject the needle into a biohazardous sharps container.

The AutoDrop blood needle holder system (Sage Products, Inc., Crystal Lake, IL) is compatible with the Venoject II blood collection system (Terumo Medical Corporation, Somerset, NJ) Fig. 4–8). It automatically drops needles safely into a sharps disposal container, eliminates manipulation of blood-drawing needles associated with other systems, and reduces contamination of a reusable needle holder.

ANTICOAGULANTS AND BLOOD COLLECTION TUBES

Many coagulation factors are involved in blood clotting, and coagulation can be prevented by the addition of different types of anticoagulants. These anticoagulants often contain preservatives that can extend the metabolism and life span of the red blood cells (RBCs) after blood collection. Anticoagulants and preservatives are used extensively in blood donations to ensure the biochemical balance of certain com-

Figure 4–7. Safety-Gard Needle Disposal Container that permits one-handed disposal of enclosed needle. *(Courtesy of Becton-Dickinson VACUTAINER Systems, Franklin Lakes, NJ.)*

Figure 4–8. Venoject II–compatible Sage AutoDrop blood needle holder system. *(Courtesy of Terumo Medical Corporation, Somerset, NJ.)*

ponents of RBCs, such as hemoglobin, pH, adenosine triphosphate (ATP), and glucose. Once transferred, anticoagulants such as **citrate–phosphate–dextrose (CPD)** and **acid–citrate–dextrose (ACD)** ensure that the RBCs provide the recipient with the means of delivering oxygen (O_2) to the tissues.

Another major use of anticoagulants and preservatives is in the collection of plasma for laboratory analysis. Specific anticoagulants or preservatives must be used depending on the test procedure ordered. Anticoagulants cannot be substituted one for another. Table 4–3 lists the various laboratory assays along with the types of anticoagulants required and the approximate milliliters of blood that must be collected for each assay.

Coagulation of blood can be prevented by the addition of **oxalates, citrates, ethylenediamine tetraacetic acid (EDTA),** or **heparin.** Oxalates, citrates, and EDTA prevent the coagulation of blood by removing calcium and forming insoluble calcium salts. These three anticoagulants cannot be used in calcium determinations; however, citrates are frequently used in coagulation blood studies. EDTA prevents platelet aggregation and is therefore used for platelet counts and platelet function tests. Fresh EDTA-anticoagulated blood allows preparation of blood films with minimal distortion of white blood cells (WBCs). Heparin, a mucopolysaccharide used in assays such as ammonia and plasma hemoglobin, prevents blood clotting by inactivating the blood-clotting chemicals—thrombin and thromboplastin.

In addition to using the correct anticoagulant for a specific laboratory assay, using the correct amount or dilution of anticoagulant in the blood specimen is important. The blood collection vacuum tubes have been designed for a certain amount of blood to be drawn into the tube by vacuum according to the amount of prefilled anticoagulant in the tube. If an insufficient amount of blood is collected in a tube with anticoagulant, the laboratory test results may be erroneous because of an incorrect blood-to-anticoagulant ratio.

Gray-Topped Tubes

Gray-topped vacuum tubes usually contain (1) potassium oxalate and **sodium fluoride** or (2) **lithium iodoacetate** and heparin. This type of collection tube is used primarily for glycolytic inhibition tests. Thus, sometimes *antiglycolytic agent* is the term for this tube's additive. Because fluoride destroys many enzymes, this additive should not be used in blood collections for enzyme determinations [e.g., creatine kinase (CK), alanine aminotransferase (ALT), aspartate aminotransferase (AST), and alkaline phosphatase (ALP) determinations]. Likewise, oxalate distorts

TABLE 4–3. LABORATORY ASSAYS AND THE REQUIRED TYPES OF ANTICOAGULANTS

Test Name	Specimen Tube (Type/Color)	Whole Blood, Minimum Volume for Adults (mL)
ABG (see Blood Gases)		
ABO group and type	Whole blood (purple) or serum (red)	5
Acetaminophen (Tylenol)	Serum (speckled)	1
Acetone	Serum (speckled)	2
Acetylcholine receptor– binding antibodies	Serum (speckled)	3
Acid hemolysis (PNH)	Plasma (light blue)	3
Acidified serum test (see Hamm's Test)		
Acid phosphatase	Serum (speckled)	2
ACTH (adrenocorticotropic hormone)	Whole blood (purple)	10
Adenovirus antibody	Serum (speckled)	3
Adrenal cortical antibody	Serum (red)	3
Albumin	Serum (speckled)	2
Alcohol (ethanol)	Whole blood (gray)	2
Aldolase	Serum (speckled)	2
Aldosterone	Serum (speckled) or plasma (purple or green) *Ice needed for transportation *Patient should be recumbent for at least 30 minutes prior to blood collection	7
Alkaline phosphatase (Alk p'tase)	Serum (speckled)	2
Alkaline phosphatase isoenzymes	Serum (speckled)	2
Alpha$_1$-antitrypsin	Serum (speckled)	1
Alpha-fetoprotein (AFP)	Serum (speckled)	3
Alpha$_2$-macroglobulin	Serum (red)	1
Aluminum	Whole blood (royal blue)	7
Amebiasis	Serum (speckled)	3
Amikacin	Serum (speckled)	1
Amino acid	Serum (speckled)	3
Amiodarone	Serum (speckled)	10
Amitriptyline	Serum (red)	3
Ammonia	Plasma (green)	3
Ampicillin	Serum (red)	5
Amylase	Serum (speckled)	2
Androstenedione	Serum (speckled) *Deliver immediately	5

(*continued*)

TABLE 4–3. (*Continued*)

Test Name	Specimen Tube (Type/Color)	Whole Blood, Minimum Volume for Adults (mL)
Angiotensin–converting enzyme (ACE)	Serum (speckled)	5
	*Ice needed for transportation	
Antibody to hepatitis A virus (anti-HAV)	Serum (speckled)	5
Antibody to hepatitis B core antigen	Serum (red)	3
Antibody to hepatitis BE antigen	Serum (red)	3
Antibody to hepatitis B surface antigen	Serum (red)	3
Antibody identification	Whole blood (red)	7
Antibody screen and blood grouping	Whole blood (red)	5
Antibody titer	Whole blood (red)	5
Anticonvulsants (Dilantin, Mysoline, phenobarbital, carbamazepine, valproic acid)	Serum (speckled)	7
Antidiuretic hormone (ADH, vasopressin)	Whole blood (purple)	3
Anti–DNase B	Serum (speckled)	3
Antinuclear antibodies, fluorescent (ANA)	Whole blood (red)	5
Anti–smooth muscle antibody (ASMA)	Serum (speckled)	3
Antithrombin III	Plasma (light blue)	1
APTT	Plasma (light blue)	1.8
Arboviruses (St. Louis encephalitis)	Serum (speckled)	3
Arsenic (As)	Whole blood (royal blue)	7
Ascorbic acid (see Vitamin C)		
ASO (anti–streptolysin O) titer	Serum (speckled)	3
Aspirin (see Salicylate)		
Autologous blood	Whole blood (red)	5
Bactrim (see Sulfonamides)		
Barbiturates	Serum (speckled)	2
B-cell antigen	Whole blood (red)	3
Benzodiazepines	Serum (speckled)	2
Beta$_2$-microglobulin	Serum (speckled)	3
Bilirubin, total and direct	Serum (speckled) *Protect blood from light	1
Blastomycosis, complement fixation (fungal serology)	Serum (speckled)	4

(*continued*)

TABLE 4–3. (*Continued*)

Test Name	Specimen Tube (Type/Color)	Whole Blood, Minimum Volume for Adults (mL)
Bleeding time	Patient	Test performed on patient's arm
Blood, packed red blood cells	Whole blood (red)	5
Blood cell count, CBC survey (WBC, RBC, Hgb, Hct, MCV, MCH, MCHC)	Whole blood (purple)	3
Blood cell count, differential	Blood smear	Blood smear
Blood cell count, eosinophil	Whole blood (purple)	3
Blood cell count, erythrocyte (RBC)	Whole blood (purple)	3
Blood cell count, leukocyte (WBC)	Whole blood (purple)	3
Blood cell count, platelets	Whole blood (purple)	3
Blood cell count, reticulocyte	Whole blood (purple)	3
Blood gases, arterial (ABG) [pH, P_{CO_2}, pO_2, HCO_3^-, base excess (BE)]	Arterial blood (heparinized syringe)	0.6
Bordetella pertussis antibody (whooping cough)	Serum (red)	3
Borrelia burgdorferi antibody (Lyme disease)	Serum (red)	3
Bromide	Serum (red)	2
Brucella	Serum (speckled)	2
BUN (blood urea nitrogen)	Serum (speckled)	1
Cadmium (Cd)	Whole blood (green, purple) *Use acid-washed syringes	2
Calcitonin	Plasma (green)	3
Calcium	Serum (speckled)	1
Calcium, ionized	Plasma (green)	3
Candida serology, qualitative	Serum (speckled)	3
Carbamazepine (see Tegretol)		
Carbon dioxide (CO_2)	Serum (speckled)	1
Carcinoembryonic antigen (CEA)	Serum (speckled)	3
Cardiolipin antibodies (anti–cardiolipin antibody IgG and IgM)	Serum (speckled)	3
Carotene	Serum (speckled)	3
Catecholamines	Whole blood (purple) *Ice needed for transportation	20
Ceruloplasmin	Serum (speckled)	3

(*continued*)

TABLE 4–3. (*Continued*)

Test Name	Specimen Tube (Type/Color)	Whole Blood, Minimum Volume for Adults (mL)
Chemistry screen (T. protein, Alb, Ca, I phos, Glu, BUN, uric acid, Creat, T. bil, Alk p'tase, LDH, ALT)	Serum (speckled)	3
Chickenpox titer	Serum (speckled)	3
Chloramphenicol	Serum (speckled)	4
Chloride	Serum (speckled)	1
Cholesterol	Serum (speckled)	1
Cholinesterase	Serum (speckled)	3
Chromium (Cr)	Serum (royal blue) *Avoid chromium-plated needles; use platinum needles and acid-washed syringes	2
Chromosome analysis	Sterile whole blood (green) (Na heparin)	7
Circulating anticoagulants	Plasma (light blue)	3
Clonazepam	Serum (red) or plasma (purple)	2
CMV, IFA serology	Serum (speckled)	3
Coccidioides immitis (San Joaquin fever)	Serum (speckled)	3
Cold agglutinins	Whole blood (speckled) *Place in warm water and deliver immediately	3
Complement, total	Serum (speckled)	5
Complement—C3	Serum (speckled)	5
Complement—C4	Serum (speckled)	5
Coombs' test, direct (direct antiglobulin test)	Whole blood (red)	3
Coombs' test, indirect (indirect antiglobulin test)	Whole blood (red)	5
Copper (Cu)	Serum (speckled) or whole blood (royal blue)	3
Cortisol	Plasma (green)	1
Coxiella burnetii (Q fever)	Serum (speckled)	3
Coxsackievirus (Bornholm disease)	Serum (speckled)	3
C-peptide	Serum (speckled)	3
CPK (CK)	Serum (speckled)	1
CPK isoenzymes (CK isoenzymes) (CK-MB)	Serum (speckled)	3
C-reactive protein	Serum (speckled)	2
Creatinine	Serum (speckled)	1

(*continued*)

TABLE 4–3. (*Continued*)

Test Name	Specimen Tube (Type/Color)	Whole Blood, Minimum Volume for Adults (mL)
Cross-match	Whole blood (red)	3
Cryofibrinogen	Plasma (green)	1
Cryoglobulin	Serum (speckled) *Immediately place in warm water and transport to lab	4
Cryptococcal antigen	Serum (red)	3
Cyclosporine	Serum (speckled)	3
Cysticercus cellulosae (pork tapeworm)	Serum (red)	3
Cytomegalovirus (CMV), IFA serology	Serum (speckled)	3
D-dimer (D-D$_1$)	Whole blood (blue)	3.5
Dengue virus antibody (breakbone fever)	Serum (speckled)	3
Deoxycorticosteroids	Serum (speckled) or plasma (green)	3
Depakene (see Valproic Acid)		
Desipramine	Serum (speckled) or plasma (green)	5
Diazepam (see Valium)		
Digitoxin	Serum (speckled)	2
Digoxin (Lanoxin)	Serum (speckled)	2
Dilantin (phenytoin)	Serum (speckled)	1
Directogen for *Haemophilus influenzae, Streptococcus pneumoniae, Neisseria meningitidis*	Serum (speckled)	3
DNA antibody (anti-DNA)	Serum (speckled)	3
Drug screen	Serum (speckled)	10
EBV–early antigen	Serum (speckled)	3
EBV-IgM	Serum (speckled)	3
EBV-NA	Serum (speckled)	3
EBV-VCA	Serum (speckled)	3
Echinococcus (hydatid disease)	Serum (red)	3
Electrolytes (Na, K, Cl, HCO$_3$)	Plasma (green) or whole blood (green)	2
Electrophoresis (hemoglobin)	Whole blood (purple)	1
Electrophoresis immuno	Serum (speckled)	3
Electrophoresis (SPE)	Serum (speckled)	3
Elution studies	Whole blood (purple)	2
Entamoeba histolytica	Serum (speckled)	3
Eosinophil count	Whole blood (purple)	1

(*continued*)

TABLE 4–3. (*Continued*)

Test Name	Specimen Tube (Type/Color)	Whole Blood, Minimum Volume for Adults (mL)
E-rosette	Whole blood (purple)	3
E-rosette receptor	Whole blood (purple)	3
Erythrocyte fragility	Whole blood (purple)	1
Erythrocyte osmotic fragility	Whole blood (green)	2
Erythromycin	Serum (speckled)	5
ESR (sedimentation rate, sed rate)	Whole blood (purple)	3
Estradiol (E_2)	Serum (speckled) or plasma (green)	3
Estriol	Serum (speckled) or plasma (green)	3
Estrogens, total	Serum (speckled)	7
Ethanol (alcohol)	Whole blood (gray)	2
Ethosuximide (Zarontin)	Plasma (green)	3
Euglobulin lysis	Plasma (blue)	4.5
Factor assays	Plasma (blue)	4.5
Fasting blood glucose (FBG)	Plasma (gray)	1
Fatty acids, free	Serum (speckled) *Transport in ice water	10
Febrile agglutinins	Serum (speckled)	7
Ferritin	Serum (speckled)	2
Fetal hemoglobin	Whole blood (purple)	2
Fibrin degradation products (FDP) (FSP)	Plasma (blue)	2
Fibrinogen	Plasma (blue)	1.8
Fibrinogen antigen	Plasma (blue)	4.5
Fibrinopeptide A	Whole blood with special tube from hematology	5
Fitzgerald factor	Plasma (blue)	4.5
Flecainide	Serum (red)	3
Fletcher factor (prekallinkrein)	Plasma (blue)	4.5
Fluorescent antinuclear antibody	Serum (speckled)	3
Fluorescent treponemal antibody test (MHA-TP)	Serum (red or speckled)	3
Fluoride	Serum (red)	6
Folate, serum	Serum (speckled)	3
Folate, whole blood (RBC and serum	Whole blood (purple)	3
Follicle-stimulating hormone (FSH)	Serum (speckled) or plasma (green)	3
Fragility, erythrocyte (RBC)	Whole blood (purple)	2

(*continued*)

TABLE 4–3. (*Continued*)

Test Name	Specimen Tube (Type/Color)	Whole Blood, Minimum Volume for Adults (mL)
Francisella tularensis antibody (tularemia)	Serum (speckled)	3
Free, T_4 (see Thyroxine, Free)		
Free thyroxine index (see Thyroid Studies)		
Fungal serology	Serum (speckled)	3
Gamma-glutamyl transpeptidase (GGT) (GT)	Serum (speckled)	3
Gastrin	Serum (speckled)	7
Gentamicin	Serum (speckled)	1
Glucagon	Whole blood (purple)	3
Glucose (FBS and tolerance)	Plasma (gray) or serum (speckled)	1
Glucose-6-phosphate dehydrogenase (G6PD), quantitative	Whole blood (green)	1
Glucose, 2-hour postprandial	Plasma (gray) or serum (speckled)	1
Glycosylated hemoglobin	Whole blood (purple)	1
Gonadotropin HCG-beta (immuno test)	Serum (speckled)	7
Growth hormone (HGH)	Serum (speckled)	1.5
Hamm's test (PNH) confirmation	Plasma (green)	5
Haptoglobin	Serum (speckled)	1
HDL (high-density lipoprotein) cholesterol	Serum (speckled)	5
Heinz body preparation	Whole blood (purple) or (green)	3
Helper T	Whole blood (purple)	2
Hematocrit	Whole blood (purple)	1
Hematology profile (Hct, Hgb, WBC, RBC, MCV, MCH, MCHC)	Whole blood (purple)	1
Hemoglobin	Whole blood (purple)	1
Hemoglobin, plasma	Plasma (purple)	1
Heparin	Plasma (blue)	3
Hepatitis A Ab IgM (Anti–HAV-IgM)	Serum (speckled)	5
Hepatitis B core antibody (HB_cAb) (Anti-HB_c)	Serum (speckled)	3
Hepatitis B surface Ab (Anti-HB_s)	Serum (speckled)	4
Hepatitis B surface antigen (HB_sAg)	Serum (speckled)	3

(*continued*)

TABLE 4–3. (*Continued*)

Test Name	Specimen Tube (Type/Color)	Whole Blood, Minimum Volume for Adults (mL)
Hepatitis C Ab (HCV)	Serum (speckled)	5
Hepatitis delta antibody and antigen	Serum (speckled)	3
Herpes simplex, virus serology	Serum (speckled)	3
Heterophile antibody (see Monospot)		
Histamine	Serum (speckled)	5
Histoplasmosis	Serum (speckled)	5
HI titer (St. Louis encephalitis)	Serum (speckled)	3
HIV antibody screen	Serum (speckled)	5
HIV antigen	Serum (speckled)	3
HLA typing (microcytotoxicity)	Whole blood (green)	5
Human growth hormone (HGH) (see Growth Hormone)		
Human T-cell lymphotropic virus type I (HTLV-I) antibody	Serum (speckled)	2
Hydroxybutyric dehydrogenase (HBD)	Serum (speckled)	5
IgA	Serum (speckled)	1
IgD	Serum (speckled)	1
IgG	Serum (speckled)	1
IgM	Serum (speckled)	1
Imipramine (Tofranil)	Serum (red)	10
Infectious mononucleosis (see Monospot)		
Inhibitor assay	Plasma (blue)	4.5
Insulin (on ice)	Plasma (purple)	4.5
Intrinsic factor antibody	Serum (speckled)	3
Iron profile (iron, TIBC, and saturation)	Serum (speckled)	3
Kanamycin	Serum (speckled)	5
Lactate dehydrogenase (LD) and LD isoenzymes (LD-1)	Serum (speckled)	3
Lactic acid (on ice)	Plasma (gray)	1
Lanoxin (see Digoxin)		
LDL (low-density lipoprotein) cholesterol	Serum (speckled)	10
Lead, blood	Blood (royal blue) or special tube from chem	2
LE cell test	Whole blood (green)	3
Legionnaires' serology	Serum (speckled)	3

(*continued*)

TABLE 4–3. (*Continued*)

Test Name	Specimen Tube (Type/Color)	Whole Blood, Minimum Volume for Adults (mL)
Leishmania antibody	Serum (speckled)	3
Leptospira agglutination	Serum (speckled)	3
Leucine aminopeptidase (LAP)	Plasma (green)	2
Leukocyte alkaline phosphatase (LAP) stain		Six fresh blood smears
LGV-psittacosis titer	Serum (speckled)	5
LH (see Luteinizing Hormone)		
Lidocaine	Serum (speckled)	5
Lipase	Serum (speckled)	2
Lipid profile	Serum (speckled)	10
Lithium	Serum (speckled)	1
Low-density lipoprotein (LDL) cholesterol	Serum (speckled)	5
Lupus anticoagulant (tissue thromboplastin inhibition test)	Plasma (blue) *Deliver immediately	5
Luteinizing hormone (LH)	Serum (speckled)	2
Lyme disease serology	Serum (speckled)	4
Lymphocyte blastogenesis (LBR)	Whole blood (green)	7
Lymphogranuloma venereum	Serum (speckled)	3
Lysozyme, serum	Serum (speckled)	2
Magnesium, serum	Serum (speckled)	1
Malaria antibody	Serum (speckled)	2
Malaria smear		Blood smear
Manganese (Mn)	Whole blood (royal blue) or serum *Use acid-washed syringes	5
Mercury (Hg)	Whole blood (royal blue)	5
Methemalbumin	Serum (speckled)	2
Methemoglobin	Serum (speckled)	3
Methicillin	Serum (speckled)	5
Methotrexate	Serum (red)	2
MHA-TP	Serum (speckled or red)	3
Monocyte antigens	Whole blood (purple)	2
Monospot (Ortho Diagnostics, Raritan, NJ) (infectious mononucleosis)	Serum (speckled)	4
Mumps serology	Serum (speckled)	3
Mycoplasma pneumoniae	Serum (speckled)	2
Myelin antibodies	Serum (speckled)	3
NAPA (see Procainamide)		

(*continued*)

TABLE 4–3. (*Continued*)

Test Name	Specimen Tube (Type/Color)	Whole Blood, Minimum Volume for Adults (mL)
Nickel (Ni)	Plasma, serum, whole blood *Must prepare collection vials by acid-washing syringes	5
5'-Nucleotidase	Serum (speckled)	2
Nutritional panel	Serum (speckled)	2
Opiates (methadone, codeine, morphine)	Serum (speckled)	3
Osmolality, serum	Serum (speckled)	2
Parathyroid hormone (PTH)	Serum (speckled)	2
Partial thromboplastin time (PTT) (APTT)	Plasma (blue)	1
Penicillin	Serum (red)	5
Pentobarbital	Serum (speckled)	5
pH, blood (see Blood Gases)		
Phenobarbital	Serum (speckled)	2
Phenylalanine	Whole blood *Filter paper with low background fluorescence	Droplets used to saturate filter paper (<0.5)
Phenytoin (Dilantin)	Serum (speckled)	1
Phenytoin (free)	Serum (speckled)	5
Phosphorus	Serum (speckled)	1
Plasminogen antigen	Whole blood (blue)	5
Platelet function profile	Whole blood (purple) Whole blood (blue)	1 7
Pneumocystic serology	Serum (red)	3
Potassium	Plasma (green)	2
Prealbumin	Serum (speckled)	3
Precursor T	Whole blood (purple)	2
Primidone (Mysoline)	Serum (speckled)	2
Procainamide, *N*-acetylprocainamide (NAPA)	Serum (speckled)	2
Progesterone	Clotted whole blood (red) *Avoid serum separator tube in speckled tube top	3
Prolactin	Serum (speckled)	2
Pronestyl (procainamide)	Serum (speckled)	2
Propranolol	Serum (speckled) or plasma (purple)	3
Protein, total	Serum (speckled)	1
Protein, total A/G ratio	Serum (speckled)	1
Proteus OX 19	Serum (speckled)	2
Prothrombin consumption time	Serum (speckled)	3

(*continued*)

TABLE 4–3. (*Continued*)

Test Name	Specimen Tube (Type/Color)	Whole Blood, Minimum Volume for Adults (mL)
Protime (International Technidyne Corporation, Edison, NJ) (prothrombin time, PT)	Plasma (blue)	2
PSA (prostatic specific antigen)	Serum (speckled)	1
PTH (see Parathyroid Hormone)		
Pyruvate	Whole blood (gray) *Transport immediately in ice water	5
Q fever antibodies	Serum (speckled)	3
Quinidine	Serum (speckled)	1
Rabies virus antibody	Serum (speckled)	3
Renin activity	Plasma (purple) *Transport immediately in ice water	2
Reptilase time	Whole blood (blue)	3.5
Reticulocyte	Whole blood (purple)	5
Rheumatoid factor assay	Serum (speckled)	2
Rickettsial *Proteus* antibodies (*Proteus* OX 19)	Serum (speckled)	3
RPR	Serum (speckled)	2
Rubella	Serum (speckled)	4
Rubeola serology	Serum (speckled)	1
Russell viper venom (RVV) time (Stypven time)	Plasma (blue)	3
Salicylate (aspirin)	Serum (speckled)	2
Salmonella antibody	Serum (speckled)	5
Sedimentation rate (ESR) (erythrocyte sedimentation rate)	Whole blood (purple)	3
Selenium (Se)	Plasma, whole blood, serum (royal blue with heparin or EDTA or no anticoagulant)	3
Serotonin blood (5-hydroxy-tryptamine)	Whole blood or special tube from chem	10
SGOT (AST)	Serum (speckled)	1
SGPT (ALT)	Serum (speckled)	1
Sickling screen	Whole blood (purple)	2
Sodium, serum	Serum (speckled)	1
SPE (serum protein electrophoresis)	Serum (speckled)	3
Special stains		
Acid phosphatase	Blood smear	
Alkaline phosphatase	Blood smear	

(*continued*)

TABLE 4–3. (*Continued*)

Test Name	Specimen Tube (Type/Color)	Whole Blood, Minimum Volume for Adults (mL)
Esterases	Blood smear	
Heinz bodies	Blood smear	
Iron	Blood smear	
Lipid	Blood smear	
PAS for glycogen	Blood smear	
Peroxidase	Blood smear	
Sudan black	Blood smear	
Toluidine blue	Blood smear	
Streptozyme (Carter-Wallace, Inc., New York, NY) (multiple strep Ab screen)	Serum (speckled)	3
Stypven time (RVV time)	Plasma (blue)	3
Sucrose presumptive (PNH)	Whole blood (blue)	3
Sulfonamides	Serum (speckled)	5
Suppressor	Whole blood (purple)	3
Syphilis (RPR)	Serum (speckled)	2
T_3 uptake	Serum (speckled)	2
Tegretol (carbamazepine)	Serum (speckled)	2
Teichoic acid antibody	Serum (speckled)	5
Testosterone	Serum (speckled)	7
Theophylline (aminophylline)	Serum (speckled)	2
Thiamine	Whole blood (green)	10
Thiocyanate	Serum (speckled) or plasma (green) or plasma (purple)	8
Thrombin time [Fibrindex (Ortho Pharmaceutical Corporation, Raritan, NJ)]	Plasma (blue)	3
Thyroglobulin	Serum (speckled)	5
Thyroid antibodies	Serum (speckled)	3
Thyroiditis, antithyroglobulin, and antimicrosomal fraction	Serum (speckled)	5
Thyroid studies (T_3, T_4, TSH)	Serum (speckled)	4
Thyroxine (T_4)	Serum (speckled)	2
Thyroxine (T_4), free	Serum (speckled)	3
Tobramycin	Serum (speckled)	1
Tofranil (see Imipramine)		
TORCH titers	Serum (speckled)	5
Total T_3 (triiodothyronine)	Serum (speckled)	2
Toxoplasmosis serological test, IFA	Serum (speckled)	3
Transaminase (ALT, SGPT)	Serum (speckled)	1
Transaminase (AST, SGOT)	Serum (speckled)	1
Transferrin	Serum (speckled)	2

(*continued*)

TABLE 4–3. (*Continued*)

Test Name	Specimen Tube (Type/Color)	Whole Blood, Minimum Volume for Adults (mL)
Trichinella agglutination	Serum (speckled)	3
Tricyclic antidepressants (amitriptyline, nortriptyline)	Serum or plasma (red, green, or purple) [a]Avoid gel separator	3
Triglycerides (fasting)	Serum (speckled)	1
TSH (thyroid-stimulating hormone, or thyrotropin)	Serum (speckled)	2
Tylenol (see Acetominophen)		
Urea nitrogen (BUN)	Serum (speckled)	1
Uric acid	Serum (speckled)	1
Valium (diazepam)	Serum (red)	2
Valproic acid (Depakene)	Serum (speckled)	5
Vancomycin	Serum (speckled)	1
Varicella-zoster immune status	Serum (speckled)	2
Varicella-zoster serology	Serum (speckled)	2
VDRL (RPR) syphilis	Serum (speckled)	2
Vitamin A	Serum (speckled) *Protect blood from light	3
Vitamin B_6	Whole blood (purple)	10
Vitamin B_{12}	Serum (speckled)	2
Vitamin B_{12} binding capacity	Serum (speckled)	3
Vitamin C (ascorbic acid)	Whole blood (green) *immediately transport in ice water	5
Vitamin D (25-OH)	Whole blood (purple)	7
Vitamin E level	Serum (speckled)	5
von Willebrand's factor assay (Ristocetin cofactor)	Whole blood (blue) *Deliver immediately	5
D-Xylose	Serum (red)	3
Zinc	Draw blood with syringe; transfer to special plastic tube from chemistry	5

[a]*Note:* For toxicology and therapeutic drugs, the speckled-topped gel serum separator tube should be evaluated to determine whether the gel serum separator interferes in test results before these tubes are used in drug analysis collections. (See Chapter 9.)

Abbreviations: A/G, albumin/globulin (ratio); Alb, albumin; Alk p'tase, alkaline phosphatase; ALT, alanine aminotransferase; APTT, activated partial thromboplastin time; AST, aspartate aminotransferase; Ca, calcium; CBC, complete blood (count); CMV, cytomegalovirus; CPK, creatine phosphokinase; Creat, creatinine; EBV, Epstein-Barr virus; ESR, erythrocyte sedimentation rate; FBS, fasting blood sugar; Glu, glucose; HB_SAg, hepatitis B surface antigen; HCG, human chorionic gonadotropin; Hct, hematocrit; Hgb, hemoglobin; IFA, indirect fluorescent antibody (test); IgA, immunoglobulin A; IgD, immunoglobulin D; IgG, immunoglobulin G; IgM, immunoglobulin M; I phos, inorganic phosphorus; LD, lactate dehydrogenase; MCH, mean corpuscular hemoglobin; MCHC, mean corpuscular hemoglobin concentration; MCV, mean corpuscular volume; PAS, periodic acid–Schiff; PNH, paroxysmal nocturnal hemoglobinuria; RBC, red blood cell; RPR, rapid plasma reagin; RVV, Russell viper venom (time); SGOT, serum glutamic oxaloacetic transaminase; SGPT, serum glutamic pyruvic transaminase; SPE, serum protein electrophoresis; T. bil, total bilirubin; TIBC, total iron-binding capacity; T. protein, total protein; VDRL, Venereal Disease Research Laboratory; WBC, white blood cell.

cellular morphological features. Thus, gray-topped tubes should not be used for hematology studies.

Green-Topped Tubes

The anticoagulants sodium heparin, ammonium heparin, and lithium heparin are found in green-topped vacuum tubes. These tubes are used in various laboratory assays requiring plasma or whole blood, mainly chemistry tests. For potassium measurement, heparinized plasma or whole blood, rather than serum, is preferred because sporadic increased potassium levels can occur in serum as a result of potassium released from platelets during blood clotting.[1] Lithium heparin tubes may be used for glucose, blood urea nitrogen (BUN), creatinine, and electrolyte studies; however, this anticoagulant is not suitable for tests involving the measurement of ionized calcium or lithium levels. Similarly, sodium heparin tubes should not be used for assays that measure the sodium concentration. In other cases, a particular procedure will require sodium heparin without lithium or vice versa.

Green-topped vacuum tubes should not be used for collections for blood smears that are to be stained with Wright's stain because the heparin causes the Wright's stain to have a blue background. When used for cytogenetic studies, these tubes must be sterile.

Purple-Topped and Light-Blue–Topped Tubes

The purple-topped vacuum tubes (containing EDTA) are used for most hematology procedures. Many coagulation procedures are done on blood collected in light-blue–topped vacuum tubes, which contain sodium citrate at a concentration of 3.8 percent.

Red-Topped, Royal-Blue–Topped, and Brown-Topped Tubes

The red-topped tubes indicate a tube without anticoagulant for collection of serum. Thus, the collected blood will clot in this tube. The royal-blue–topped tubes are used to collect samples for nutritional studies, therapeutic drug monitoring, and toxicology. The royal-blue–topped tube is the trace element tube. The brown-topped tube contains heparin or no additive and is used for blood lead values.

Black-Topped Tubes

From certain manufacturers, a black-topped tube with buffered sodium citrate is available for blood collections used to determine the ESR.

Blood Culture Collection Tubes

Sterile blood specimens are also ordered for blood cultures when the patient is suspected of having septicemia (symptoms of sepsis). A major problem with collecting blood for culture is that the patient's sample can become contaminated with microorganisms from the skin. Thus, the blood must be collected in a sterile container (vacuum vial or syringe) under aseptic conditions.

As shown in Figure 4–9, blood can be collected directly into vacuum vials that contain culture media. This type of collection minimizes the risk of specimen contamination. The vacuum vials can be purchased with different types of culture media, an unplugged venting unit for aerobic incubation, or a plugged venting unit for anaerobic incubation.

Separation Tubes (Mottled-Topped Tubes)

Another collection method is to draw blood into a serum separation tube such as the Monoject Corvac (Sherwood Medical Monoject Division, St. Louis, MO). Blood is collected in the vacuum Monoject Corvac tube by conventional blood-collecting means. As illustrated in

Figure 4–9. BACTEC culture vials. *(Courtesy of Becton-Dickinson Diagnostic Instrument Systems, Sparks, MD.)*

Figure 4–10, this tube contains a gel in a cup-shaped plastic "energizer" containing microscopic glass particles. As blood enters the tube, the glass particles go into suspension and accelerate clotting by providing an increased surface area. As shown in Figure 4–11, when the blood in the Monoject Corvac tube is centrifuged, the energizer cup displaces the gel and forces it from the bottom to the sides of the tube. The gel's specific gravity is intermediate to that of serum and clotted blood. Thus, the gel stops moving when the equilibrium point is reached. At this

Figure 4–10. Monoject Corvac tube. *(Courtesy of Sherwood Medical Monoject Division, St. Louis, MO.)*

1. The CORVAC tube utilizes traditional phlebotomy techniques.

2. Powdered glass suspended throughout the sample accelerates coagulation.

3. Centrifugal force drives the gel energizer into the silicone gel at the base of the tube.

4. The energizer controls the flow of the gel up the sides of the tube.

5. The gel continues to move up the sides of the tube, seeking an equilibrium between serum and coagulum.

6. The gel reaches an equilibrium between serum and coagulum.

7. The gel forms a stable barrier between serum and coagulum.

Figure 4–11. How the Monoject Corvac works. *(Courtesy of Sherwood Medical Monoject Division, St. Louis, MO.)*

point, the gel forms a positive, stable, chemical and physical barrier between the clotted blood and the serum for as long as 24 hours after centrifugation.

Blood-collecting vacuum tubes can be ordered in different sizes to allow for the different amounts of blood needed for various types of clinical laboratory assays.

SYRINGES

Some patients' veins are too fragile for blood collection with vacuum tubes. Thus, syringes must be used for the collection process. A syringe, without the needle, consists of the barrel, the plunger, and the tip. The barrel and the plunger are made to fit together tightly so that when the plunger is in the barrel and drawn back, a vacuum is created. This vacuum allows blood or other fluids to be aspirated, or sucked, into the barrel as the plunger is pulled back. The barrel of the syringe has graduated measurements in milliliter increments. Sizes range from approximately 0.2 to 50.0 mL; however, for specimen collection purposes, 5- to 20-mL syringes are used most often. A needle is usually attached directly on the smooth tip of the syringe. Some syringes have Luer-Lok tips (Becton-Dickinson VACUTAINER Systems, Franklin Lakes, NJ), which lock the needle onto the tip for a firm hold. In addition, the health care worker should ensure that the syringe is the correct size for the amount of blood to be collected.

Although disposable plastic syringes are used most frequently, on occasion a glass syringe may be needed for blood collection for a special procedure. In such cases, the glass plunger and barrel should be inspected carefully before use to check for possible cracks or chips.

NEEDLES

The gauge and length of a needle used on a syringe or a vacuum tube is selected according to the specific task. For example, larger (18-gauge) needles are used for collecting donor units of blood (450 mL or less), whereas smaller (21- and 22-gauge) needles are used for collecting specimens for laboratory assays. When blood is collected from children, a 21- to 23-gauge needle is usually used with a tuberculin, or 3-mL, syringe, or with a winged infusion set. The **gauge number** indicates the diameter of the needle; the smaller the number, the larger the needle. The length of the needle depends on the depth of the vein to be punctured.

Needles are sterilized and packaged by vendors in sealed shields that maintain sterility. These shields are packaged in individual containers that are color coded according to the gauge size of the needles and must be twisted apart before the needles are used in blood collection.[2] Terumo Medical Corporation has introduced the Venoject II ultrathin wall needle, which allows the use of a smaller-gauge needle without compromising the rate of blood flow into the collection tube.

The tip of each needle should be checked for damage. A blunt or bent tip can be harmful to the patient's vein and may result in failure to collect blood.

Different types of needles are used for single- and multiple-sample collections. **Multiple-sample needles** are used with vacuum collection tubes and the holder to allow for multiple tube changes without blood leakage within the plastic holder. The multiple-sample needle has a plastic cover over the tube-top puncturing portion of the needle; this cover creates a leakage barrier. The **single-sample needle** is usually used for collecting blood with a syringe.

One type of needle that has been introduced to help prevent not only accidental needle sticks, but also the transmission of acquired immunodeficiency syndrome (AIDS) and other infectious diseases is the High Risk (HR) needle (ICU Medical, Inc., Mission Viejo, CA). Because the used HR needle is covered permanently at the point of injection, the hazards of recapping or disassembling the needle are eliminated.

The Butterfly Needle (Winged Infusion Set)

The butterfly needle (winged infusion set) is the most commonly used intravenous device. It is a stainless steel beveled needle and tube with attached plastic wings. The most common butterfly needle sizes are 21 and 25 gauge. The butterfly needle is sometimes used in the collection of blood from patients who are difficult to stick by conventional methods (e.g., geriatric patients, cancer patients, pediatric patients).

Numerous types of safety butterfly needles are now available. These safety needles each have a shield that automatically covers the contaminated needle point upon withdrawal from the patient's vein. One example is the Angel Wing blood collection set (Fig. 4–12) from Sherwood Medical Monoject Division (St. Louis, MO). It has a stainless steel safety shield that automatically resheaths the needle during withdrawal from the patient. The system includes multisample needle-shielded tube holders and sets for use in drawing blood specimens directly into blood collection tubes and blood culture bottles, as well as multisample needle-shielded transfer tube holders and sets for transferring blood from syringes into collection tubes and blood culture bottles.

The Shamrock safety winged set (Ryan Medical, a division of

Figure 4–12. Angel Wing blood collection set. *(Courtesy of Sherwood Medical Monoject Division, St. Louis, MO.)*

Winfield Industries, San Diego, CA) has a luer hub that can be connected to a syringe or a multiple-sample luer adapter with a preattached Saf-T Holder (Ryan Medical, a division of Winfield Industries, San Diego, CA) (Fig. 4–13). Another example of a winged infusion set is the Luer-Lok blood collection device (Fig. 4–14) manufactured by Becton Dickinson VACUTAINER Systems.

Needle Disposal

As shown in Figure 4–15, Datar, Inc., (Long Lake, MN) produces a phlebotomy resheather and tube holder. This system allows needles to be resheathed safely, and it acts as a holder for vacuum tubes. Because

Figure 4–13. Shamrock safety winged set. **A.** The luer hub can be connected to a syringe or a multiple-sample luer adapter with a preattached Saf-T Holder. **B.** After withdrawal from the patient's vein, the needle is simply and securely pulled back into its protective shield. **C.** The audible click and the visual indicator ensure that the needle has been locked into its protective shield for safe disposal. *(Courtesy of Ryan Medical, a division of Winfield Industries, San Diego, CA.)*

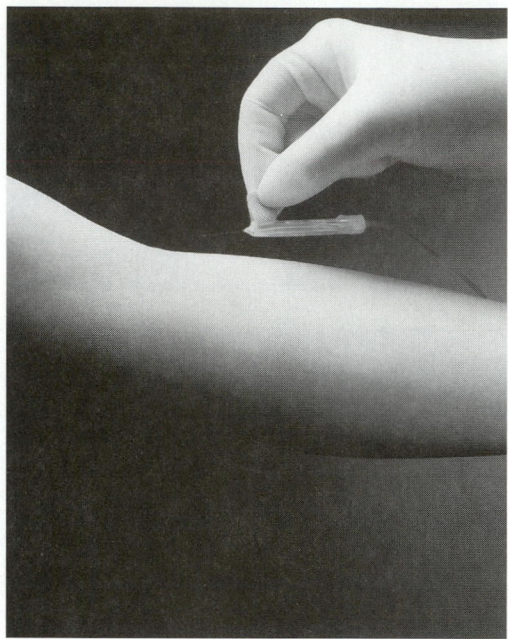

Figure 4–14. Luer-Lok blood collection device. *(Courtesy of Becton-Dickinson VACUTAINER Systems, Franklin Lakes, NJ.)*

the unit can be autoclaved, it can be reused. In addition, Datar, Inc., offers a pocket resheather (Fig. 4–16) that allows the phlebotomist to resheath needles safely with the "one-handed technique." The IV Pole Resheather (IV-R), also by Datar, Inc., provides a safe one-handed method (Fig. 4–17) for recapping needles from intermediate intravenous (IV) tubing and syringes. It can connect directly to an IV pole or be used as a portable stand-alone resheather.

Datar, Inc., also produces several sizes of needle-disposal containers (Fig. 4–18) for use at the bedside, on the cart, in isolation, during surgery, on home health care trays, and so on. Needles and syringes must be discarded in rigid plastic containers, which reduce the possibility of needle sticks for the phlebotomist. Each unit is disposable as biohazardous waste.

SAFE ACCESS TO BLOOD SAMPLES

After blood collection, the health care worker must gain access to the blood in the vacuum tube for testing purposes. To protect laboratory personnel against blood exposure during this hazardous step, manufacturers recently developed several different types of items.

Figure 4–15. Phlebotomy resheather and tube holder. *(Courtesy of Datar, Inc., Long Lake, MN.)*

An example is the Becton Dickinson VACUTAINER tube with Hemogard. This device is a vacuum blood collection tube with a plastic shield over the stopper. The shield protects the health care worker from splattering blood when the stopper is removed from the tube.

The Pumpette (Helena Laboratories, Beaumont, TX) is a device that can provide access to the needed blood sample without uncapping the blood collection tube. The sample is aspirated by pressing the accordion-style pump on top of the stopper. Safety and efficiency are increased by using this device.

Terumo Medical Corporation offers Venoject II plastic evacuated blood collection tubes (Fig. 4–3) that have UltraSeal closure seals. The UltraSeal closure seal reduces the potential for splatter contamination, and the thin septum of this seal may easily be pierced by the automated hematology analyzer.

Figure 4–16. Pocket resheather. *(Courtesy of Datar, Inc., Long Lake, MN.)*

Figure 4–17. IV Pole Resheather. *(Courtesy of Datar, Inc., Long Lake, MN.)*

Figure 4–18. Needle disposal system. *(Courtesy of Datar, Inc., Long Lake, MN.)*

Another device that was developed to reduce the possibility of infection, contamination, and aerosol spray is the Aerotrap (Innovative Laboratory Products, Ltd., Citrus Heights, CA, distributed by Fisher Scientific, Citrus Heights, CA). It is used in laboratories to remove the stopper from vacuum tubes. The Aerotrap allows laboratory personnel to handle the vacuum tubes without touching the stoppers, and it reduces the amount of contamination that is hand carried throughout the laboratory.

After blood is drawn by syringe, it should immediately be transferred to a dry, chemically clean tube. The blood should be allowed to clot for a minimum of 15 minutes at room temperature, or longer if it is refrigerated. If the clot is allowed to retract for a longer period, the chances for hemolysis are decreased and the yield of serum is enhanced. The longer the blood cells remain in contact with the serum, the greater the shift of substances from blood cells to serum through the metabolic process of glycolysis.

TOURNIQUETS

The tourniquet is a key to successful venipuncture: it provides a barrier against venous flow. Tourniquets are used in specimen collection to apply enough pressure to the arm to slow the return of venous blood to the heart. This slowing of venous return causes pooling of blood in the veins, which makes the veins more visible and easier to feel and find. A tourniquet should *not* restrict arterial blood flowing into the arm. Blood should enter the arm at a normal rate and, with the use of a tourniquet, return to the heart at a slower rate.

Tourniquets that are usually used include the pliable strap, the Velcro type, and the blood pressure cuff. The blood pressure cuff can be used successfully when veins are difficult to find. The most efficient blood barrier provides a resistance that is less than systolic blood pressure but greater than diastolic; or, stated another way, blood flows in but not out. The blood pressure cuff can determine these pressures; consequently, it is a perfect tourniquet.[3]

Another type of tourniquet is the Seraket (Propper Manufacturing Co., Inc., Long Island City, NY), which uses a seat-belt design. It allows the phlebotomist to partially release the venous pressure by using a lever that releases some pressure, but not all. Thus, if the phlebotomist needs to tighten the tourniquet again, the lever can be used to adjust the tourniquet. Because errors in laboratory test results can occur from prolonged tourniquet pressure, the Seraket provides a solution to this problem. However, one drawback of this type of tourniquet is the difficulty in cleaning and decontaminating it if it is soiled with blood.

Velcro-type tourniquets are popular because they are easy to apply and comfortable for the patient. Alternatively, because of major concern for infection control in health care institutions, many facilities now use a disposable natural latex tourniquet strap (The Hygenic Corp., Akron, OH) to help prevent cross-contamination. If the tourniquets used in the health care facility are not disposable, they must be wiped frequently with 70 percent isopropyl alcohol.

BLEEDING-TIME EQUIPMENT

Bleeding time is an assay used to assess the contributions of platelet function and blood vessel integrity to primary blood-clotting abilities.[4] The test is performed by making a minor standardized incision in the forearm or earlobe and recording the length of time required for bleeding to stop. Many procedures have been used to measure bleeding time. Recent advances have led to the development of mechanical devices that are used to create uniform skin incisions for bleeding-time determination. One such device is the Hemalet (Medprobe Laboratories, New York, NY), which has an automatic blade-retraction mechanism. Another such device is the Surgicutt (International Technidyne Corporation, Edison, NJ), which provides a uniform surgical incision. The procedure for determining bleeding time is provided in Chapter 9.

GLOVES FOR BLOOD COLLECTION

Safety guidelines have been established for health care workers to help them prevent the possibility of acquiring infections such as hepatitis or those associated with AIDS. These guidelines include the use of gloves during collection of blood from patients. Examples of gloves being used by health care workers include Ultraderm sterile surgeon's gloves (Baxter Travenol Laboratories, Inc., Deerfield, IL), talc-free Eudermic surgical gloves (Becton, Dickinson and Company, Franklin Lakes, NJ), Medi-Pak latex gloves (General Medical Corp., Richmond, VA), and Lab Safety Supply nonirritating surgical gloves (Lab Safety Supply, Janesville, WI), which are made without talc. It is recommended that phlebotomists not use gloves with talc powder containing calcium because tubes of patients' blood may become contaminated with this powder, and such contamination can result in falsely elevated calcium values. Researchers have found that latex gloves provide better protection than vinyl gloves.[5] The Safeskin hypoallergenic latex glove (Safeskin Corporation, Coral Gables, FL) outperformed all other brands in the referenced study. However, phlebotomists should not use petroleum products or other skin protectants when wearing latex gloves because these substances break down the latex and decrease the active barrier.[6] If a health care worker develops allergenic dermatitis to gloves, she or he should try other brands of gloves or wear cotton gloves under the latex gloves. Stahmer Weston Scientific (Portsmouth, NH) developed UltraFIT glove liners (Fig. 4–19) for individuals who are extrasensitive to latex. These liners are made with 100 percent durable nylon material and can be washed several times for reuse. Another approach suggested by the US Food and Drug Administration (FDA) is to wear latex gloves between two vinyl gloves.[7]

If the patient is allergic to latex, the phlebotomist should wear non-latex gloves or latex gloves between two vinyl gloves. Also, in such cases, latex bandages or tourniquets should not be used on the patient. Instead, a cloth tourniquet and latex-free tape should be used.

Glove liners have also been developed that provide hand protection from cuts, nicks, and abrasions (Vigard Medical Products, Lovell-

Figure 4–19. UltraFIT glove liner. *(Courtesy of Stahmer Weston Scientific, Portsmouth, NH.)*

Schenck, Inc., Charlotte, NC). These glove liners are available in three styles—reusable, disposable, and clinical.

Uarco Inc. (Barrington, IL) developed adhesive labels that do not stick to gloves. These Glove-Free labels adhere firmly to glass, plastic, and paper, but they do not stick to vinyl or latex gloves. The labels, coated with a special adhesive, aid laboratory safety by eliminating the problem of torn gloves caused by trying to remove an adhering label.

ANTISEPTICS, STERILE GAUZE PADS, AND BANDAGES

✔ The health care worker needs **antiseptics, sterile gauze pads,** and bandages for blood collection by either venipuncture or microcollection. Therefore, 70 percent isopropyl alcohol preparation and povidone–iodine (Betadine) swab sticks or pads (for blood cultures) are essential items for blood collection.

MICROCOLLECTION EQUIPMENT

Usually, skin puncture blood-collecting techniques are used on infants because venipuncture is excessively hazardous. Skin puncture collection is also indicated for adults and older children when they are severely burned, have veins that are difficult to stick because of their small size or location, must undergo bedside clinical testing, are extremely obese, or must perform home glucose testing.

The volume of plasma or serum that generally can be collected from a premature infant is approximately 100 to 150 µL, and about two times that amount can be taken from a full-term newborn. Larger volumes are obtained from older children and adults.[8]

A **disposable sterile lancet** should be used to puncture the skin for skin puncture collection. For newborns, lancets with tips 2.4 mm or less in length, such as the **Microtainer** safety flow lancet (Becton-Dickinson VACUTAINER Systems, Franklin Lakes, NJ) (Fig. 4–20), are required to avoid penetrating bone.[9] Research indicates that for some infants (including premature infants) a puncture depth of 2.4 mm may be excessive and that the appropriate puncture depth for infants requires more study.[10] The Monolet OPD lancet (Sherwood Medical Monoject Division, St. Louis, MO), as shown in Figure 4–21, is a lancet available for safe skin puncture of neonates. In addition, Sherwood Medical manufactures Monolet lancets for adults and children.

International Technidyne Corporation (Edison, NJ) has produced fully automated, single-use, automatically retracting, disposable devices that provide safety both for the neonate and for the health care worker. Tenderlett jr. for children. Tenderlett for adults, and Tenderlett toddler for infants and toddlers are engineered to incise to the least invasive but most effective depth for optimal blood flow. The Tenderlett incises

Figure 4–20. Microtainer safety flow lancet. *(Courtesy of Becton-Dickinson VACUTAINER Systems, Franklin Lakes, NJ.)*

Figure 4–21. Monolet and Monojector lancet device. *(Courtesy of Sherwood Medical Monoject Division, St. Louis, MO.)*

1.75-mm deep, Tenderlett jr. incises 1.25-mm deep, and Tenderlett toddler incises only 0.85-mm deep. The retracting blade of each of these devices eliminates potential injury from an exposed blade contaminated with blood.

The Unistik 2 (Owen Mumford Inc., Marietta, GA) is a safe, single-use, capillary blood–sampling device. This microcollection lancet is available in two penetration ranges (2.4 and 3.0 mm) and automatically retracts after incision.

Other devices for microcollection are the Autolet II Clinisafe (Fig. 4–22) and the Autolet Lite Clinisafe (Fig. 4–23), both by Ulster Scientific, Inc., New Paltz, NY. The Autolet II Clinisafe is a spring-activated puncture device that allows easy ejection of the lancet and platform, providing safety for both patient and phlebotomist. The Autolet platform can be chosen for the patient's level of comfort and the needed blood volume. These platforms are available in three color-coded depths: white (1.8 mm) for shallow penetration, yellow (2.4 mm) for normal penetration, and orange (3.0 mm) for deeper incisions.

The Autolet Lite Clinisafe features a safety mechanism that inhibits the use of the device unless it is first reloaded with a new lancet and platform. Complying with FDA and Centers for Disease Control and Prevention (CDC) guidelines, both the lancet and the platform can be used only *once* and are simultaneously ejected at the touch of a button.

Superfine lancets have been developed with a slimmer needle and a new bevel to allow for smooth and easy skin penetration, which pro-

Figure 4–22. Autolet II Clinisafe blood-drawing device. *(Courtesy of Ulster Scientific, Inc., New Paltz, NY.)*

vides more comfort for the patient. Blades that do not provide appropriate control of the cutting edge and depth of puncture should not be used.

The **microcontainers** recommended for use for collections for blood gas, electrolyte, and general chemistry analyses are described in Table 4–4. Usually, microspecimens for blood gas analysis are collected in

Figure 4–23. Ulster Scientific blood collection products. *(Courtesy of Ulster Scientific, Inc., New Paltz, NY.)*

TABLE 4–4. CONTAINERS FOR BLOOD COLLECTION

Container[a]	Remarks
Blood gases (pH, P_{CO_2}, P_{O_2}):	
Natelson glass collecting pipettes, 250-µL volume, lithium heparin; heparinized glass capillary tubes, 100 to 250 µL.	To mix, insert metal "fleas," or mixing bars, after filling.[b] Seal with plastic caps or sealing wax. Mix by use of a magnet. Source: many laboratory suppliers.
Blood-collecting pipette kits and component parts, supplied by manufacturers of blood gas apparatus.	Kits containing glass capillaries, sealing wax, metal mixing bars, and magnets. Source: laboratory suppliers of Corning, IL, and radiometer equipment.
Caraway glass tubes, 370-mL volume, sodium or lithium heparin.	Mix and seal as above, or by inversion. Source: many laboratory suppliers.
Electrolytes (CO_2, Cl, K, Na) and general chemistry:	
Microhematocrit glass capillary tubes 1.1– 1.2 mm inner diameter, 75-mm long, ammonium heparin; other sizes.	Plasma obtained. Mix and seal as above.
Microsample tubes, polyethylene, 300 µL, lithium heparin; larger sizes (400 to 550 µL) for general chemistry, with and without heparin.	Plasma obtained. Seal with attached cap. Mix by inversion.[c] Source: Kew Scientific and Beckman Instruments, Inc., Fullerton, CA.
Microtainer, polypropylene, 600 and 700 mL, silicone separator, with and without lithium heparin.	Serum obtained. Seal with accompanying cap. Centrifuge at 6000 x *g*. Source: Becton, Dickinson VACUTAINER Systems, Franklin Lakes, NJ.

[a]Containers listed here are all commercially available.
[b]Mixing without a flea is also possible by gently inverting the capillary before sealing.
[c]Shake the first drop entering the tube to its bottom. All further drops should then flow along the path of the first drop if the tube is held in a nearly vertical position.
From Meites S (ed): Pediatric Clinical Chemistry, *3rd ed. Washington, DC, American Association for Clinical Chemistry, 1989, p 10, with permission.*

heparinized glass Natelson tubes. These tubes may have a color band indicating the presence and type of anticoagulant. The band also identifies the top part of the pipette in reference to sample handling. A red band indicates an ammonium heparin coating in the tube, and a green band indicates a sodium or lithium heparin coating. Because ammonium ions can falsely change the blood pH of the collected blood, sodium or lithium heparin should be used in collections for blood gas analysis. The blood collected in these tubes must be mixed with the heparin by a small metal "flea," or bar, with a magnet. After mixing, the ends are sealed with sealing wax or plastic caps.

AVL Scientific Corporation (Graz, Austria) has developed the AVL microsampler for collection of two 120-µL **arterial blood gas** samples from children or adults. It has a 26-gauge microneedle, which reduces the chances of puncture pain and hematoma formation. The tubes are coated with heparin to prevent clotting, and they automatically fill without bubble formation. This microsampler is used on the radial, brachial, or femoral artery.

Microhematocrit **capillary tubes** are disposable narrow-bore pipettes that are used for packed red cell volume in microcentrifugation. These tubes also have colored bands; a red band indicates a heparin-coated tube, and a blue band indicates no anticoagulant.

Plastic microcollection devices for general laboratory collections (e.g., chemistry, immunology) are usually color coded according to the established protocol for blood collection vacuum tube stoppers. Thus, purple-topped (lavender-topped) tubes contain EDTA, green-topped tubes contain heparin, red- or pink-topped tubes have no additive, and gray-topped tubes have sodium fluoride to inhibit blood enzymes that destroy glucose.

Sherwood Medical Company (St. Louis, MO) manufactures the Samplette capillary blood collector (Fig. 4–24), which is offered with a full range of anticoagulants and serum and plasma separation gels. One

Figure 4–24. Samplette capillary blood collector. *(Courtesy of Sherwood Medical Monoject Division, St. Louis, MO.)*

of their collectors is an amber capillary blood separator that provides protection for light-sensitive analytes (e.g., bilirubin).

Electrolytes and general chemistry microspecimens can be collected in the Microtainer tube (Becton-Dickinson VACUTAINER Systems, Franklin Lakes, NJ), which has its own capillary blood collector, self-contained serum separator, and plastic top (Fig. 4–25). This system can collect as much as 600 µL of blood. Alternatively, two or more capillary tubes can be used for electrolyte and general chemistry collection. One advantage of these tubes is that if blood hemolyzes in one capillary tube, another capillary tube containing the patient's sample can be used for the chemical analyses.

The Microvette capillary blood collection system (Sarstedt, Inc., Princeton, NJ) is another microcollection system that is offered with a full range of anticoagulants and serum separation gel. This system can be used to collect, store, and separate samples in the same unbreakable, disposable container (Fig. 4–26).

Figure 4–25. Microtainer tube. *(Courtesy of Becton-Dickinson VACUTAINER Systems, Franklin Lakes, NJ.)*

Figure 4–26. Microvette capillary blood collection system. *(Courtesy of Sarstedt, Inc., Princeton, NJ.)*

RAM Scientific Co. (Princeton, NJ) has developed an unbreakable plastic capillary-receptacle system. The device consists of a plastic capillary inserted into a microtube receptacle. With the attached receptacle, blood flows directly to the bottom of the tube. This system makes the blood drawing safe and clean. The capillary can then be removed, and the tube is closed with the appropriate color-coded cap.

For most chemical assays, lithium and ammonium salts of heparin are the anticoagulants of choice for microcollections. They have rarely been reported to interfere with the determination of electrolytes and most other chemical assays.[9]

Another type of microcollection device is the Unopette (Becton-Dickinson VACUTAINER Systems, Franklin Lakes, NJ), shown in Figure 4–27. This device serves as a collection and dilution unit for blood samples and thus increases the speed and simplicity of laboratory procedures. These devices are prefilled with specific amounts of diluents or reagents, or both, for different types of laboratory assays. Some of the more prevalent procedures in which Unopette devices are used include the WBC count, RBC count, platelet count, hemoglobin, RBC fragility, sodium and potassium, and lead determinations.

The standard Unopette test comprises (1) a disposable, self-filling diluting pipette consisting of a straight, thin-walled, uniform-bore, glass capillary tube fitted into a plastic holder and (2) a plastic reservoir containing a premeasured volume of reagent for diluting. For quick and easy visual identification, each capillary pipette is color coded according to its capacity. Color coding for all disposable self-filling Unopette cap-

Figure 4–27. Unopette, a collection and dilution unit for blood samples. *(Courtesy of Becton-Dickinson VACUTAINER Systems, Franklin Lakes, NJ.)*

illary pipettes is as follows: 3 µL—green, 3.3 µL—gray, 10 µL—pink, 20 µL—yellow, 25 µL—blue, and 44.7 µL—black.

Sealing Items for Microcollection Tubes

For capillary pipettes and tubes, sealing wax or caps are necessary when the blood is drawn into the tube. Puttylike sealants and plastic closures are available from various manufacturers. The phlebotomist must be sure to follow the instructions with the sealant in order to provide safe sealing during microcentrifugation. A capillary tube device that was developed to reduce the opportunity for blowout of the sealant during microcentrifugation is the Safecap capillary and Safeplug (Safe-Tec, Inc.). Safecap capillary has a self-sealing plug called *Safeplug* that was manufactured to permit a more accurate measurement of the packed cell volume and to decrease biohazardous risk to blood splatters and aerosol spray during microcentrifugation.

Transporting Microspecimens

Glycolysis in RBCs and WBCs causes a decrease in blood pH that can be detected after a blood gas sample has been stored at room temperature for approximately 20 minutes. Therefore, blood gas microsamples should be immersed in a slurry of ice water from the time of collection until they are delivered to the clinical laboratory. Plastic containers that are small enough to hold these specimens with ice and water should be carried on the specimen collection tray. Ice is usually available on the patient ward. Other items to be carried on a microcollection tray include the following:

1. Seventy percent isopropyl alcohol and Betadine pads
2. Marking pens for labels
3. Microtainer blood serum separator tubes (600 µL)
4. Microtainer capillary whole blood cell collectors with 0.23 mg of EDTA (200 µL)
5. Lancets for skin puncture
6. Sterile gauze pads or bandages
7. Unheparinized plastic microcentrifuge tubes
8. Heparinized plastic microcentrifuge tubes (250, 400, and 500 µL)
9. Heparinized Natelson tubes (75 µL)
10. Unopette devices for collection and dilution procedures
11. Disposable gloves
12. Cloth towel or washcloth
13. Thermometer
14. Biohazardous waste containers for sharps
15. Glass microscope slides
16. Capillary tube sealer

BLOOD-DRAWING CHAIR

In an outpatient clinic that requires blood collections, a **blood-drawing chair** must be available for patients. The chair is designed for maximum safety and comfort of the patient plus easy accessibility to either arm of the patient. The chair should have an armrest for the patient's use during blood drawing. The armrest should lock in place so that the patient cannot fall from the chair if he or she becomes faint. Also, the armrest should adjust in an up-and-down position so that the best venipuncture position for each patient can be achieved.

SPECIMEN COLLECTION TRAYS

The health care worker needs a specimen tray (Fig. 4–28) to take on blood-collecting rounds. The tray is usually made of plastic and must be amenable to sterilization. The tray should include all necessary collection equipment, and its contents usually differ from one hospital or clinic to another, depending on the patient population. For example, if

Figure 4–28. Specimen collection tray. *(Courtesy of Becton-Dickinson VACU-TAINER Systems, Franklin Lakes, NJ.)*

the phlebotomist works in a children's hospital, he or she needs micro-collection trays containing equipment such as that described earlier. For home health care providers and reference laboratory couriers, the necessary collection supplies, equipment, and collected blood must be carried in an enclosed container with the biohazard symbol shown on the outside. For example, the Loc-Top Lab Tray (Healthmark Industries Co., Detroit, MI), shown in Figure 4–29, is lockable to protect the contents from tampering or accidental contamination. It also has a tight seal to reduce the risk of infection from bloodborne pathogens due to spills or accidents.

Health care workers who collect blood from adults usually have the following equipment on their trays or in their safety container:

1. Marking pens or pencils
2. Vacuum tubes containing the anticoagulants designated in the clinical laboratory blood collection manual
3. Holders for vacuum tubes
4. Needles for vacuum tubes and syringes
5. Syringes
6. Tourniquet

7. Seventy percent isopropyl alcohol, iodine, and Betadine pads or swab sticks
8. Sterile gauze pads
9. Bandages
10. Biohazardous waste containers for used needles and lancets
11. Lancets for skin puncture
12. Unopette devices for finger-stick blood collection
13. Microtainer blood serum separator tubes (600 µL)
14. Microtainer capillary whole blood collectors with 0.23 mg of EDTA (200 µL)
15. Disposable gloves
16. Cloth towel or washcloth
17. Thermometer

TRANSPORTING AND PROCESSING PATIENT SPECIMENS

Every health care facility has a specific protocol for specimen transportation and processing. Many institutions require the use of a leakproof plastic bag for insertion of the specimen container. This bag

Figure 4–29. Loc-Top Lab Tray. *(Courtesy of Healthmark Industries, Co., Detroit, MI.)*

protects the phlebotomist from pathogenic (disease-producing) organisms during transportation of the specimen. This special transport bag should have a pouch on the outside for the laboratory request slip so that the request slip does not become contaminated.

For special types of specimens, the clinical laboratory has special handling steps. For example, if a health care worker is requested to transport an arterial specimen to the laboratory for blood gas analysis, he or she should be aware that the specimen must be transported in an airtight heparinized syringe and packed in ice with water. The airtight container and the ice water decrease the loss of gases from the specimen. Speed is essential to prevent loss of gases from the blood.

Because glycolytic action from the blood cells interferes in the analysis of various chemicals (e.g., glucose, calcitonin, aldosterone, phosphorus, enzymes), the blood samples should be transported to the clinical laboratory within 45 minutes of collection so that the serum or plasma can be separated from the blood cells. The serum or plasma that is separated from the cells must be handled according to the laboratory procedure; therefore, it may remain at room temperature, be refrigerated, be stored in a dark place, or be frozen, depending on the prescribed laboratory method.

Some chemical constituents in blood, such as bilirubin, are light sensitive and decrease in value if exposed to light. Thus, blood collected for chemical analysis should be protected from bright light with an aluminum foil wrapping around the tube.

Blood specimens for microbiology must also be transported to the laboratory as quickly as possible so that the blood can be transferred to culture media.

The blood vacuum tubes and Microtainer tubes should be maintained in a vertical position to promote complete clot formation, if required, and to reduce the possibility of hemolysis. The health care worker must also transport the blood specimens in a gentle manner to prevent hemolysis of the specimens.

Processing specimens may occur in one location of the clinical laboratory or in each section (e.g., hematology, clinical chemistry, clinical immunology, blood bank, coagulation), depending on the organization of the laboratory. The health care worker must learn the processing requirements of the clinical laboratory so that specimens are transported and processed as quickly as possible. As discussed earlier in this chapter, safety devices should be used to gain access to the blood so that splashing and aerosol spray from the blood sample do not contaminate the health care worker. Efficient and safe processing of the specimens leads to better clinical laboratory results and thus better patient care. In many laboratories, the specimen collection area has a medical technologist (clinical laboratory scientist) or a medical laboratory technician who centrifuges the specimens and makes the appropriate aliquots for each section. These aliquots are then distributed to the clinical laboratory sections for testing. Some specimens must be prepared for shipping to referral laboratories. Sometimes, this preparation involves special packaging requirements, such as freezing the specimen to maintain stability and packaging it in a Styrofoam mailing container. (See Chapter 14 for more information on shipping laboratory specimens to reference laboratories.)

✔ Key Terms

ACID–CITRATE–DEXTROSE (ACD)

ANTICOAGULANTS

ANTISEPTICS

ARTERIAL BLOOD GAS

BLOOD-DRAWING CHAIR

CAPILLARY TUBES

CITRATES

CITRATE–PHOSPHATE–DEXTROSE (CPD)

DISPOSABLE STERILE LANCET

ETHYLENEDIAMINE TETRAACETIC ACID (EDTA)

GAUGE NUMBER

HEPARIN

HOLDER (ADAPTER)

LITHIUM IODOACETATE

MICROCONTAINERS

MULTIPLE-SAMPLE NEEDLES

OXALATES

SINGLE-SAMPLE NEEDLES

SODIUM FLUORIDE

STERILE GAUZE PADS

VACUUM (EVACUATED) TUBE

Study Questions

1. Which of the following anticoagulants prevent coagulation of blood by removing calcium through the formation of insoluble calcium salts?

   a. EDTA
   b. ammonium oxalate
   c. sodium citrate
   d. sodium heparin

2. Which of the following anticoagulants is found in a green-topped blood-collection vacuum tube?

   a. EDTA
   b. ammonium oxalate
   c. sodium citrate
   d. sodium heparin

3. For capillary collection from newborns, a lancet of which of the following lengths should be used to avoid penetrating bone?

   a. 2.40 mm
   b. 2.75 mm
   c. 3.00 mm
   d. 3.25 mm

4. Which of the following blood chemical constituents is light sensitive?

   a. glucose
   b. bilirubin

   c. phosphorus
   d. blood gases

5. When blood is collected from a patient, the serum should be separated from the blood cells as quickly as possible to avoid

   a. hemoconcentration
   b. hemolysis

   c. glycolysis
   d. hemostasis

6. The color coding for needles indicates the

   a. length
   b. gauge

   c. manufacturer
   d. anticoagulant

7. From the listed needle gauges, which one has the largest diameter?

   a. 19
   b. 20

   c. 21
   d. 23

8. Which of the following is/are skin puncture equipment?

   a. Tenderlett
   b. Autolet Lite

   c. Samplette
   d. AVL microsampler

9. Which of the following laboratory tests requires that the blood be transported in a slurry of ice water to the laboratory?

   a. bilirubin
   b. CK

   c. blood gas analysis
   d. complete blood cell (CBC) count

REFERENCES

1. Hyman D, Kaplan N: The difference between serum and plasma potassium (letter). *N Engl J Med* 313:642, 1985.
2. National Committee for Clinical Laboratory Standards (NCCLS): *Procedures for the Collection of Diagnostic Blood Specimens by Venipuncture,* 3rd ed. Approved Standard, NCCLS Document H3-A3, Villanova, PA, NCCLS, 1991.
3. Scranton PE: *Practical Techniques in Venipuncture.* Baltimore, Williams & Wilkins, 1977, p 66.
4. Harker LA, Slichter SI: The bleeding time as a screening test for evaluation of platelet function. *N Engl J Med* 287:155, 1972.
5. Brown JW, Backwell H: Putting on gloves in the fight against AIDS. *Med Lab Observ* November:47, 1990.
6. Personius CD: Patients, health care workers and latex allergy. *Med Lab Observ* March:30–32, 1995.
7. Strickland DA: Latex sensitivity prompts alert. *Med World News* April:13, 1991.

8. National Committee for Clinical Laboratory Standards (NCCLS): *Procedures for the Collection of Diagnostic Blood Specimens by Skin Puncture.* NCCLS Document H4-A3, Villanova, PA, NCCLS, 1991.

9. Meites S (ed): *Pediatric Clinical Chemistry,* 3rd ed. Washington, DC, American Association for Clinical Chemistry, 1989.

10. Reiner CB, Meites S, Hayes J: Optimal sites and depths for specimens by skin puncture of infants and children as assessed from anatomical measurements. *Clin Chem* 36:574, 1990.

five

5

VENIPUNCTURE PROCEDURES

Chapter Outline

Chapter Objectives

Upon completion of Chapter 5, the learner is responsible for the following:

1. Describe the patient identification process for inpatients, emergency room patients, and ambulatory patients.

2. List essential information for test requisitions.

3. List supplies that would be used in a typical venipuncture procedure.

4. Identify the most common sites for venipuncture, and describe situations when these sites might not be acceptable sites for venipuncture. Identify alternative sites for the venipuncture procedure.

5. Describe the process and the time limits for applying a tourniquet to a patient's arm.

6. Describe the decontamination process and the agents used to decontaminate skin for routine blood tests and blood cultures.

7. Describe the actual venipuncture procedure and the steps that are different using the evacuated tube method, the syringe method, and the butterfly method.

8. Describe the order of draw for collection tubes when using the evacuated tube method, the syringe method, and the butterfly method.

9. List examples and explain reasons for the importance of collecting "timed specimens" at the requested times.

10. Describe the proper method for hand washing.

11. Describe what the terms *fasting* and *STAT* mean when referring to blood tests.

BLOOD COLLECTION

In preparing for blood collection, each health care worker generally establishes a routine that is comfortable for him or her. However, several essential steps are part of every successful collection procedure. This chapter discusses the following steps in which a health care worker would progress through the blood collection process.

1. Assessing the patient's physical disposition[1] (see Chapter 7)
2. Identifying the patient
3. Approaching the patient
4. Selecting and preparing equipment and supplies
5. Finding a puncture site
6. Preparing the puncture site
7. Choosing a venipuncture method
8. Collecting the samples in the appropriate tubes and in the correct order
9. Labeling the samples
10. Considering any special circumstances that occurred during the phlebotomy procedure
11. Assessing criteria for sample re-collection or rejection
12. Prioritizing patients and sample tubes

IDENTIFICATION

Patient Identification Process

Prior to any specimen collection procedure, the patient must be correctly identified by using a two-step process:

1. The patient should be asked to state his or her first and last names.
2. More important, a confirmatory match should be made among the patient's response, the test requisition form, and some type of identification such as a hospital identification bracelet, a driver's license, or another identification card.

Inpatient Identification

A hospitalized patient should always wear an identification bracelet indicating his or her first and last names and a designated hospital number (often called a *unit number*). Hospital identification numbers help hospital personnel to distinguish between patients with the same first or last names. To practice the two-step identification process, the health care worker should, upon entering the room, ask the patient what his or her name is. The health care worker should *not* ask, "Are you Ms. Doe?" because an ill patient on medication may mistakenly utter something, nod, or answer yes. Consequently, the best tactic is to ask, "What is your name?" and let the patient reply. *The patient* must *be correctly identified by his or her identification bracelet.* Information on the bracelet may also include the patient's room number, bed assignment, and physician's name (Fig. 5–1). A three-way match should be made

TEST REQUEST SLIP	HAPPY HOSPITAL			DATE REQUESTED **5/22/95**		TIME REQUESTED **7 /AM**
	Department of Laboratory Medicine			DATE COLLECTED **5/22/95**		TIME COLLECTED **7 /AM**
	TEST	RESULT	PERFORMED BY	NAME **Peter McLaughlin**		
				ADDRESS **4129 University Blvd.**		
				Houston, Texas		
				PATIENT ROOM NO. **1708**	BED NO. **2**	
				AGE **35** SEX **M**	HOSPITAL I.D. NO. **601537**	
				PHYSICIAN **Dr. McGarry**		
				TODAY ☐		ROUTINE ☐
				EMERGENCY ☐	SIGNED **DG**	

Sample Requisition Form

Sample Identification Bracelet

Printed information should include the following: patient's name, hospital number, room number, and patient's physician.

Labeled Specimen

Printed information should include the following: patient's name, hospital number, date, time, and phlebotomist's initials.

Figure 5–1. Identification bracelet, requisition form, specimen labeling. *(Adapted from College of American Pathologists: So You're Going to Collect a Blood Specimen: An Introduction to Phlebotomy, 6th ed. Northfield, IL, Author, 1994, with permission.)*

with the identification bracelet, the test requisition form, and the patient's statement of his or her name. The name card on the bed or door should never be used for confirming identity because it is often the last to be changed when patients are discharged and new patients are admitted.

If the patient does not have an identification bracelet, the nurse responsible for the patient must be asked to make the identification. In such cases, the situation and the nurse's name should be documented on the requisition form. Specimens should *not* be collected until a positive identification can be made and documented. Drawing blood from the wrong patient can lead to serious consequences such as incorrect treatment or therapy, and it is a violation for which the health care worker may be counseled or dismissed.

Identification of Infants and Young Children

See Chapter 8, Pediatric Phlebotomy.

Emergency Room Patient Identification

Health care workers must also be careful when identifying emergency room patients. Often, when patients come to the emergency room, they are unconscious and unidentified. Each hospital has policies and procedures for dealing with these cases. Usually, standard procedure involves assigning the patient an identification tag with a hospital or medical record number. This tag may be a multipart form that can be used by health care workers who need some type of temporary identification. The temporary identification number will be cross-referenced with the permanent identification number when the patient's identity is confirmed.

Ambulatory Patient Identification

Patient identification for ambulatory patients is usually more difficult to monitor. However, most outpatient clinics distribute identification cards to patients before any specimens are collected. If this is the case and the patient has the card available, positive identification can occur in the same manner as with hospitalized patients. These cards can also be used to make an imprinted label for the specimen if an Addressograph machine (Addressograph Company, Chicago, IL) is used. Alternatively, some ambulatory clinics issue identification bracelets to patients. If the patient does not have a patient identification bracelet or card, it is *strongly recommended* that another form of identification (e.g., driver's license) be checked and documented prior to specimen collection.

Some patients, infants or children, may not have any form of identification. In this situation, someone else, for example, the nurse or a parent should be asked to confirm the identification, verify the birth date, and document the identification process prior to specimen collection. Misidentification of patients' specimens can result in serious medical consequences, including patient death.

Test Requisitions

Laboratory tests must be ordered by physicians. The documented requests are usually transmitted in the form of a requisition form or by computer. Computer-generated requests contain the same required information as paper requisition forms. In either case, the requisition should contain the following information:

1. Patient's full name
2. Patient's identification (or medical record) number
3. Patient's date of birth
4. Types of tests to be performed
5. Date of test
6. Room number and bed
7. Physician's name and/or code
8. Test status (timed, **stat,** fasting, etc.)
9. Billing information (optional)
10. Special precautions (potential bleeder, faints easily, etc.)

When requisitions are received in a centralized laboratory department, computer-generated labels that, in some laboratories, also serve as the requisition are often printed (Fig. 5–2). The numerous types, colors, and styles of labels and requisitions are discussed further in Chapter 14.

Regardless of whether the requisitions are computer-generated or multipart forms, the health care worker should be familiar with the forms and with the procedures for generating, printing, and using the forms properly. Collection requests should be checked prior to the venipuncture procedure to ensure that there are no discrepancies or duplicates in the test orders. If the health care worker does not understand the test ordered, a supervisor, a laboratory technologist, or a nurse should be consulted prior to the phlebotomy procedure. Knowing which tests are requested helps the health care worker to prepare the patient appropriately and to collect the specimen in the appropriate tubes and in the correct order.

Figure 5–2. Labels and requisition forms.

PERFORMING THE PHLEBOTOMY

Health Care Worker Preparation

Prior to performing any type of specimen collection, the health care worker should have all protective equipment, supplies, forms, and so forth ready for the procedure. If patient information is incomplete on test requisitions, the health care worker may not be able to correctly identify the patient or may not know in which tubes to collect the blood. In such cases, assistance from a laboratory supervisor or a nurse is required.

Exercising Universal Precautions

All health care workers must be familiar with current recommendations and hospital policies on precautions for handling blood and body fluids. *All specimens should be treated as if they are hazardous and infectious,* according to the universal precautions described in detail in Chapters 12 and 13 (Fig. 5–3). Hands should be washed before and after specimen collection procedures (Fig. 5–4). A clean pair of gloves should be put on in the presence of the patient;[2] this is a safety-conscious, reassuring gesture for the patient and the health care worker. A clean, pressed uniform

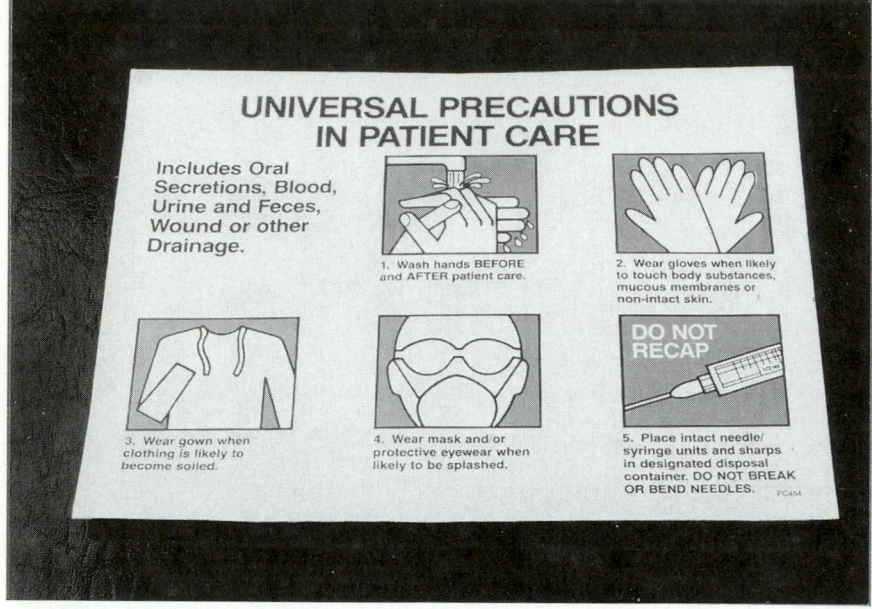

Figure 5–3. Universal precautions.

with a laboratory coat also instills a sense of commitment to safety and cleanliness, which is gratifying to patients and promotes a safer work environment for health care workers.

Approaching the Patient

In addition to being prepared with the proper equipment and supplies, and safety precautions, the health care worker must be emotionally prepared. Such preparation involves adopting a professional appearance and behavior, as well as exercising good communication skills, both as a listener and as a speaker.

Several professional and courteous behaviors and phrases can help make the patient–health care worker encounter a smooth interaction. The first of these is a polite knock on the patient's door prior to entering the patient's room. The health care worker should introduce him- or herself and state that he or she is from the laboratory and has come to collect a blood sample. As stated previously, making a correct identification is crucial. Once this has occurred, the process may continue. Sometimes, the health care worker may need to explain to the patient that the physician ordered the laboratory test or tests. The health care worker may also need to explain the procedure as supplies are being set up. During setup, the specimen collection tray should *not* be placed on

Figure 5–4. Hand-washing technique. **A.** Hand-washing techniques should involve soap lather, friction between hands, and thorough washing between fingers. Foot pedals are preferable for controlling the flow of water. **B.** Washing should include the wrist areas. **C.** Lather should be rinsed. Rinsing should continue until all soap is removed. If the water must be turned off by hand, a clean paper towel should be used to grab the faucet.

Knock on the patient's door.

Health care worker: Good morning. I am Ms. Smith from the laboratory. I have come to collect a blood sample.

Pause to give the patient an opportunity to speak. If the lights are off or dimmed, explain that you need to turn the lights on. Doing so gives the patient a moment to adjust to the idea of bright lights if he or she has been asleep.

Health care worker: What is your name, please? (*In general, it is not wise to ask a patient, "How are you?" because most patients in the hospital do not feel well.*)

Patient: I am John Jones.

Health care worker: May I please see your identification (ID) armband?

Check armband against laboratory requisitions and patient's verbal identification. If all three match, proceed.

Health care worker: This will take only a few minutes.

Patient: Will it hurt?

Health care worker: It will hurt a little, but it will be over soon. Please allow me to look at your arm veins.

Proceed with the remainder of the procedure, maintaining a highly professional atmosphere and a respectful attitude.

For certain tests, you may need to ascertain whether the patient has been fasting.

Health care worker: Mr. Jones, when was the last time you ate or drank anything? (*Do not use the term* fast *because some patients may not understand it completely.*)

At the end of the procedure, say the following:

Health care worker: Thank you, Mr. Jones.

Figure 5–5. Typical health care worker–patient interaction.

the patient's bed or eating table. As supplies are being readied and the vein is being palpated, the health care worker may try to alleviate some of the patient's fears. Chapter 16 covers verbal and nonverbal cues for detecting apprehension in patients. Figure 5–5 presents a typical scenario of a health care worker–patient interaction.

EQUIPMENT SELECTION AND PREPARATION

Supplies for Venipuncture

Supplies for venipuncture differ according to the method used (i.e., **syringe method** or **evacuated tube system**). Both methods of venipuncture involve the use of gloves, a **tourniquet,** alcohol pads or disinfectants, cotton balls, bandages or gauze pads, glass microscope slides, needles, syringes or evacuated tube holders, capillary tubes, tube sealer, blood collection tubes, laboratory request slips or labels, marking pens, and discard buckets, (Fig. 5–6). Supplies should be readily available and selected just prior to the procedure. These supplies are discussed in more detail in Chapter 4.

Positioning of the Patient and Venipuncture Sites

It is important to choose the least hazardous site for blood collection by skin puncture or venipuncture. Several techniques can facilitate the selection of a suitable site.

Proper positioning is important to both the health care worker and the patient for a successful venipuncture or skin puncture, and efforts to make sure that the patient is comfortable are worthwhile. Patients should *not* stand or sit on high stools during the procedure because of the possibility of fainting. A reclining (supine) position is preferred;

Figure 5–6. Supplies for venipunctures.

A.

B.

Figure 5–7. Differences in the visibility of veins. **A.** Veins are easily visible on a 45-year-old healthy male. **B.** On a 50-year-old healthy female, the veins are more difficult to visualize.

however, sitting in a sturdy, comfortable chair with arm supports is also acceptable. The health care worker can position him- or herself in front of the chair to protect the patient from falling forward in the event of fainting. A slight rotation of the patient's arm or hand may help expose a vein and prevent it from rolling as the needle is inserted. The visibility of veins varies with each individual, skin color, weight, physiological conditions, gender, and physical features (Fig. 5–7). Therefore, the health care worker must rely on the sense of touch (palpation) to locate the vein. A pillow may be used for arm support of a bedridden patient if the patient is too weak to hold the arm in one position. Equipment should be placed in an accessible spot where it is unlikely to be disturbed by the patient.

The most common sites for venipuncture are in the antecubital area of the arm, where the median cubital, cephalic, and basilic veins lie close to the surface of the skin and are most prominent. Palpating this area usually helps the health care worker get an idea of the size, the angle, and the depth of the vein. The patient can assist in the process by opening and closing the fist tightly.[2]

The dorsal side of the hand or wrist, ankle, and foot veins should be used only after arm veins have been determined unsuitable (Figs. 5–8

Figure 5–8. Hand and foot veins.

Figure 5–9. Differences in the patterns of hand veins. **A.** Male. **B.** Female.

and 5–9). Reasons for not using arm veins include the following: the patient has intravenous (IV) lines in both arms, is burned, has a cast, has thrombosed veins, or has edematous arms. Hand veins or the veins on the posterior surface of the wrist are preferred over foot or ankle veins because coagulation and vascular complications tend to be more troublesome in the lower extremities. The posterior surface of the wrist is preferred to the palmar venous network in the wrist because nerves lie very close to the palmar venous network. Veins in the wrist or ankle tend to move, or "roll," aside as the needle is inserted; therefore, it may be helpful to have the patient extend the foot or hand into a position that helps hold the vein taut (see Figure 5–9). However, veins of the extremities should be avoided if they are edematous. Some hospitals do not allow health care workers to use the lower extremities for blood-sampling sites. Other hospitals allow sampling from these sites only after permission is granted from the patient's physician. Venipuncture in small veins may be facilitated by the use of a 21- to 25-gauge butterfly needle (or winged infusion set) (Fig. 5–10).

Warming the Puncture Site

Warming the puncture site helps facilitate phlebotomy by increasing arterial blood flow to the area and, in some cases, by making the veins

Figure 5–10. Winged infusion set, or butterfly needle. *(Courtesy of The University of Texas, M.D., Anderson Cancer Center.)*

more prominent. Although several methods of warming are available commercially, a surgical towel or a washcloth heated with warm water to 42°C will not burn the skin. When the towel or cloth is wrapped around the site for 3 to 5 minutes, the skin temperature can increase several degrees. The wrap can be encased in a plastic bag to help retain heat and to keep the patient's bed dry. The health care worker may leave the warm wrap on the patient while he or she collects specimens from other patients, and then can return to the original patient after several minutes.

Tourniquet Application

A tourniquet or blood pressure cuff may be used to help find a site for venipuncture. A soft rubber tourniquet about 1-in. (2.5-cm) wide and about 15- to 18-in. (45-cm) long is most comfortable. To apply it, the health care worker should stretch the ends around the patient's arm about 3 in. (7.6 cm) above the venipuncture area; both ends of the tourniquet can be held in one hand while the other hand grasps a section next to the skin and makes a partial loop with the tourniquet. The tourniquet should be tight but not painful to the patient (Fig. 5–11). It should not be placed over sores or burned skin. The partially looped tourniquet should allow for easy release by the health care worker during the venipuncture procedure. During the venipuncture, the health care worker should be able to release the tourniquet with one hand because the other hand will be holding the needle and tubes. The tourniquet should not be left on for more than 1 minute because it becomes uncomfortable and causes **hemoconcentration**—that is, increased blood concentration of large molecules such as proteins, cells, and coagulation factors. The patient may be asked to clench and unclench the fist only a *few* times because excessive clenching also results in hemoconcentration. If no vein becomes apparent or "pops up," the patient may be asked to dangle the arm for 1 to 2 minutes, then the tourniquet may be reapplied and the area palpated again. The health care worker should *never* stick a vein unless it can be felt. It is better to defer the patient to someone else who can search for the vein than to take a blind chance.

Decontamination of the Puncture Site

Once the site is selected, it should be **decontaminated** with a sterile swab or sponge soaked in 70 percent isopropanol (isopropyl alcohol), or with a commercially packaged alcohol pad (see Figure 5–11F). The health care worker should rub the site, working in concentric circles from the inside out. If the skin is particularly dirty, the process should be repeated. The health care worker should also decontaminate his or her own gloved finger if he or she intends to palpate the site again. The decontaminated area should never be touched with any nonsterile object. The alcohol should be allowed to dry (approximately 30 to 60 seconds) or should be wiped off with sterile gauze or cotton after the site is prepared; otherwise, the puncture site will sting, and the alcohol can interfere with test results such as blood alcohol levels. Blowing on the site to hasten the drying process is not advised because doing so may recontaminate the site.[2]

Povidone–iodine (Betadine) preparations are primarily used for drawing blood for blood gas analysis and blood cultures (see Chapter 9, Arterial and Special Collection Procedures). For some patients, iodine causes skin irritation. Efforts should be made to remove iodine from the skin with sterile gauze after decontamination because excess iodine can interfere with some laboratory tests.

VENIPUNCTURE METHODS

Venipuncture

Once the puncture site is cleansed, the health care worker may hold the patient's arm below the site, pulling the skin tightly with the thumb. A syringe, butterfly, or VACUTAINER (Becton, Dickinson and Company, Franklin Lakes, NJ) assembly can be used for venipuncture. (If a syringe is used, before the needle is inserted the plunger should be moved back

A. B.

Figure 5–11. Performing a venipuncture procedure. **A.** Greeting the patient and confirming identification. **B.** Equipment preparation. **C.** Site selection. **D.** Tourniquet application. **E.** Palpating the site. **F.** Decontamination with alcohol. **G.** The venipuncture procedure. **H.** Removal of tourniquet. **I.** Tube and needle removal. **J.** Application of pressure. **K.** Waste disposal. **L.** Application of bandage. **M.** Immediate labeling of tube. **N.** Adding initials, time, and date.

Figure 5–11. *(continued)*

Figure 5–11. *(continued)*

and forth to allow for free movement and to expel all air.) The whole assembly can be held between the thumb and the third or fourth finger. (The index finger may rest on the hub of the needle to guide the needle entry.) The needle should run in the same direction as the vein and should be inserted quickly and smoothly at approximately a 15-degree angle with the skin.[3] Just before inserting the needle, the health care worker should mention to the patient that he or she will "feel a stick." This warning cautions patients and usually alerts them to be still. The health care worker may also need to tell the patient, "Please be very still." The needle should be inserted with the bevel side upward and directly above a prominent vein or slightly below the palpable vein. The health care worker may need to palpate with one hand after needle insertion if the vein has not been hit. Often, the health care worker can feel a slight "pop" when the needle enters the vein. As the blood begins to flow, the patient may open the fist. The tourniquet can be released immediately, or after the blood has been collected, but before needle withdrawal. (Refer to Figure 5–11G–I.)

Figure 5–12 describes the specific laboratory procedure used to perform a routine venipuncture.

Evacuated Tube System

If the evacuated tube (e.g., VACUTAINER) system is used, the test tube should be pushed *carefully* into the holder so that the test tube cap is punctured by the inside needle and blood can enter the evacuated tube. If multiple sample tubes are to be collected, each tube should be *gently removed* from the VACUTAINER holder and replaced with another tube. Experienced health care workers are able to mix a full tube in one hand while holding the needle apparatus and waiting for another tube to fill. Some health care workers use the dominant hand to change tubes while the other hand keeps the needle apparatus steady. This approach may require the health care worker to switch hands after needle insertion. The position that is the most comfortable for the patient and the health care worker should be used while the needle is simultaneously kept as stable and motionless as possible during tube fillings. Multiple tubes can be filled in less than 1 minute if the needle remains stable in the vein and the vein does not collapse. So that the proper dilution of blood and additive in the tube is ensured, each tube should be allowed to fill until the blood flow stops. Tubes do not fill completely, so the health care worker must be attentive to when the blood flow ceases. To change tubes, the health care worker should remove the full one from the needle apparatus with a gentle twist-and-pull motion, then replace it with an empty tube, using a gentle push onto the needle apparatus. During the tube exchange, the needle apparatus should be held firmly so that the needle remains in the vein and is not pushed through or pulled out of the vein.

Syringe Method

If a syringe is used, the same approach to needle insertion should take place as used for the evacuated tube method. Once the needle is in the vein, the syringe plunger can be drawn back slowly until the required amount of blood is drawn. (It may be helpful to turn the syringe slightly so that the graduated markings are visible.) Care must be taken not to accidentally withdraw the needle while pulling back on the plunger and not to pull hard enough to cause hemolysis (e.g., rupture of the cells) or collapse of the vein.

After tourniquet release and collection of the appropriate amount of blood, the entire needle assembly should be withdrawn quickly. A

Performance of a Venipuncture

1. Greet the patient in a friendly, professional manner.

   In an outpatient setting:

   Ask the patient a direct question, "What is your name, sir/madam?" "What is your date of birth?" Compare the name and date of birth stated by the patient with information on the identification card, computer labels, and laboratory request slips. When a blood specimen is required for blood components, an identification bracelet must be worn by the patient.

   In a hospital setting (inpatients):

   Knock on the patient's door and enter the room. Compare your request slip or computer labels with the patient's name and hospital number found on the door of the patient's room to make sure you are in the right room. Identify yourself to the patient, stating that you have come to draw blood for some laboratory tests ordered by his or her physician. Compare information on the patient's identification bracelet with that on your computer labels and laboratory request slips. **This information must be identical.** Request a nurse to identify a patient who does not have an identification bracelet. The nurse should also place a bracelet on the patient's wrist except in cases when this is not feasible. Sometimes a patient cannot wear an ID bracelet because his or her wrist is irritated or too edematous for an ID bracelet to fit.

   If this is the case, on the requisition make a note of the nurse who identified the patient.

2. Try to gain the patient's confidence and remind the patient that the venipuncture may be slightly painful. Patient's should never be told, "This will not hurt." Exercise Universal Precautions, including use of gloves.

3. Position the patient:

   Procedure for seating the patient (usually outpatients):

   The patient should be seated comfortably in a chair and should position his or her arm on an armrest, extending the arm so as to form a relatively straight line from the shoulder to the wrist. The arm should be supported firmly by the armrest and should be only slightly bent at the elbow.

Figure 5–12. Sample procedure for performance of a routine venipuncture.

Procedure for having the patient lie down (usually inpatients):

The patient lies comfortably on his or her back. If additional support is needed, a pillow may be placed under the arm from which the specimen is to be drawn. The patient extends the arm so as to form a relatively straight line from the shoulder to the wrist.

4. Assemble the following supplies for collecting a blood specimen: gloves, blood-collecting tubes, needles, syringe or Vacutainer holder, tourniquet, 70 percent isopropyl alcohol, and gauze pads or alcohol preparation, pads, povidone–iodine and acetone alcohol swab sticks (if blood cultures are to be drawn), and gauze bandage rolls, or paper tape and cotton balls.

5. Select a vein site. Place a tourniquet on the patient's arm. Choose the vein that feels fullest. Look at both arms. Ask the patient to make a fist that makes the veins more prominent and easier to enter. Vigorous hand excercise "pumping" should be avoided because it may affect some test values. Use your index finger to palpate and trace the path of the vein. Thrombosed veins lack resilience, feel cordlike, and roll easily. Feel firmly, but do not tap or rub your finger lightly over the skin because you may feel only small surface veins. Always feel for the median cubital vein first; it is usually bigger and anchored better, and it bruises less. The cephalic vein (depending on size) is the second choice over the basilic vein because it does not roll and bruise as easily. The bend of the elbow is the best place to make a puncture. When this is not possible, other sites include the surface of the forearm, dorsal wrist area above the thumb, volar area of the wrist, knuckle of the thumb or index finger, back of the hand, and back of the lower arm. If a "good" vein cannot be found, try the following:

   • Try the other arm unless otherwise instructed.
   • Ask the patient to make a fist again.
   • Apply the tourniquet, remembering that the tourniquet should never be left on the arm for more than 2 minutes.
   • Massage the arm from wrist to elbow.
   • Tap a few times at the vein site with your index finger.
   • Apply heat to the vein site.
   • Lower the arm over the bedside or venipuncture chair.

6. Cleanse the venipuncture site. Using an alcohol preparation pad or cotton ball saturated with alcohol, cleanse the area by moving the pad in a circular motion from the center of the vein site outward.

Figure 5–12. *(continued)*

The area must be allowed to dry. *Never* touch the skin after the site is cleansed unless you have prepared your gloved finger.

7. Inspect the needle, syringe, or evacuated tube before performing the venipuncture. The appropriate needle is attached to the syringe or the evacuated tube holder and threaded into the holder until it is secure; the needle sheath will lock onto the holder. The cover of the needle must not be removed until you are ready to draw blood so that the needle does not become contaminated. If the needle touches anything but the sterile site, it should be changed.

8. Perform the venipuncture:

Evacuated tube method:

Grasp the patient's arm firmly, using your thumb to draw the skin taut. The vein is entered with the bevel of the needle upward. One hand should hold the evacuated tube while the other depresses the tube to the end of the holder.

The tube should be filled until the vacuum is exhausted and the blood flow ceases, to ensure a correct ratio of anticoagulant to blood. After each tube is drawn, an additive should be mixed immediately by inverting the tube at least five times. Gentle inversion will prevent hemolysis. *Never* shake a tube of blood after collecting a blood specimen.

Occasionally, a faulty tube will have no vacuum. If a tube is not filling and the needle is inside the vein, another tube should be used. If a tube starts to fill but then stops, the needle should be moved slightly forward or backward. Usually, this adjustment will increase the blood flow. The needle can then be rotated half a turn, and the tourniquet, which may have been applied too tightly, is loosened. Probing is not recommended because it is painful to the patient. If none of these procedures is helpful, the needle should be removed and an alternate site used.

Syringe method:

A syringe and needle should be used to collect blood from patients with more difficult veins. If the puncture has been made and the blood is not flowing, determine whether you are pulling too hard on the plunger and collapsing the vein. The needle should be drawn back while the plunger is being pulled slightly. Make sure that the bevel is covered by the skin. With the syringe

Figure 5–12. *(continued)*

in the right hand, you can use the index finger of the left hand to feel for the vein. After the vein is relocated, keep your finger gently on the vein, and guide the needle to that point. Then, pull gently on the plunger. As soon as the blood starts to flow into the syringe, the needle should not be moved.

Other methods:

A winged infusion set with leur adapters can be used instead of a syringe and needle for very difficult veins. The winged collection set is a closed system. Blood flows from the vein, through the set directly into a Vacutainer tube.

If all possibilities have been exhausted, and you have not successfully performed a venipuncture on a patient after two attempts, enlist the aid of a co-worker or a supervisor. Inform the nurse caring for the patient that you have made two unsuccessful attempts to draw blood from the patient. Make a notation of the circumstances on a worksheet.

9. The tourniquet is released after the blood is drawn and the patient has opened his or her hand. Releasing the tourniquet allows for normal blood circulation and a reduction in the amount of bleeding at the venipuncture site. Fold a gauze pad or place a cotton ball over the needle, then gently remove the needle. The gauze pad or cotton ball should be held firmly over the venipuncture site.

10. All tubes should be appropriately mixed and labeled at the patient's bedside. Labels must include the patient's first and last names and ID number, the date, the time of collection, and the phlebotomist's initials.

11. Dispose of contaminated materials and supplies in designated containers.

12. Deliver specimens to the appropriate laboratory.

   Summary of steps in performing a venipuncture:

   - Ensure identification of patient.
   - Reassure patient and ensure that the patient is properly positioned.
   - Assemble supplies, wear protective equipment (eg, gloves)
   - Verify paperwork and tube identification.

Figure 5–12. *(continued)*

- Select vein site.
- Apply tourniquet.
- Cleanse venipuncture site.
- Perform venipuncture.
- Release tourniquet.
- Remove needle.
- Bandage arm.
- Fill tubes (when syringe and needles are used).
- Label tubes.
- Dispose of contaminated supplies.
- Chill specimen, if necessary.
- Distribute specimen(s) to the appropriate laboratory section

Figure 5–12. *(continued)*

dry, sterile cotton ball or piece of gauze should be applied with pressure to the puncture site for several minutes or *until bleeding has ceased.* If the patient has a free hand, he or she may be asked to apply the pressure. The patient's arm may be kept straight, slightly bent at the elbow, or elevated above the heart.

Winged Infusion System, or Butterfly Method

A winged infusion set, or butterfly needle, can be used for particularly difficult venipunctures in smaller veins (hand or wrist) or in pediatric phlebotomies (Fig. 5–13). The use of this system has also been reported to be less painful to patients. The needle ranges from 1/2 in. to 3/4 in. in length and from 21 gauge to 25 gauge in diameter. Attached to the needle is thin tubing with a Luer adapter at the end so that it can be used on a syringe or an evacuated tube system. Thus, the order of the tube draw should correspond with the adapter type (evacuated tube or syringe) used with the butterfly needle.

Health care workers should be cautious of the needle once it is removed from the patient because it tends to hang loose on the end of the tubing. Most manufacturers now make retractable safety enclosures for butterfly needles; these enclosures allow the health care worker to cover the needle immediately after it is withdrawn. (Refer to Chapter 4, Blood Collection Equipment.)

Figure 5–13. Performing a venipuncture procedure with the combination butterfly (double-pointed) needle and evacuated tube system.

Proper Disposal

All disposable or contaminated equipment should be discarded into appropriate containers. Paper and plastic wrappers can be thrown into a wastebasket. However, needles and lancets should *not* be thrown into a wastebasket, but into a sturdy, puncture-proof, disposable container to be autoclaved or incinerated (see Figure 5–11K). Any items that have been contaminated with blood should be disposed of in biohazardous disposal containers as explained in the universal precautions (see Chapter 12, Infection Control).

Order of Tube Collection

Very often, multiple blood assays are ordered on patients. Whether the health care worker chooses to use a multiple-draw evacuated tube collection system or a plastic syringe, there are certain guidelines for delivery of blood into the proper collection tubes.

Evacuated Tube Collection System. **The National Committee for** **Clinical Laboratory Standards (NCCLS)** recommends this order of draw[2]:

1. Blood culture tubes (yellow stopper) or culture bottles
2. Nonadditive or serum tube (red stopper)
3. Coagulation tube (light-blue stopper)
4. Additive tube(s) (green, lavender, or gray stoppers)

Becton-Dickinson, the tube manufacturer, recommends the following specific order for collection of tubes. Although steps 1–3 are the same, their recommendation specifically states the order of collection for tubes with additives.[4] (It may be helpful to check with the manufacturer about their recommendations for the order of tube draw if using other brands of tubes.)

1. Blood culture tubes (yellow stopper), or culture bottles
2. Nonadditive or serum tube (red stopper)
3. Citrate (light-blue Hemogard)
4. Heparin (green or light-green Hemogard)
5. EDTA (lavendar Hemogard)
6. Gel separator tubes and PLUS serum tubes containing silica clot activators (mottled-gold Hemogard closure or PLUS red-top tube)
7. Other additives

The blood cultures are always drawn first to decrease the possibility of bacterial contamination. The procedure for collection of blood cultures is discussed in Chapter 9 in greater detail. Whenever coagulation studies are ordered, at least one other tube of blood should be drawn before the coagulation test specimen. This diminishes contamination with tissue fluids, which may initiate the clotting sequence. Any tube that has an anticoagulant in it should be drawn last so that it can be mixed as soon after collection as possible. Care should be taken so that the anticoagulant present in the tube does not come into contact with the multisample needle when changing tubes, as some may be carried into the next tube and cause erroneous test results. For example, it is recommended that blood for serum iron be drawn before other specimens with chelating anticoagulants (e.g., EDTA) are collected in tubes. This will avoid interference in testing the serum iron level. Also, electrolyte determinations include measurement of potassium (K) and sodium (Na). Since the chelating anticoagulant EDTA is usually bound to potassium as $EDTA(K_3)$ or to sodium (Na) as $EDTA(Na_2)$, it is important to collect specimens that require EDTA after a specimen is collected in heparin for electrolytes. The K_3 and Na_2 from the EDTA may falsely elevate the patient's K or Na values. To minimize transfer of anticoagulants from tube to tube, holding the tube horizontally or slightly downward during blood collection is recommended.

Plastic Syringe Collection. When a health care worker chooses to use a syringe, the order of delivery of blood into the tubes changes. It should be as follows:

1. To minimize contamination, blood culture tubes are filled first.
2. Before proceeding, tubes for coagulation studies are filled and mixed.
3. Other anticoagulated tubes then are filled and mixed as quickly and safely as possible.
4. Lastly, tubes without anticoagulants are filled. (See Fig. 5–14.)

Again, care should be taken not to transfer anticoagulants from one tube to another. Blood should always be delivered gently to the tubes to avoid hemolyzing the cells. This is done by directing the flow from the needle or the syringe hub along the side of the tube without allowing the blood to foam or without putting extra pressure on the plunger. Remember that evacuated tubes fill themselves; therefore the blood does *not* need to be forcefully ejected from the syringe.

Sometimes, when a large volume (more than 20 mL) of blood has been drawn, there is a possibility that some of the blood may be clotted. If this occurs, the needle can be *carefully* removed from the hub of the syringe, the top can be removed from the tube, and then the blood can be *carefully* expelled into the tube. Again, it is suggested that the tube be filled by letting the blood run *gently,* not forcefully, down the inside

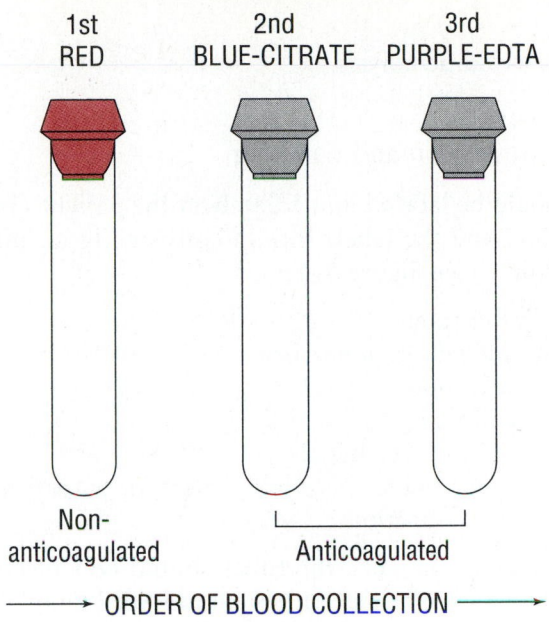

Evacuated tube method

1st	2nd	3rd
RED	BLUE-CITRATE	PURPLE-EDTA

Non-anticoagulated

Anticoagulated

⟶ ORDER OF BLOOD COLLECTION ⟶

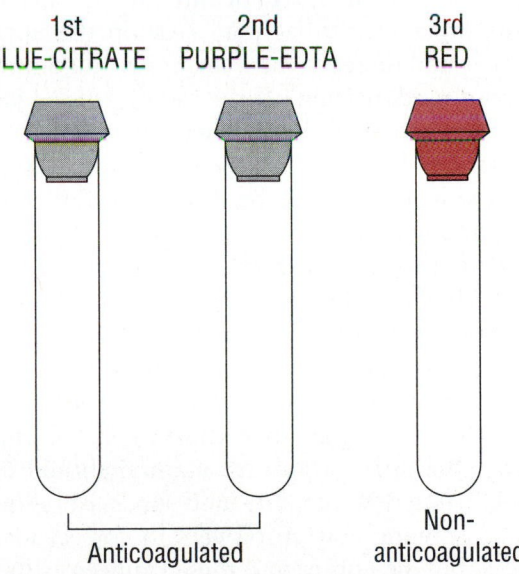

Syringe deposit method

1st	2nd	3rd
BLUE-CITRATE	PURPLE-EDTA	RED

Anticoagulated

Non-anticoagulated

→ ORDER OF BLOOD DEPOSITED FROM SYRINGE −

Figure 5–14. Collection priority. Depending on the method used, the order of tube collection changes. When the evacuation tube method is used, the plain red-topped tube is used first, followed by the light-blue–topped tube, the purple-topped tube, and any others that are needed. When the syringe deposit method is used, the blood should be expelled into the light-blue–topped tube first, followed by other anticoagulated tubes, and finally the plain red-topped tube.

of the tube to avoid hemolysis.

Specimen Identification and Labeling

Specimens should be labeled immediately at the patient's bedside or ambulatory setting, and the labels should consistently include the following information[2,3] (see Figure 5–1):

1. Patient's full name
2. Patient's identification number
3. Date of collection
4. Time of collection
5. Health care worker's initials
6. Patient's room number, bed assignment, or outpatient status is optional information

For hospitalized patients, the tubes should be labeled immediately after the specimen is collected. Tubes should *not* be prelabeled because they may not be used, then they might be erroneously picked up and used for another patient. Also, a different health care worker may complete the venipuncture if the initial health care worker is unsuccessful. In that case, the prelabeled tubes may contain the initials of the first health care worker and therefore be inaccurate. In addition, if the prelabeled tubes are not used, tearing off the old or unused label may be difficult because of the adhesive; thus, either a new label (from a different patient) would have to be placed on the tube with a partially torn label, *or* the unused tube would have to be discarded. Either option is unsatisfactory, messy, and wasteful.

For the ambulatory care setting, there are mixed opinions about when to label the blood collection tube. The NCCLS suggests that the health care worker "must apply a label to each of the necessary tubes" prior to the actual collection process.[2] However, many health care workers (the authors included) believe that the same risks exist with prelabeled tubes in the outpatient setting as in the inpatient setting. Therefore, each laboratory procedure manual should contain explicit instructions on labeling requirements, and supervisors should spend ample time not only training new employees in correct identification and labeling practices, but also observing these trainees as they employ such practices.

For unidentified or unconscious patients who come to a hospital through the emergency room or other unusual circumstances, a temporary identification number can be assigned. The identification tag should be a multiple-part form with the same identification number on each part. One part can be attached to the patient's arm, and the other can be used for the specimens. When the hospital's permanent identification number is assigned to the patient, it can be cross-referenced to the temporary number.

The health care worker should confirm all the information before leaving the patient's hospital room or before drawing blood from another clinic outpatient. The date and time are necessary because requisition forms may indicate the date and time when a laboratory test was *ordered,* rather than the date and time when it was *collected.* For timed specimens (e.g., specimens for glucose tolerance testing), the actual collection time is critical to the test. The health care worker's initials are necessary to help clarify questions about the specimen if any arise during laboratory processing or testing.

No foolproof method exists for labeling specimens. The health care worker may write directly on the container. Alternatively, many commercial collection tubes have blank affixed labels for this purpose. Similarly, hospitals often use computer-generated labels for collection tubes. However, capillary tubes, microcollection tubes and vials, or other containers without labels must be identified, either by labeling them directly with a permanent felt-tipped pen, by wrapping an adhesive label around them, or by placing them into a larger labeled test tube for transport. In some cases, small computerized adhesive labels with printed information are available with and detachable from the requisition form.

Other Considerations

Because the health care team members (including doctors, medical technologists, clerks, secretaries, and nurses) are all working for the welfare of the patient, they should strive to reduce the total number of daily phlebotomies. To do this, all health care workers involved in patient care duties could follow these suggestions: Doctors could write orders on the same line on the chart rather than scattered throughout the page, and orders could be coordinated among all staff physicians working with the patient. Furthermore, the laboratory could be notified when multiple timed tests are ordered. If a patient needs a hemoglobin test at 2:00 PM and a glucose test at 3:00 PM, coordinating the times and drawing both specimens during one venipuncture may be possible. Laboratory testing for therapeutic drug monitoring should be coordinated among laboratory, nursing, and pharmacy personnel. Nurses and ward secretaries could organize laboratory orders as much as possible to avoid sending frequent requests minutes apart. When orders are transcribed, all of them should be requested at the same time. The laboratory should be notified of patient transfers. An up-to-date log of room numbers and patients' names should be available on the ward as a resource for laboratory personnel.

Health care workers collecting blood specimens should organize requisition forms by patient and by floor. Any identification discrepancies should be communicated to a nurse.

One hospital has suggested several slogans for their health care personnel regarding phlebotomy:

- A stick in time saves nine.
- We care—several pokes are no joke.
- For their sake, let's stick together.

Other items that should be considered for inclusion in policies and procedures are as follows:

1. The number of times that a patient can be punctured by the same health care worker. Generally, a health care worker should not puncture a patient more than twice before calling for a second opinion.
2. The number of times that a patient can be punctured in 1 day. Staff physicians, nurses, and health care workers should coordinate their efforts to minimize the number of patient venipunctures.
3. The total volume of blood that can be drawn daily from a patient, especially a patient in pediatrics or in the nursery (see Table 5–1).
4. The type of information that a health care worker may provide to the patient about the laboratory tests ordered. In general, the use of good judgment is required. Providing basic information about the tests that have been ordered is acceptable *if* the health care worker is knowledgeable. However, the health care worker should always emphasize that the patient's physician ordered the tests.
5. The steps to take if a patient refuses to have blood collected. All patients have a right to refuse treatment. In these cases, the health care worker should use good, sound judgment in explaining to the patient that laboratory results are used to help the physician make an accurate diagnosis, establish proper treatment, and monitor the patient's health status. The health care worker should explain that the patient's cooperation would be greatly appreciated. If the patient continues to refuse, the health care worker must remain professional and acknowledge the right to refuse. The health care worker should indicate to the patient that he or she will make a note of the refusal and notify the patient's physician.

TABLE 5–1. MAXIMUM AMOUNTS OF BLOOD TO BE DRAWN FROM PATIENTS YOUNGER THAN 14 YEARS

Patient's Weight		Maximum Amount to Be Drawn at Any One Time (mL)	Maximum Amount of Blood (Cumulative) to Be Drawn During a Given Hospital Stay (1 Month or Less) (mL)
lb	kg (approx)		
6–8	2.7–3.6	2.5	23
8–10	3.6–4.5	3.5	30
10–15	4.5–6.8	5	40
16–20	7.3–9.1	10	60
21–25	9.5–11.4	10	70
26–30	11.8–13.6	10	80
31–35	14.1–15.9	10	100
36–40	16.4–18.2	10	130
41–45	18.6–20.5	20	140
46–50	20.9–22.7	20	160
51–55	23.2–25.0	20	180
56–60	25.5–27.3	20	200
61–65	27.7–29.5	25	220
66–70	30.0–31.8	30	240
71–75	32.3–34.1	30	250
76–80	34.5–36.4	30	270
81–85	36.8–38.6	30	290
86–90	39.1–40.9	30	310
91–95	41.4–43.2	30	330
96–100	43.6–45.5	30	350

Adapted from Becan-McBride K: Textbook of Clinical Laboratory Supervision. New York, Appleton-Century-Crofts, 1982.

Leaving the Patient

Before leaving the patient's side, the health care worker must check the puncture site to make sure that the bleeding stopped. All tubes must be appropriately labeled and the information on the labels confirmed. All supplies and equipment that were brought in should be removed or discarded appropriately, and the health care worker should thank the patient. An adhesive bandage may be applied. However, such bandages are not recommended for infants or young children because of possible irritation and the potential of swallowing or aspirating a bandage.

SPECIMEN REJECTION

Each clinical laboratory should establish its own guidelines for specimen rejection. In general, the following factors should be considered[5]: discrepancies between requisition forms and labeled tubes (names, dates, times); unlabeled tubes; hemolyzed specimens (except for tests in which hemolysis does not interfere); specimens in the wrong collection tubes; use of outdated equipment, supplies, or reagents; and contaminated specimens. (See Chapter 7, Table 7–5.)

When a problem arises, the appropriate investigational channels should be followed. The health care worker who drew the specimen and his or her supervisor should try to solve the problem initially. Errors should be acknowledged and documented with corrective actions. Other personnel may be involved as needed. Communication, honesty, and ethical professional behavior are the keys to an efficient and reliable health care environment.

PRIORITIZING PATIENTS

In the course of a day's work at a busy hospital or clinic, a health care worker may have to make decisions about the order in which blood work is obtained. Priorities must be set and adhered to, whether they concern the order in which certain blood tests are drawn on a particular patient or which patients are to be drawn from first among a group. If these distinctions are not made properly, test results can be affected and interpretation of the results may be difficult.

Patient Priorities

Timed Specimens. Whenever a test is ordered to be drawn at a particular time, the health care worker is responsible for drawing the blood as near to the requested time as possible. The most common requests for timed specimens are for glucose level determination for which blood should be drawn 2 hours after a meal. The glucose value in the blood is constantly changing, so the blood must not be drawn too early, which yields a falsely elevated result, or too late, which yields a falsely normal result.

Other timed specimens may be used for determining peak and trough levels of certain drugs. Often, patients on drug therapy must be monitored to ensure that effective therapeutic levels are being given. If the trough level is too high, the drug may be discontinued for a period until blood drug level returns to lower and safer levels. Again, the timing of drawing blood from these patients can be critical and must be scheduled as close as possible to the time ordered. If a time delay is unavoidable, the actual time of the collection must be indicated on the requisition form.

Certain natural hormone levels, such as cortisol, increase and decrease with the time of day. For instance, a sample of blood taken at

8:00 AM shows the highest value for cortisol during the day, whereas a sample taken at 8:00 PM usually shows approximately two thirds the value of the morning sample. Therefore, if a health care worker has difficulty obtaining a blood specimen on a patient at 8:00 AM, someone else should try as soon as possible thereafter, or the test may be canceled until the following day at the discretion of the attending physician. Obtaining a specimen at noon for cortisol level determination may give the physician little information on which to base treatment.

Another hormone, aldosterone, requires another type of timing for blood collection and analysis. The patient must be in a recumbent position for at least 30 minutes prior to blood collection. Serum or plasma can be used in the analyte determination, but heparin or EDTA should be the anticoagulant if plasma is preferred. Because glass interferes in the aldosterone determination, the collecting container should be made of plastic.

To collect blood for a renin-activity test, the health care worker must collect an anticoagulated blood specimen from the patient after a 3-day special diet. In addition, the health care worker must be sure to note whether the patient is in an upright position or a supine (prone) position when blood is drawn. For this analyte, the blood should be collected from a peripheral vein (e.g., antecubital vein).

Fasting Specimens. When a health care worker works at an institution where inpatients are treated, care should be taken that the patient is not unduly inconvenienced by an order for fasting blood tests [i.e., tests performed on blood taken from a patient who has abstained from eating and drinking (except water for a particular period of time)]. Fasting levels of glucose, cholesterol, and triglycerides can be important in diagnosing patients and monitoring their progress during the hospital stay. If the health care worker finds that a patient has not been fasting, the health care worker should consult with a physician to determine whether a nonfasting level will be of benefit. The requisition should then indicate that the patient is nonfasting.

Stat Specimens. The term *stat,* which means "immediately," has come to indicate a patient whose medical condition suddenly may become critical and who must be treated or responded to as a medical emergency. When blood work is ordered stat, usually a specimen must be drawn and analyzed *immediately* so that a critically ill patient can be handled properly. Consequently, the health care team should be prepared for immediate response, employ effective technique, and have personnel constantly available for stat blood collections. The health care worker not only should draw the blood quickly and properly, but also should ensure its timely delivery to the laboratory for stat analysis. Regardless of the patient's physical state, the health care worker must adhere to the proper procedure for obtaining the best possible specimen from the patient. Despite the emergency situation that may be in progress, no shortcuts can be allowed. The health care worker has a responsibility to the patient to obtain a properly labeled, correct specimen for the test that is ordered; if this responsibility is not carried out, precious time for the patient who is being treated may be lost while another specimen is collected.

✔ Key Terms

DECONTAMINATE

EVACUATED TUBE SYSTEM

FASTING BLOOD TESTS

HEMOCONCENTRATION

HEMOLYSIS

NATIONAL COMMITTEE FOR

CLINICAL LABORATORY STANDARDS (NCCLS)

STAT

SUPINE

SYRINGE METHOD

TOURNIQUET

Study Questions

1. A patient may be identified by which of the following means?
   a. patient's chart
   b. nurse
   c. patient's armband
   d. ward clerk

2. Identification procedures for outpatients may include asking for which of the following?
   a. photo identification
   b. birth date
   c. employer's name
   d. identification by a family member

3. The most common sites for venipuncture are in which of the following areas?
   a. the dorsal side of the wrist
   b. the antecubital area of the arm
   c. the middle finger
   d. the middle forearm

4. Palpating the venipuncture site serves what purpose(s)?
   a. provides an indication of the size of the vein
   b. distracts the patient from the discomfort of the procedure
   c. provides an indication of the depth of the vein
   d. helps the phlebotomist determine what angle to insert the needle

5. When is using a butterfly needle beneficial? For
   a. heel puncture
   b. veins in the wrist or hand
   c. veins in the ankle
   d. finger stick

6. What effect does warming the site have on venipuncture?
   a. prevents veins from rolling
   b. makes veins stand out
   c. causes hemoconcentration
   d. increases localized blood flow

7. How long should the tourniquet be placed around the patient's arm?
   a. Approximately 4 minutes
   b. Until the needle is removed
   c. Until the entire venipuncture is completed
   d. No more than 1 minute

8. What is the best angle for needle insertion during venipuncture?
   a. 15 degrees
   b. 30 degrees
   c. 45 degrees
   d. 80 degrees

9. The suggested order of draw for the evacuated tube system should be
   a. blood culture
   b. lavender-topped tube
   c. light blue–topped tube
   d. red-topped tube

10. Containers for the disposal of needles and syringes should have which of the following features?
    a. be puncture resistant
    b. be labeled with a "biohazard" sign
    c. have yellow and black markings
    d. contain antiseptic solution

REFERENCES

1. Henry JB: *Todd, Sanford, Davidsohn—Clinical Diagnosis and Management by Laboratory Methods,* 18th ed. Philadelphia, W. B. Saunders, 1991.
2. National Committee for Clinical Laboratory Standards (NCCLS): *Procedures for the Collection of Diagnostic Blood Specimens by Venipuncture.* Approved standard, H3-A3, Villanova, PA, Author, 1991.
3. College of American Pathologists (CAP): *So You're Going to Collect a Blood Specimen: An Introduction to Phlebotomy,* 6th ed. Northfield, IL, Author, 1994.
4. Becton-Dickinson Systems, Personal communication, July 1995.
5. Richael JL, Naples MF: Creating a workable specimen rejection policy. *Med Lab Observ* March:37–42, 1995.

six

SKIN PUNCTURE PROCEDURES

Chapter Outline

Chapter Objectives

Upon completion of Chapter 6, the learner is responsible for the following:

1. Describe reasons for performing a skin puncture procedure.

2. Identify the proper sites for performing a skin puncture procedure.

3. Explain why controlling the depth of the puncture is necessary.

4. Describe the process of making a blood smear.

5. Explain why blood from a skin puncture procedure is different from blood taken by venipuncture.

INDICATIONS FOR SKIN PUNCTURE

Skin punctures are particularly useful for both adult and pediatric patients when small amounts of blood can be obtained and adequately tested. In contrast, venipuncture in children can be hazardous and difficult because of the risk of complications such as anemia, cardiac arrest, hemorrhage, venous thrombosis, reflex arteriospasm, gangrene of an extremity, danger to surrounding tissues or organs, infections, and injuries from restraining the child during the procedure. It is particularly important to withdraw only the smallest amounts of blood necessary from neonates, infants, and children so that the effects of blood-volume reduction are minimal. A 10-mL blood sample, which could be tolerated by most adults, would represent 5 to 10 percent of the total blood volume in a neonate's body. Sample sizes and procedures for obtaining specimen collections from children are covered in Chapter 8, Pediatric Phlebotomy.

Skin punctures are also useful for the following adult patients:

- Patients with severe burns
- Obese patients
- Patients with thrombotic tendencies
- Oncology patients whose veins are being "saved" for therapy
- Geriatric patients
- Those who have fragile veins
- Patients doing home testing (e.g., blood glucose screening)

Sometimes, skin puncture cannot be used because testing may require larger amounts of blood, interstitial fluids dilute the blood to some extent, and/or a patient has poor peripheral circulation. Specific tests for which skin punctures are not recommended include coagulation studies (because of the interstitial fluid), blood cultures, and erythrocyte sedimentation rate (ESR) determinations.

COMPOSITION OF SKIN PUNCTURE BLOOD

The composition of skin puncture blood is significantly different from that of venous blood acquired by venipuncture. It is composed of blood from arterioles, venules, and capillaries, as well as some tissue (interstitial) fluid, which is released during the sticking process. The content of arterial blood is greater because the arterial pressure in the capillaries is stronger than the venous pressure. Therefore, skin puncture blood is actually more like arterial blood than venous blood.

PREPARATION FOR SKIN PUNCTURE

Skin puncture procedures involve the same preparation steps as discussed for venipuncture procedures. Such steps include greeting the patient to put him or her at ease, ensuring proper patient identification, following universal precautions, labeling procedures appropriately, and practicing the correct hand-washing techniques. For additional discussion of these issues, see Chapter 5.

SUPPLIES FOR SKIN PUNCTURE

As mentioned in Chapter 4, Blood Collection Equipment, supplies for skin puncture include the following: disposable gloves, lancets or automatic puncture devices, micropipettes, disinfectant pads, cotton balls, sterile bandages or gauze pads, glass microscope slides, diluting fluids, microcollection tubes or capillary tubes, capillary tube sealer, laboratory request slips or labels, a marking pen, and a discard bucket.

SKIN PUNCTURE SITES

Skin puncture in adults most often involves one of the fingers. The fleshy surface of the distal portion of the second, third, or fourth finger can be used for puncture. Patients generally prefer their nondominant hand. The fifth, or pinky, finger is not recommended because the tissue of this finger is considerably thinner than that of the others.[1] The second, or index, finger and the middle, or third, finger are used most often.

The heels of infants and neonates are good sites for skin puncture if the procedure is performed properly. The most medial or lateral sections of the plantar, or bottom, surface of the heel should be used. (Refer to Chapter 8 for additional information regarding pediatric phlebotomies.) The thumb, great toe, and earlobe are rarely used as sites for skin puncture. Swollen or edematous areas should not be used for venipuncture or skin puncture because body fluids can contaminate the specimen. Fingers that are cyanotic, swollen, cold, or inflamed should also be avoided.

WARMING THE SKIN PUNCTURE SITE

Warming the skin puncture site helps facilitate phlebotomy by increasing arterial blood flow to the area. Although several easy-to-use methods of warming are available commercially, a surgical towel or a wash-

Procedure for Finger Puncture

1. Remember the following supplies: gloves, sterile cotton balls or gauze sponges (2 x 2), alcohol swabs, sterile lancets, pipettes, capillary tubes, microcollection tubes, glass tubes, diluting fluids, marking pen or pencil, and bandages. Exercise universal precautions, including the use of gloves.
2. Choose a finger that is not cold, cyanotic, or swollen. If possible, the stick should be at the tip of the fourth, or ring finger of the nondominant hand.
3. *Gently* massage the finger five or six times from base to tip to aid blood flow.
4. With an alcohol swab, cleanse the ball of the finger. Allow to air dry.
5. Remove the lancet from its protective paper without touching the tip.
6. Hold the patient's finger firmly with one hand and make a swift, deep puncture with the lancet halfway between the center of the ball of the finger and its side. The cut should be made across the fingerprints to produce a large, round drop of blood.
7. Wipe the first drop of blood away with clean gauze.
8. *Gently* massage the finger from base to tip to obtain the proper amount of blood for the tests required.
9. Each type of microsample has different collection tube and blood volume requirements. Follow the appropriate manufacturer's instructions.

Notes

If the patient's hands are cold, wrap one of them in a warm-to-hot towel 10 to 15 minutes before the puncture is performed.
A free-flowing puncture is essential to obtain accurate test results. *Do not use excessive squeezing or massaging to obtain blood.*

Figure 6–1. Sample procedure for performance of a finger puncture.

cloth heated with warm water to 42°C will not burn the skin. When the towel or cloth is wrapped around the site for 3 to 10 minutes, the skin temperature can increase several degrees.[1]

CLEANING THE SKIN PUNCTURE SITE

The skin puncture site should be cleaned with 75 percent isopropanol and thoroughly dried before being punctured because residual alcohol causes rapid hemolysis and may contaminate glucose determinations. Furthermore, alcohol prevents round drops of blood, which are needed for blood smears, from forming. Povidone–iodine (Betadine) preparations are not recommended for use on skin puncture sites because these preparations can falsely elevate potassium, phosphorus, and uric acid determinations.[1]

SKIN PUNCTURE PROCEDURE

Microcollection by skin puncture involves many of the same steps used during venipuncture. If the phlebotomist is performing a heel stick, the infant's heel should be held firmly, with the forefinger at the arch of the foot and the thumb below and away from the puncture site (see Chapter 8). If a finger stick is being performed, the patient's finger should be held firmly, with the phlebotomist's thumb away from the puncture site (Figs. 6–1 to 6–3). The puncture should be done in one sharp continuous movement, almost perpendicular to the site and across the fingerprint.

THIS   **NOT THIS**

Figure 6–2. The finger puncture should involve a quick, deep puncture across the fingerprints, not parallel to them.

Figure 6–3. Skin puncture procedure. **A,B.** Decontamination of the site. **C.** The first drop of blood is wiped off with sterile gauze. **D.** Blood is collected into an Unopette capillary tube by capillary action. **E.** Blood is collected into a microcollection tube. **F.** The patient presses sterile gauze on finger to stop the bleeding. **G.** The Unopette capillary tube is inserted into the vial and the specimen is mixed thoroughly.

Figure 6–4. The blood smear. Blood smears can be made from venous or capillary blood. In both cases, the smears should be made from fresh drops of blood. With the capillary method, the finger puncture should be made in the usual way and the first drop of blood wiped away. The slide can be touched to the second drop. It should be touched approximately ½ to 1 in. (1.3 to 2.5 cm) from the end of the slide. **A.** A second (spreader) slide should be placed in front of the drop of blood. **B.** The blood collector should pull the spreader slide into the drop, allowing blood to spread along the width of the slide. When the blood spreads almost to the edges, the spreader slide should be quickly and evenly pushed forward at an angle of approximately 30 degrees. The only downward pressure should be the weight of the spreader slide. The slide should be allowed to air dry. It should *not* be blown on. If the venous method is being used, the needle should be touched to the slide immediately after it has been withdrawn. A drop about 1 to 2 mm in diameter will suffice. From this point on, the procedure is the same as for capillary blood smears. **C.** Good smears should have a **feathered edge** and should cover approximately half the surface of the glass slide. No ridges, lines, or holes should be visible in the smear. Errors are often the result of too large a drop, too long a delay in making the smear, or using a chipped slide. **D.** Blood smears should be allowed to air dry after they are labeled.

If the puncture is made along the lines of the fingerprint, the blood tends to run down the finger. The average depth of a skin puncture should be 2 to 3 mm to avoid hitting a bone. Special lancets that control the depth of the puncture are available commercially. If the bone is repeatedly punctured it can lead to **osteomyelitis,** which is an inflammation of the bone due to bacterial infection. Pressure from the phlebotomist's thumb may be eased and reapplied as the drops of blood appear. However, the area should not be massaged or milked excessively because doing so causes hemolysis and contamination of the blood specimen with tissue and intracellular fluids. The first drop of blood should be removed with a dry, sterile pad, then capillary tubes [e.g., Unopette tubes (Becton, Dickinson and Company, Franklin Lakes, NJ)] can be filled and blood smears can be made from subsequent drops of blood. Capillary tubes are filled by **capillary action,** whereby blood flows freely into the tube on contact, without suction.

Figures 6–3 and 6–4 indicate methods for making blood dilutions and blood smears with capillary pipettes. (Chapter 4 provides illustrations of different types of microcollection tubes.) When filling the capillary tubes, the phlebotomist must not allow air bubbles to enter the tubes because air bubbles can cause erroneous results in many laboratory tests. Blood flow is better and air bubbles are less likely if the puncture site is held downward and gentle pressure is applied. Scooping up blood from the skin surface is not advised.

Hands should be washed after contact with each patient. *Before leaving the patient's side,* the phlebotomist must check the puncture site to make sure that the bleeding stopped. All tubes must be appropriately labeled and the information on the labels confirmed. All supplies and equipment that were brought in should be removed or discarded appropriately, and the phlebotomist should thank the patient. An adhesive bandage may be applied. However, such bandages are not recommended for infants or young children because of possible irritation and the potential of swallowing or aspirating a bandage.

✔ Key Terms

CAPILLARY ACTION   OSTEOMYELITIS

DIFFERENTIAL   TISSUE (INTERSTITIAL) FLUID

FEATHERED EDGE

Study Questions

1. Which of the following are *not* sites for skin puncture?

    a. wrist   c. ankle
    b. vein   d. heel

2. Controlling the depth of lancet insertion during skin puncture prevents which of the following?

    a. puncturing a vein   c. excessive bleeding
    b. bacterial contamination d. osteomyelitis

3. A finger puncture should involve which of the following steps?

    a. puncturing parallel to the   c. puncturing across the
       fingerprint   fingerprint
    b. collecting the first drop   d. wiping away the first drop

4. Skin puncture is useful for patients who have which of the following conditions?

    a. obesity   c. fragile veins
    b. burns   d. thrombotic tendencies

5. Which fingers are used most often for skin puncture?

    a. thumb   c. third, or middle, finger
    b. second, or index, finger d. fifth, or pinky, finger

6. Test(s) for which skin puncture cannot be used are

    a. routine hematology tests c. coagulation studies
    b. blood cultures   d. erythrocyte sedimentation rate
                                   (ESR) determinations

7. Blood from skin puncture is more like arterial blood than venous blood for which of the following reasons?

   a. the skin has more arterioles
   b. arterial pressure is stronger in capillaries
   c. more arterial blood flows in capillaries
   d. venous pressure is greater in capillaries

8. Capillary or microcollection tubes should be filled with blood in which of the following ways?

   a. using a syringe to fill the tube
   b. allowing tube to fill by itself using capillary action
   c. using suction to pull blood into the tube
   d. using the tube to carefully scoop droplets off the skin

9. Alcohol should be allowed to dry completely prior to skin puncture

   a. to prevent stinging
   b. to prevent dilution of sample
   c. to prevent lysis of red blood cells
   d. to allow formation of a round drop of blood

10. The best angle for using two glass slides to make a blood smear is approximately

   a. 10 degrees
   b. 15 degrees
   c. 30 degrees
   d. 90 degrees

REFERENCE

1. National Committee for Clinical Laboratory Standards (NCCLS): *Procedures for the Collection of Diagnostic Blood Specimens by Skin Puncture,* 3rd ed. Villanova, PA, NCCLS, 1991.

seven

COMPLICATIONS IN BLOOD COLLECTION

Chapter Outline

Chapter Objectives

Upon completion of Chapter 7, the learner is responsible for the following:

1. Describe the potential physiological and other complications related to phlebotomy procedures.

2. Explain how to prevent complications in blood collection and how to handle the complications that do occur.

3. List the effects of physical disposition on blood collection.

4. Discuss the types of substances that can interfere in clinical analysis of blood constituents and the methods used to prevent these occurrences.

Because complications can occur in blood collection, it is extremely important for the health care provider who is collecting the sample to know how to avoid complications if at all possible. If the complications are unavoidable, the health care worker must be knowledgeable of methods that will decrease the negative impact of the complication on the patient, on the quality of the blood sample, or on both.

COMPLICATIONS ASSOCIATED WITH BLOOD COLLECTION

Fainting (Syncope)

Many patients become dizzy and faint at the thought or sight of blood. Consequently, the health care worker should be aware of the patient's condition throughout the collection procedure. This can be done by asking ambulatory patients if they tend to faint or if they ever previously fainted during blood collections. If so, they should be moved from a seated position to a lying position. Even for an ambulatory patient without a history of fainting, it is still extremely important to use a blood collection chair with a "locked" arm rest to avoid the possibility of a fall if he or she faints. If a seated patient feels faint, the needle should be removed, the patient's head should be lowered between the legs, and the patient should breathe deeply. If possible, the health care worker should ask for help and move the patient to a lying position. Talking to patients can often reassure them and divert their attention from the collection procedure. Bed-bound patients also experience fainting, or **syncope,** during blood collection, although rarely. In any case, however, the health care worker should stay with the patient at least 15 minutes until he or she recovers. A wet towel gently applied to the forehead or a glass of juice or water may help the patient feel better.

If a patient faints during or after the procedure, the health care worker should try to terminate the venipuncture procedure immediately and make sure that the patient does not fall or become injured. Sometimes, controlling the situation is difficult because of the patient's physical size; however, the health care worker should use common sense about the safest position for a patient. If a patient has fainted and is in a secure position, the health care worker should quickly request assistance from the nursing staff or a physician. A patient who has fainted should recover fully before being allowed to leave and should be instructed not to drive a vehicle for at least 30 minutes. An incident report must be filed with the health care facility regarding the fainting incident and the immediate precautions and instructions provided to the patient to prevent the possibility of long-term complications (e.g., car accident after fainting incident).

Failure to Draw Blood

Several factors may cause the health care worker to "miss the vein." These factors include not inserting the needle deep enough, inserting the needle all the way through the vein, holding the needle bevel against the vein wall, or losing the vacuum in the tube (Fig. 7–1). During needle insertion, the health care worker's index finger can be used to help locate the vein. The needle may need to be moved or withdrawn somewhat, and redirected. In the geriatric patient, the vein may be "tough" during needle entry and may roll; such rolling can cause the needle to slip to the side of the vein instead of properly puncturing it. Thus, the health care worker must securely anchor the vein prior to blood collection.

On occasion, a test tube will have no vacuum because of a manufacturer's error or tube leakage after a puncture. Consequently, the health care worker should carry an extra set of tubes in his or her pocket in case this happens during venipuncture. Also, needles for evacuated tube systems have been known to unscrew from the barrel during venipuncture. If this happens, the tourniquet should be released immediately and the needle removed.

Hematomas

When the area around the puncture site starts to swell, usually blood is leaking into the tissues and causing a **hematoma.** This complication can occur when the needle has gone completely through the vein, the bevel opening is partially in the vein, or not enough pressure is applied to the site after puncture. This swelling results in a large bruise after several days (Fig. 7–2). If a hematoma begins to form, the tourniquet and the

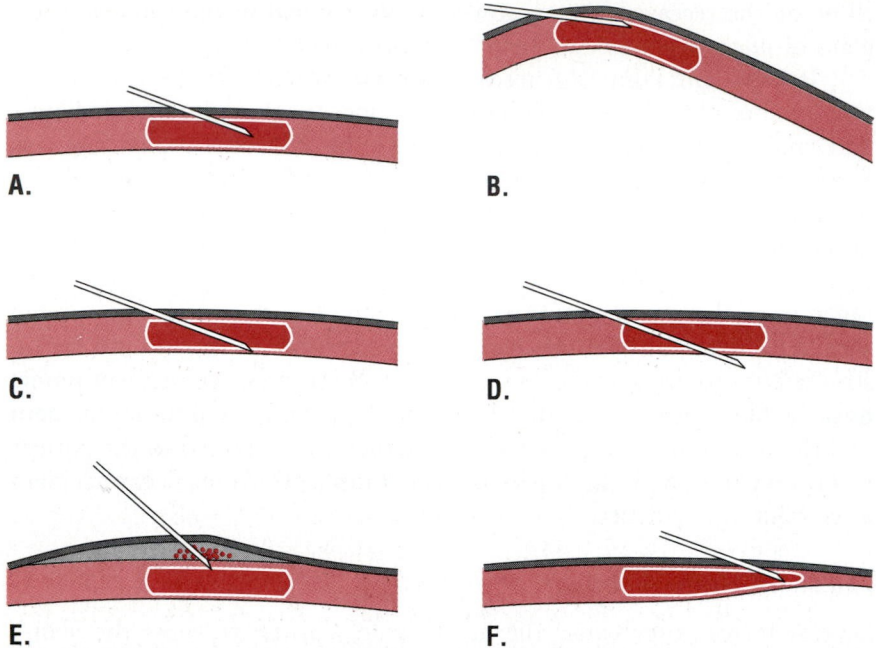

Figure 7–1. Needle positioning and failure to draw blood. **A.** Correct insertion technique; blood flows freely into needle. **B.** Bevel on vein upper wall does not allow blood to flow. **C.** Bevel on vein lower wall does not allow blood to flow. **D.** Needle inserted too far. **E.** Needle partially inserted, which causes blood leakage into tissue. **F.** Collapsed vein.

needle should be *removed immediately,* and pressure should be applied to the area for approximately 2 minutes. If the bleeding continues, a nurse should be notified.

Petechiae

✔ **Petechiae,** small red spots appearing on a patient's skin, indicate that minute amounts of blood have escaped into skin epithelium. This complication may be a result of coagulation problems, such as platelet defects, and should caution the health care worker that the patient's puncture site may bleed excessively.

Excessive Bleeding

A patient usually stops bleeding at the venipuncture site within a few minutes. However, patients on anticoagulant therapy, and/or those taking high dosages of arthritis medication or other medication, may bleed for a longer period. Thus, anytime a venipuncture is performed, pressure must be applied to the venipuncture site until the bleeding stops. The health care worker *must not* leave the patient until the bleeding stops or a nurse takes over to assess the patient's situation.

Seizures

One rare complication that may occur during blood collection is seizures. If a patient begins to have a seizure, the health care worker should immediately release the tourniquet, remove the needle, attempt to hold pressure over the blood collection site, and call for help from the nursing station. No attempt should be made to place anything in the patient's mouth.

Mastectomy

A woman who has had a **mastectomy** (removal of a breast) may also have **lymphostasis** (no lymph flow) due to lymph node removal adjacent to the breast. Without lymph flow on that particular side of the body, the patient is highly susceptible to infection. Thus, venipuncture should not be performed on the same side as that of a mastectomy. Also, the pressure from the tourniquet could lead to injuries in a patient who has had this type of surgery.

Edema

Some patients develop an abnormal accumulation of fluid in the intercellular spaces of the body. This swelling can be localized or diffused over a larger area of the body. The health care worker should avoid collecting blood from these sites because veins in these areas are difficult to palpate or stick, and the specimen may become contaminated with fluid.

Figure 7–2. Patient's hematoma several days after a venipuncture.

Obesity

Obese patients generally have veins that are difficult to visualize and palpate. If the vein is missed, the health care worker must be careful not to probe excessively with the needle because doing so ruptures red blood cells (RBCs), increases the concentration of intracellular contents, and releases some tissue clotting factors.

Intravenous Therapy

Every time a catheter is used, vein damage occurs. Circulatory blood is rerouted to collateral veins and can result in hemoconcentration. Consequently, patients on intravenous (IV) therapy for extended periods often have veins that are palpable and visible but damaged or occluded (blocked). Whenever a patient has an IV line, the arm with the IV line should not be used for venipuncture because the specimen will be diluted with IV fluid. Instead, the other arm or another site should be considered. Alternatively, sometimes the nurse or the physician can disconnect the IV line and draw blood from the needle that is already inserted. In this situation, the first few milliliters of the specimen should be discarded to remove the IV fluid, and a note should be made on the laboratory requisition form that this step was performed.

Damaged, Sclerosed, or Occluded Veins

✔ Obstructed, or occluded veins, do not allow blood to flow through
✔ them; sclerosed, or hardened, veins are a result of inflammation and disease of the interstitial substances; and patients' veins that have been repeatedly punctured often become scarred and feel hard when palpated. Because blood is not easily collected from these sites, they should be avoided.

Hemoconcentration

An increased concentration of larger molecules and formed elements in
✔ the blood is called hemoconcentration. Several factors can cause this complication, including prolonged tourniquet application; massaging, squeezing, or probing a site; long-term IV therapy; and sclerosed or occluded veins.

Hemolysis

When RBCs are lysed, hemoglobin is released and serum, which is normally straw colored, becomes tinged with pink or red. If a specimen is

grossly hemolyzed, the serum appears very dark red. **Hemolysis** can be ✔
caused by improper phlebotomy techniques such as using a needle that
is too small, pulling a syringe plunger back too fast, expelling the blood
vigorously into a tube, and shaking or mixing tubes vigorously. These
problems can easily be prevented with appropriate handling. Hemolysis
may also be the result of physiological abnormalities. The health care
worker should make a note on the requisition form whenever he or she
notices that a specimen is hemolyzed.

Collapsed Veins

If a syringe plunger is withdrawn too quickly during venipuncture, or
the vacuum draw of a tube is too great, the vein may collapse, especially
when blood is being collected from smaller veins (see Figure 7–1F) and
veins in geriatric patients. Thus, the blood collector should pull slowly
on the syringe plunger or use an evacuated tube with a smaller volume
during the collection process on patients with smaller veins and geriatric
patients. A collapsed vein should *not* be probed with the needle.

Allergies

Some patients are allergic to iodine or other solutions used to disinfect
a puncture site. If a patient indicates that he or she is allergic to a solution, all efforts should be made to use an alternative method.

Thrombosis

Thrombi are solid masses derived from blood constituents that reside in ✔
the blood vessels. A thrombus may partially or fully occlude a vein (or
an artery), and such occlusion will make venipuncture more difficult.

Burned or Scarred Areas

Areas that have been burned or scarred should be avoided during phlebotomy. Burned areas are very sensitive and susceptible to infection,
whereas veins under scarred areas are difficult to palpate.

Infections

The health care worker should remember at all times that many patients
have transmittable diseases (e.g., hepatitis) and that likewise, he or
she can pass an infection to a patient. (For precautionary techniques,
refer to Chapter 12, Infection Control, and Chapter 13, Safety and
First Aid.)

EFFECTS OF PHYSICAL DISPOSITION ON BLOOD COLLECTION

Basal State

Blood specimens that will be used to determine the concentrations of body constituents such as glucose, cholesterol, triglycerides, electrolytes, and proteins should be collected when the patient is in a **basal state**—that is, in the early morning, approximately 12 hours after the last ingestion of food. The results of laboratory tests on basal state specimens are more reliable because normal values are most often determined from specimens collected during this time. Several factors such as diet, exercise, emotional stress, obesity, menstrual cycle, pregnancy, *diurnal variations,* posture, tourniquet application, and chemical constituents (alcohol or drugs) cause changes in the basal state.

Diet

To ensure that the patient is in the basal state, the physician must require the patient to fast overnight. The term **fasting** refers to abstinence from food and beverages (except water). The required time period necessary for abstaining varies with the test procedure or procedures to be performed. Before collecting a specimen, the health care worker should ask the patient if he or she has eaten. Blood composition is significantly altered after meals and consequently is unsuitable for many clinical chemistry tests. If the patient has eaten, and the physician still needs the test, the word *nonfasting* must be written on the requisition form.[2]

Inadequate patient instructions are often the cause of mistakes in specimen collection. The health care worker may be asked to explain fasting restrictions to a patient. In such cases, these restrictions must be explained clearly and in detail. Some patients assume that the term *fasting* refers to abstaining from food *and* water. Abstaining from water can result in dehydration, which can alter test results. Thus, the health care worker must ensure that the patient understands what is required of him or her. Written instructions can be given, if available.

Gaining the patient's understanding and cooperation is important and is determined by the professional behavior and the degree of confidence displayed by the health care worker. Casual instructions are apt to be taken lightly by the patient or even forgotten. A health care worker who is organized, attentive, and skilled and who emphasizes important points of the procedure is more likely to get patient cooperation and an accurate test result, and to make the patient more comfortable.

If a procedure involves some discomfort or inconvenience, the patient should be informed. For example, if blood is to be drawn for a timed blood glucose level determination, the patient needs to fast for 8 to 12 hours. However, prolonged fasting has been shown to falsely alter blood test results.[2] The health care worker can inform the patient that several specimens will be collected at timed intervals and that he or she may drink water, but that coffee and tea should be avoided because they cause a transitory fluctuation in the blood sugar level.

Normally, serum is clear, light yellow, or straw colored. Turbid serum appears cloudy or "milky" and can be a result of bacterial contamination or high lipid levels in the blood. Turbidity is caused primarily by ingestion of fatty substances such as meat, butter, cream, and cheese. If a patient has recently eaten these substances, he or she may have a temporarily elevated lipid level, and the serum will appear lipemic, or cloudy. Because lipemic serum does not represent a basal state, and may indicate some chemical abnormalities,[2] a note on the requisition form about the appearance of the serum may be useful to the physician.

Exercise

Muscular activity, as a result of moderate or excessive exercise, has a marked effect on laboratory test results, especially when the levels of lactic acid, creatinine, fatty acids, some amino acids, proteins, and some enzymes are being tested. Most of these values, except certain enzyme levels, return to baseline shortly after the exercise stops. However, the levels of enzymes such as creatine phosphokinase (CPK), aspartate aminotransferase (AST), and lactate dehydrogenase (LD) can remain elevated as long as 24 hours after a person engages in 1 hour of moderate-to-strenuous exercise.[2]

Research suggests that exercise also has some effects on hemostasis. Some reports indicate that physical exercise activates coagulation, fibrinolysis, and platelet formation. Because different types of exercise were studied, other reports cite conflicting results or no changes in measured hemostatic parameters. Nevertheless, most researchers conclude that some hemostatic changes do occur after strenuous exercise.[3]

Stress

Patients are often frightened, nervous, and overly anxious. These emotional stresses can cause a transient elevation in the white blood cell (WBC) count, a transient decrease in serum iron levels, and abnormal adrenal hormone (e.g., cortisol) values.[3,4] Newborns who have been crying violently will have WBC counts that are 140 percent above resting baseline counts. Even mild crying has been shown to increase WBC counts 113 percent. These elevated counts return to baseline values within 1 hour. Consequently, blood samples for WBC counts should be taken approximately 1 hour after a crying episode.[5] Anxiety that results in hyperventilation also causes acid–base imbalances, increased lactate levels, and increased fatty acid levels.[2]

Diurnal Rhythms and Posture

✔ **Diurnal rhythms** are body fluid fluctuations during the day. Certain hormone levels decrease in the afternoon [e.g., cortisol, adrenocorticotropic hormone (ACTH)], whereas eosinophil counts and serum iron levels increase. Thus, collecting specimens during the designated time periods is important for proper clinical evaluation.

Posture changes are also known to vary laboratory test results of some chemical constituents (e.g., aldosterone). This consideration is important when inpatient and outpatient results are being compared. ✔ Changing from a **supine** (or lying) position to a sitting or standing position causes body water to shift from intravascular to interstitial compartments (in tissues). Certain larger molecules cannot filter into the tissue; therefore, they concentrate in the blood. Enzyme, protein, lipid, iron, and calcium levels are significantly increased with changes in position.[6]

Age

Laboratory test results vary considerably during the stages of life: infancy, childhood (pediatric population), adulthood, and older adulthood (geriatric population). For example, blood cholesterol and triglyceride values increase as a person ages. Various hormone levels, such as estrogen and growth hormone (GH) levels, decrease in geriatric women. GH levels are also decreased in geriatric men.

Testing Interference from Tourniquet Pressure

Laboratory test results can be falsely elevated or decreased if the tourniquet pressure is too tight or is maintained too long. The pressure from the tourniquet causes biological analytes to leak from the tissue cells into the blood, or vice versa. For example, plasma cholesterol, iron, lipid, protein, and potassium levels will be falsely elevated if the tourniquet pressure is too tight or prolonged. Significant elevations may be seen with as short as a 3-minute application of the tourniquet.[6] In addition, some enzyme levels can be falsely elevated or decreased because of tourniquet pressure that is too tight or prolonged.

Other Factors Affecting the Patient

Many other factors can affect laboratory test results. Gender and pregnancy have an influence on laboratory testing; thus, reference ranges are often noted according to gender. Geographic factors such as altitude, temperature, and humidity also affect normal baseline values. Therefore, normal reference values must be established for each clinical laboratory according to its patient population and its location.

Medications may also alter laboratory test results significantly. Consequently, physicians must work closely with pharmacy and laboratory staff to rule out laboratory test results that are altered because the patient is taking medication.

INTERFERENCE OF DRUGS AND OTHER SUBSTANCES IN BLOOD

Many prescribed drugs can interfere with clinical laboratory determinations or can physiologically alter the levels of blood constituents measured in the clinical laboratory. The interference of drugs and other substances is so complicated and dependent upon the chemical procedures used that only general recommendations are described in this section.

The direct analytical interference of drugs is decreasing with the advent of more specific and sensitive chemical procedures. However, the physiologically induced abnormalities from various types of drugs are the major causes of interference from medications. Drugs administered to alleviate an illness can induce physiological abnormalities in one or more of the following systems: hepatic, hematologic, hemostatic, muscular, pancreatic, and renal. The result is obscuration of the clinical diagnosis.

Prior to laboratory measurement of chemical constituents, the attending physician should take the necessary precautions in prescribing drugs to the patient. If the patient must be maintained on medication that may cause interferences in laboratory assays, the medication name should be written on the laboratory request form. Unless interference of medications can be avoided by ordering different laboratory assays, medications should be discontinued if possible, and assays should be repeated when false laboratory values are suspected.

Direct analytical interference in laboratory determinations is least likely to occur in blood assays because drug concentrations are usually low. However, some drugs or drug metabolites in blood can directly cause falsely decreased or falsely elevated values in laboratory analyses.

Drug interferences leading to falsely decreased values in blood specimens may be caused by inhibition of the chromogenic or fluorescent reaction. Examples of drugs that cause such inhibition are indicated in Table 7–1. A more complete list of such drugs can be found in Hansten's *Drug Interactions*.[7] These drugs can do the following:

1. Diminish fluorescence of the blood analyte by quenching the fluorescent energy and thus falsely decrease the analyte concentration
2. Compete with the blood analyte for a chromogenic reagent and thus falsely decrease the resultant color and concentration of the analyte
3. Compete with the chromogenic reagent for peroxide in a peroxide-generating reaction and thus falsely decrease chromogen oxidation and the concentration of the blood analyte

The falsely decreased values of the blood analyte can be mistakenly interpreted as normal or subnormal if the blood analyte was truly in an elevated range or a normal range, respectively.

Drug interferences leading to falsely elevated values of blood analytes may be caused by increasing the color or fluorescence produced in the laboratory analysis, altering the binding characteristics in radioimmunoassays and enzyme immunoassays, or both. Examples of drugs that do this are shown in Table 7–2.

Interference from medications usually causes falsely elevated values rather than falsely decreased values. Some drugs, such as acetaminophen (Tylenol) and erythromycin, can increase serum AST and

TABLE 7–1. DRUG INTERFERENCES LEADING TO FALSELY DECREASED RESULTS IN BLOOD SPECIMENS

Analyte	Method	Drug Interference
Albumin	Colorimetric	Aspirin[8]
Bilirubin	Colorimetric (diazo reaction)	Ascorbic acid[9] (vitamin C)
Cholesterol	Colorimetric	Thiouracil[10]
Glucose	Colorimetric	Ascorbic acid[11]
	Chromogenic oxidation (hexokinase reaction)	L-Dopa[12]
	Chromogenic oxidation (oxidase reaction)	Tetracycline[13]
Phosphate	Colorimetric	Phenothiazine[14]
Protein	Colorimetric	Cytarabine[10]
Uric acid	Colorimetric (phosphotungstic acid)	Salicylates[15]
	Enzymatic	Lithium[10]
		Ascorbic acid[16]

TABLE 7–2. DRUG INTERFERENCES LEADING TO FALSELY ELEVATED RESULTS IN BLOOD SPECIMENS

Analyte	Method	Drug Interference
Aspartate aminotransferase (ALT)	Colorimetric	Erythromycin[15]
Catecholamines	Fluorescent	Ampicillin[13] Ascorbic acid[13]
Cholesterol	Colorimetric	Corticosteroids[10] Salicylates[10]
Creatine kinase (CK)	Colorimetric	D-Penicillamine[17]
Creatinine	Colorimetric	Dexamethasone[17]
Iron	Colorimetric	Dextran[15]
Protein	Colorimetric	Sulfobromophthalein[10] Phenazopyridine[10] Tetracycline[10]
Total leukocytes count	Automated counting system	Azathioprine[17]
Triglycerides	Enzymatic with color development	Aspirin[18]
Uric acid	Colorimetric (phosphotungstic acid)	Ascorbic acid[10] Caffeine[10]

bilirubin levels and thus falsely create a clinical interpretation of hepatic dysfunction without the true presence of hepatic abnormality.[19] Drug-induced elevations of blood constituents can be mistakenly interpreted as falsely increased or normal, when the true values are in the normal range or the subnormal range, respectively.

In addition to prescribed oral medications, intravenous injections of medications and dyes can interfere with laboratory test results. For example, the results of laboratory tests performed after fluorescein angiography may be erroneous owing to interference by the intravenous fluorescein.[20] The results for blood creatinine, cortisol, and digoxin determinations are altered by this dye. Consequently, if the health care worker, nurse, or clinical assistant collects blood in a cardiology section or a specialized health care institution for heart patients, he or she needs to be alert to this potential for laboratory test interference. If he or she is aware of collecting blood from a patient who just had a dye injection, this information must be communicated promptly to the specimen collection supervisor.

Physiologically, drugs can alter blood analytes through various metabolic reactions; the production of blood cells and platelets, as well as their survival times, can be changed. Chemotherapeutic drugs can lead to a decrease in all forms of blood cellular elements and, thus, their metabolic and immunologic processes.

A variety of medications are toxic to the liver (Table 7–3) and thus can lead to acute hepatic necrosis.[19] In turn, the hepatic dysfunction leads to an increase in the concentration of blood liver enzymes such as alanine aminotransferase (ALT), alkaline phosphatase (ALP), and LD. Also, the production of globulins and clotting factors is decreased in patients with drug-induced hepatotoxicity.

Patients receiving medications that may result in renal impairment should be monitored for a possible electrolyte imbalance and elevation of blood urea nitrogen (BUN) levels. Antihypertensive agents given for a long period to lower high blood pressure can lead to kidney damage if the patient is not monitored closely.

Pancreatitis can be caused by corticosteroids, estrogens, and diuretics and causes elevations of serum amylase and lipase values. Aspirin causes hypobilirubinemia (a decrease in bilirubin) by expelling bilirubin from the plasma to the surrounding tissue cells.[21]

Because many metabolic activities can be altered by medications, as described in the preceding examples, the attending physician must note on the laboratory request form all medications that the patient is taking. As a general rule, the College of American Pathologists (CAP)[22] recommends that medications that might interfere in laboratory assays be discontinued for at least 4 to 24 hours prior to blood studies and 48 to 72 hours prior to urine studies. However, this recommendation should be followed only if the patient will not be at risk or experience serious discomfort.

The health care worker collecting the blood specimen is the link between the clinical laboratory and the patient. Laboratory tests are often ordered without knowledge of the drugs taken by a person. Yet, as discussed previously, these drugs will lead to falsely elevated or decreased values. Sometimes during blood collection, a patient will mention that he or she has taken over-the-counter drugs such as Tylenol. It is impor-

TABLE 7–3. DRUGS TOXIC TO THE LIVER

Salicylates	Penicillin	Acetaminophen
Mitomycin	Isoniazid	Chlorpromazine
Actinomycin	Halothane	Methyldopa
Thiazides	Chloramphenicol	Acetohexamide
Trifluoperazine	Sulfamethoxazole	Chlorpropamide
Sulfachlorpyridazine	Tetracycline	Paramethadione
Phenytoin		

Adapted from Sher PP: Drug interferences with clinical laboratory tests. Drugs 24:24, 1982; and Sherlock S: Progress report: Hepatic reaction to drugs. Gut 20:634, 1979.

TABLE 7–4. COMPLICATIONS LEADING TO BLOOD SPECIMEN REJECTION

Hemolyzed specimen (except for tests in which hemolysis does not interfere)
Anticoagulated blood containing clots
Improper specimen transportation (e.g., blood gas specimen not transported in slurry of ice water)
Improper blood collection tube
Lipemic specimen
Insufficient quantity of blood in collection tube
Discrepancies between requisition form and labeled tube (e.g., names, dates, times)
Unlabeled tube
Outdated equipment, supplies, or reagents
Contaminated specimen

tant for the health care worker to communicate the patient's name and the possible drug interference to the clinical laboratory supervisor in charge of specimen collection. The supervisor can then communicate with the attending physician and determine whether the medication will interfere in the laboratory assays. The follow-up communication can lead to better patient care by preventing the presence of interfering substances in laboratory specimens.

SPECIMEN REJECTION

Each department or section in the clinical laboratory should establish its own guidelines for specimen rejection. In general, the factors shown in Table 7–4 should be considered.

When a problem arises, the appropriate investigational channels should be followed. The health care provider who drew the specimen and his or her supervisor should try to solve the problem initially. Other personnel may be involved as needed. Communication and honesty are the keys to an efficient and reliable health care environment.

✔ Key Terms

BASAL STATE

DIURNAL RHYTHMS

FASTING

HEMATOMA

HEMOCONCENTRATION

HEMOLYSIS

HYPOBILIRUBINEMIA

LIPEMIC

LYMPHOSTASIS

MASTECTOMY

OCCLUDED VEINS

PETECHIAE

SCLEROSED VEINS

SUPINE

SYNCOPE

THROMBI

TURBID

Study Questions

The following questions may have one or more answers.

1. Which of the following factors result in failure to draw blood during venipuncture?

    a. losing the vacuum in the tube

    b. tying the tourniquet too tightly

    c. inserting the needle through the vein

    d. puncturing a sclerosed vein

2. Hematomas during venipuncture result from which of the following?

    a. needle bevel is against the vein wall

    b. needle bevel is partially inserted in the vein

    c. needle is occluded

    d. patient has coagulation problems

3. Hemoconcentration can be caused by which of the following?

    a. long-term IV therapy

    b. lengthy tourniquet application

    c. excessive needle probing

    d. sclerosed or occluded veins

4. Which of the following is a solid mass derived from blood constituents and can occlude a vein (or an artery)?

   a. hemolyzed RBC   c. thrombus
   b. hemolyzed WBC   d. triglyceride

5. If blood is to be drawn for a timed blood glucose level determination, the patient must fast for

   a. 4 to 6 hours   c. 8 to 12 hours
   b. 6 to 8 hours   d. 14 to 16 hours

6. Which of the following laboratory test results are affected most if the patient is not fasting?

   a. AST and CPK   c. cortisol and testosterone
   b. triglycerides and glucose   d. complete blood cell (CBC)
                                  count and prothrombin time

7. An abnormal accumulation of fluid in the intercellular spaces of the body that is localized or diffused is referred to as

   a. hemoconcentration   c. atherosclerosis
   b. edema   d. hemolysis

8. If a patient is taking high doses of Tylenol, which of the following analyte results is most likely to be affected?

   a. serum bilirubin   c. blood glucose
   b. CPK   d. blood cholesterol

9. If the tourniquet is applied for longer than 3 minutes, which of the following analytes will most likely become falsely elevated?

   a. potassium   c. GGT
   b. bilirubin   d. parathyroid hormone

10. Emotional stress, such as anxiety or fear, can lead to alterations of which of the following analytes?

   a. serum iron   c. cortisol
   b. WBCs   d. RBCs

REFERENCES

1. Larson JM: A stick in time saves nine. *Med Lab Observ* April: 109, 1981.
2. Statland BE, Winkel P: Preparing patients and specimens for laboratory testing, in Henry JB (ed): *Clinical Diagnosis and Management by Laboratory Methods*. Philadelphia, WB Saunders, 1991.
3. Rudmann SV: The effects of exercise on hemostasis: A review of the literature and implications for research. *Am J Med Technol* 4(5):215, 1987.

4. Damon Corporation: *Handbook of Specimen Collection and Preparation.* Damon Co, 1977.
5. Becton, Dickinson and Company: *Blood Specimen Collection by Skin Puncture in Infants.* East Rutherford, NJ, Becton, Dickinson and Company, 1982.
6. Statland BE, Winkle P, Bokelund H: Factors contributing to intra-individual variation of serum constituents. 4. Effects of posture and tourniquet application on variation of serum constituents in healthy subjects. *Clin Chem* 20:1513, 1974.
7. Hansten PD: *Drug Interactions.* Philadelphia, Lea & Febiger, 1981.
8. Sunderman FW: Drug interference in clinical biochemistry. *Crit Rev Clin Lab Sci* 1:427, 1970.
9. Panek E, Young D, Bente J: Analytical interference of drugs in clinical chemistry. *Am J Med Technol* 44:217, 1978.
10. Sher PP: Drug interferences with clinical laboratory tests. *Drugs* 24:24, 1982.
11. Romano AT: Automated glucose methods: Evaluation of glucose oxidase–peroxidase procedure. *Clin Chem* 19:1152, 1973.
12. Neely WE: Simple automated determination of serum or plasma glucose by a hexokinase/G6PD method. *Clin Chem* 18:509, 1972.
13. Garb S: *Clinical Guide to Undesirable Drug Interactions and Interferences.* New York, Springer, 1971.
14. El-Dorry HF, Medina H, Bacila M: Interference of phenothiazine compounds in colorimetric determination of inorganic phosphate. *Anal Biochem* 47:329, 1972.
15. Young DS: *Effects of Drugs on Clinical Laboratory Tests.* Washington, DC, AACC Press, 1990.
16. Siest G, Galteau M: *Drug Effects on Laboratory Test Results.* Littleton, MA, PSG Publishing Co, 1988, p 433.
17. Siest G (ed): *Drug Effects on Laboratory Test Results.* The Hague, Martinus Nijhoff, 1980.
18. Letellier G, Desjarlais F: Analytical interference of drugs in clinical chemistry: I. Study of twenty drugs on seven different instruments. *Clin Biochem* 18:345, 1985.
19. Sherlock S: Progress report: Hepatic reaction to drugs. *Gut* 20:634, 1979.
20. Elin RJ, Bloom JN, Herman DC, et al: Interference by intravenous fluorescein with laboratory tests. *Clin Chem* 35(6):1159, 1989.
21. Routh J, Paul W: Assessment of interference by aspirin with some assays commonly done in the clinical laboratory. *Clin Chem* 22:837, 1976.
22. College of American Pathologists (CAP): *Standards for Accreditation of Medical Laboratories.* Skokie, IL, CAP, 1974.

Phlebotomy Case Study

HOME CARE COLLECTIONS

Mr. Albert A. Thomson, a 55-year-old white male, was released from Nicholson Community Hospital on March 25. He had been in the hospital for 14 days as a result of undergoing cardiac bypass surgery and experiencing some complications. On March 29, Ms. Terry Alright, a home health care phlebotomist from Nicholson Community Hospital saw that her schedule included a visit to Mr. Thomson for blood collection for the following laboratory tests:

Chemistry screen
Protime
CBC
APTT
Calcium, ionized

When she arrived at Mr. Thomson's home and began her preparations for blood collection, she noticed that Mr. Thomson had hematomas in both antecubical fossa areas of the left and right arms. Thus, she checked the right hand and found a vein that looked suitable for collecting blood with a safety winged infusion set with small blood collection vacuum tubes. She prepared the site for blood collection, and using a 23-gauge safety winged infusion needle, she inserted the needle into the vein and first collected blood in a red-speckled-topped vacuum tube, followed by a purple-topped tube, two light blue–topped tubes, and then a green-topped tube. As she collected each tube, she mixed the blood and additive in the blood collection tube. After completing the blood collection, she labeled the tubes, discarded the biohazardous blood collection items in her biohazardous disposal container, and left Mr. Thomson's home with the collected blood and her blood collection items.

She traveled next to Ms. Jennifer Smith's home to collect blood from Ms. Smith for a digoxin assay and a plasma potassium level determination. Ms. Smith, an 85-year-old black female, was homebound because of arthritis and a cardiac arrhythmia problem. Collecting blood from the median cubital vein in Ms. Smith's left arm, the phlebotomist used a syringe because of the fragility of the vein. After collecting 5 mL of blood in the syringe, Ms. Alright placed 2 mL of blood in a small red-speckled-topped blood collection tube and 3 mL of blood in a small purple-topped blood collection tube. She labeled the tubes, discarded the biohazard blood collection items, and left Ms. Smith's house to travel to the hospital laboratory and drop off the blood specimens.

Questions:

1. For each of the following laboratory tests, what color should the top of the blood collection tube be?

Laboratory Assay	Color of Blood Collection Tube Top
Calcium, ionized	_____
APTT	_____
CBC count	_____
Protime	_____
Chemistry screen	_____
Digoxin	_____
Plasma potassium	_____

2. Did the home health care phlebotomist use the proper order of draw for Mr. Thomson's laboratory tests? If not, what was the proper order of draw?

3. Did the phlebotomist use the proper order of draw for Ms. Smith's laboratory tests? If not, what was the proper order of draw?

SPECIAL PROCEDURES

III

*T*he practice of phlebotomy involves specialized duties and functions in certain circumstances. Part III describes the special procedures that are becoming part of the expanding role of health care workers. Each new activity can be learned alone or along with other, more routine duties. For some health care workers, a procedure that was previously special is now routine.

Chapter 8, Pediatric Phlebotomy, focuses on the special attention and technical skills necessary for dealing with infants and children. The chapter describes effective communication with children and parents; different procedures for blood collection, including heel sticks, neonatal screening procedures, and the dorsal hand vein technique; and special concerns regarding diagnostic testing for children.

Chapter 9, Arterial and Special Collection Procedures, covers site selection and puncture procedures for blood collection for arterial blood gas determinations; the Allen test; bleeding-time tests; blood cultures; glucose, lactose, and other tolerance tests; and therapeutic drug monitoring (TDM) tests. Also discussed are blood collections through a central venous catheter, blood donor room collections, and emergency room blood collections.

Chapter 10, Home, Hospital Bedside, and Nursing Home Collections, highlights procedures that are becoming more routine in the care and monitoring of patients in these settings. Emphasis is on point-of-care testing such as glucose monitoring, blood gas and electrolyte analysis, and cholesterol screening.

Chapter 11, Urinalysis and Body Fluid Collections, describes the various alternative procedures for urine and other body fluid collections, including cerebrospinal fluid, seminal fluid, amniotic fluid, and specimens for microbiological cultures. Emphasis is on proper collection and safe handling of the specimens.

eight

8

PEDIATRIC PHLEBOTOMY

Chapter Outline

Chapter Objectives

Upon completion of Chapter 8, the learner is responsible for the following:

1. Explain how child development relates to blood collection from neonates, infants, children, and teenagers.

2. Identify puncture sites for a heel stick on an infant and demonstrate the procedure.

3. Describe the venipuncture sites for infants and young children.

4. Discuss the types of equipment and supplies that must be used during microcollection and venipuncture of infants and children.

✔ Drawing blood from a pediatric patient requires much expertise and knowledge. Not all **pediatric phlebotomies** are capillary work, so the novice health care worker must study anatomy and physiology, be familiar with the types of equipment that are available, observe the various techniques as they are performed by an experienced health care worker, and practice the techniques to develop the necessary skills.

Performing venipunctures on young patients is challenging for the health care worker, not only technically, because of these patients' small size, but also because children are less emotionally and psychologically developed than adults. Therefore, a successful outcome requires the use of good interpersonal skills in dealing with ill children and their concerned, apprehensive parents.[7]

With proper training in technique and an understanding of pediatric psychological development, the delicate task of drawing blood from a frightened child need not strike fear or dread in the heart of the health care worker. Skills should be perfected on older children first, then, when confidence is attained, venipunctures can be attempted on younger children. When learning the techniques, the health care worker should remember to ask for help if needed and to allow adequate time to develop the necessary skills.

CHILD DEVELOPMENT

✔ The model of **child development,** shown in the table on page 231, describes not only the fears and concerns of the pediatric patient at various ages, but also subtested parental involvement at each stage.

PREPARING CHILD AND PARENT

Preparing the child and the parent for the blood collection procedure involves the following steps:

1. Introduce yourself. Be warm, friendly, establish eye contact, and show that you are concerned about the child's health and comfort. When you interact with a pediatric patient and his or her parent, you should instill a sense of trust and confidence in the parent and the child. A calm, confident

Stage (Age)	Fears and Concerns	Proper Parent Behavior
Newborns (0–12 months)	Totally dependent on parents and other adults Trust that adults respond to basic needs	Parent should hold infant as an aid to collector and to comfort child
Infants and toddlers (12–24 months)	Little fear of danger Fear of separation from mother Limited language and understanding	Parent should assist in holding, explaining to, and comforting child
Preschoolers (3–6 years)	Greater body awareness Fear of injury to body Play years Puppets = "play"	Parent may be present to provide emotional support and to assist in obtaining the child's cooperation
School-age, preadolescents (7–12 years)	Fear loss of self-control Less depedent on parent— more autonomous More willing to participate	Child may ask parent to leave room
Teenagers (13–18 years)	Actively involved in anything concerning the body Embarrassed to show fear May act hostile to mask fear	Child may not want parent to be present
Special problems Mentally retarded	Fears similar to age-appropriate behaviors above, based on developmental level Need relaxed, gentle approach	Parent should stay with patient and assist if necessary.

Adapted from Erickson EH: Childhood and Society, *2nd ed. New York, Norton, 1963.*

approach is the first step in limiting their anxiety and obtaining their cooperation.

2. Correctly identify the patient. A hospitalized infant usually has an identification bracelet on his or her ankle. Newborns who are not yet named are usually referred to by their last names (e.g., Baby Boy Smith, Baby Girl Jones). If the mother is still in the hospital after delivery, the baby may wear a bracelet that is cross-referenced to the mother for breast-feeding times and so forth. Keeping identifications straight is always crucial, but especially so when specimens from twin babies must be collected and labeled.

3. Find out about the child's past experience with blood drawing. This can be accomplished easily by asking whether the child has ever had blood drawn. The child and the parent

can then tell about their experiences with past procedures and provide you with valuable information about the approaches that worked effectively for them and those that were not as successful.

4. Develop a plan. Asking the parent how cooperative his or her child will be is a simple and accurate means of predicting the level of the child's distress. Usually, the younger child with poor venous access will experience more distress. A successful plan involves not only the parent's ability to make educated choices about what will be most helpful, but also your knowledge of pediatric phlebotomy techniques. If possible, allow the child to have some control by asking him or her from which arm or finger he or she prefers blood to be taken. After assessing the experiences, anxiety, and fears of the parent and the child, you can tailor the procedure for optimal success.

5. Explain and demonstrate the procedure. When explaining what you will be doing, use words appropriate for the child's age. Children interpret words literally, so be careful of your choice of words. Use of a doll, a puppet, or a stuffed animal in the demonstration can help you relate to the child in a nonthreatening manner. If the child has a favorite doll, blanket, or toy, he or she should be encouraged to hug it for comfort and support.

6. Establish guidelines. Tell the child and the parent that you will most likely be successful on the first attempt, but if not, you only will try once more. Then another health care worker will be called in to complete the procedure.

7. Be honest with the child who asks whether the puncture will hurt. Some children cannot separate pain from fear. Instructing the child to tell you when he or she feels pain will help the child to make this distinction. The child should be told that saying "ouch" or making faces is acceptable, but that he or she must make an effort to keep the arm absolutely still. Also tell the child that if the procedure hurts too much, you will momentarily stop; but that the quicker the procedure is performed, the less painful it will be. Reassure the child that you will draw the blood as quickly as possible so that the pain will be brief.[2]

8. Encourage parent involvement. Most recent research demonstrates that **parental involvement**—the parent's presence and support—has the most beneficial effect on the child's anxiety.[4] However, some parents may be reluctant to be present because they do not understand how they can assist or because they do not want to be a part of a

procedure that will cause their children pain. You must assess each parent's ability to assist, and if after discussing his or her role, the parent is still reluctant to participate, his or her wishes should be respected.

Studies have shown that parental behavior influences the child's behavior during the procedure. The following parental behaviors and examples will have a positive effect on relieving the child's distress.[4,5]

Behavior	Example
Distraction	"Look at Mommy"; "Tell the nurse about your doll"
Emotional support	Hugging, stroking hair, patting, and saying soothing words
Explanation	"We need to take a tiny bit of blood from your finger"; "Mommy will help you hold your arm so that we can finish quickly"

Psychological Response to Needles and Pain

Children especially fear needles, and an emotionally distraught child has difficulty separating fear from actual pain. Many children perceive that a "shot," or needle, hurts more than anything else that has ever happened to them. Children's drawings of hospital procedures often depict huge needles that go entirely through the limb.[2] Nevertheless, with proper preparation, the child and the parent can develop coping skills to help alleviate the fear and thereby diminish the "hurt."

Location for Phlebotomy

For psychological reasons, the best location for a painful procedure is a treatment room away from the child's bed or playroom. For a hospitalized child, the bed should be a safe, secure place to rest and sleep, not a place associated with pain. If the child shares a room with another child, performing the procedure at the bedside can upset the roommate as well. If the child cannot be moved to a treatment room, privacy should be maintained by drawing a curtain between the beds.

Equipment Preparation for a Friendlier Environment

Just the sight of needles, syringes, and a person in a white laboratory coat can be frightening to a child. Nurses and other health care providers working with children frequently wear bright, colorfully printed uniforms or smocks to create a friendlier environment. Equipment, too, can be modified to appear less threatening. As an example, prepare the phlebotomy equipment and supplies prior to entering the room in which the child is located so that the child does not become even more anxious in the health care environment. Use shorter needles if possible, and keep threatening-looking supplies (e.g., needles) covered and out of sight. If your hospital policy requires goggles or face shields for blood-exposure precautions, put this equipment on after you have greeted the child. At the completion of the procedure, reward the child with praise, a special Band-Aid with cartoon characters, a sticker, an age-appropriate toy, or, with parental permission, a lollipop. If no parent is present to assist in relieving the child's anxiety, you may cuddle and offer a pacifier to an infant, or stroke or talk softly to sooth a small child.

Positions for Restraining a Child

To ensure that a child does not move the limb during venous access, physical restraint may be required. A supportive parent can assist with restraining while providing comfort to the child.

Two preferred methods of restraining a child to immobilize the arm are the vertical position and the horizontal, or supine, position.[2,14] The vertical technique, which works well for toddlers, requires the parent to hold the child on the lap. As the parent hugs and holds the child's body and the arm not being used, the health care worker can firmly hold the other arm to perform the procedure (Fig. 8–1).

In the horizontal position, the child lies supine, with the health care worker on one side of the bed and the parent on the opposite side. The parent gently but firmly leans over the child, restraining the near arm and the body while holding the opposite extended arm securely for the health care worker (Fig. 8–2).

Neonates and infants younger than 3 months usually do not require restraint. Consequently, they can be managed by the health care worker alone.

Combative Patients

At times, a child will become uncooperative even after the proper steps have been followed to elicit cooperation. Children may become combative—kicking and thrashing—if force is used. Because sharps are involved in blood collection, you must be certain that the procedure can be performed safely. Using force to the point of potential physical injury is unethical and unprofessional. Therefore, if you feel that the risk of injury to yourself or the child is likely, you should discontinue the blood collection attempt, and notify the nurse or the physician.[16] In such instances, alternative coping measures or pharmacological intervention may be necessary prior to the next attempt.

Figure 8–1. Vertical position for restraining a child to perform a phlebotomy.

Interventions to Alleviate Pain

Depending on the anticipated duration of the procedure, the severity of the child's illness, and the anxiety of the child, pharmacological intervention may be used to alleviate pain and anxiety. In May 1993, the US Food and Drug Administration (FDA) approved a topical anesthetic, **EMLA (eutectic mixture of local anesthetics),** which is an emulsion of lidocaine and prilocaine that can be applied to intact skin. This local anesthetic is ideal for use on children prior to venipuncture or starting intravenous (IV) therapy because it does not require a needle. EMLA has minimal side effects—pallor at the application site or erythema due to the adhesive covering—and penetrates both the epidermal and dermal layers, anesthetizing to a depth of 5 mm. It is applied to the skin as a patch or a cream that is then covered with a transparent occlusive dressing. Optimal anesthesia occurs after 60 minutes and may last as long as 2 to 3 hours. Drawbacks to the use of EMLA are cost, the need to apply it 60 minutes prior to the procedure, and having to know in advance the location of the vein to be used. Two separate locations may be anesthetized if the child has difficult venous access. However, EMLA should not be used if the child is allergic to local anesthetics or is younger than 1 month.[2,8]

Figure 8–2. Horizontal, or supine, position for restraining a child to perform a phlebotomy.

Sucrose Nipple or Pacifier

✔ Giving an infant a sucrose nipple or pacifier to suck during and immediately after phlebotomy offers some degree of comfort, although it does not alleviate the pain. Once the infant is crying vigorously and the heart and respiratory rates have increased, a pacifier has no significant effect on changing the rates. However, infants given pacifiers or sucrose nipples have been shown to be more alert following the procedure and to be less fussy and to cry for a shorter duration.[6]

PREVENTION OF DISEASE TRANSMISSION

If a child is in isolation, a sign posted on the door will describe the type of isolation and the personal protective equipment (PPE) to be worn. Isolation categories are based on the mode of transmission (see Chapter 12, Infection Control).[15] All necessary supplies; a gown, gloves, and a mask should be available at the room. Always wash your hands according to policy before and after gloving. Usually, an anteroom is available before the isolation room, where you may wash and put on the protective equipment.

Universal or Standard precautions should be followed throughout pediatric phlebotomy procedures. All children should be treated as if they could be potentially infectious. To prevent transmission of blood-borne pathogens, you should always use standard precautions in addition to transmission category isolation precautions.[15] (See Chapter 12, Infection Control, and Chapter 13, Safety and First Aid.)

Precautions to Protect the Child

Premature babies, newborns, infants and children who are chronically ill, immunocompromised, or have extensive burns are more likely to be susceptible to environmental microorganisms. To protect these children, some hospitals may require PPE, gowns, gloves, and masks to be worn as indicated before entering the room. Remove your PPE according to policy and dispose of them in the appropriately marked container. Wash your hands and put on a clean gown and gloves before attending to the next child or infant.

Latex Allergy or Alert

Some children and health care workers may be allergic to latex. Usually, a sign posted on the door will note the child's allergy, or the child may wear a bracelet indicating a **latex allergy** or a latex alert. Several brands of nonlatex gloves should be available for use with children who have this allergy. Children with spina bifida and those with congenital urinary tract abnormalities or neurogenic bladders are particularly sensitive to latex.[12,13]

PEDIATRIC PHLEBOTOMY PROCEDURES

Two methods are used to obtain blood from infants and children: microcapillary skin puncture and venipuncture. The previously described steps for preparing the child and the parent should be taken before you perform the procedure.

Microcapillary Skin Puncture

Skin punctures are particularly useful for pediatric phlebotomy when only small amounts of blood need to be obtained and can be adequately tested. It is particularly important to withdraw only the smallest amounts of blood necessary from neonates, infants, and children so that the effects of blood-volume reduction are minimal. A 10-ml sample taken from a premature or newborn infant is equivalent to 5 to 10 percent of the infant's total blood volume (see Table 7–1).

Figure 8–3. Sites for heel stick on an infant. (*From Ball J, Bindler R:* Pediatric Nursing: Caring for Children. *Norwalk, CT, Appleton & Lange, 1995, p 814, with permission.*)

When performing skin punctures, the hematology specimens are collected first to minimize platelet clumping, then chemistry and blood bank specimens. Each laboratory has approved procedures for phlebotomy; these procedures should always be followed.

Sites. The heel of the infant or neonate is the most desirable site for skin puncture to obtain capillary blood. The most medial or lateral section of the plantar, or bottom, surface of the heel should be used (Fig. 8–3). For children older than 1 year, the palmar surface of the tip of the third or fourth finger may be used instead (see Chapter 6, Skin Puncture Procedures). The plantar surface of the great toe is rarely used and only for children older than 1 year.

Equipment for Microcapillary Sampling. The following equipment is necessary for pediatric skin puncture procedures:

1. Sterile automatic pediatric lancet device—disposable
2. Seventy percent alcohol swab in a sterile package
3. Sterile cotton balls or gauze sponge
4. Capillary collection tubes and sealer

5. Microcollection tubes
6. Glass slides for smears
7. Puncture-resistant sharps container
8. Disposable gloves
9. Compress (towel or washcloth) to warm heel if necessary
10. Marking pen
11. Laboratory request slips or labels

Special Equipment for Capillary Blood Gas Collection. See Chapter 9, Arterial and Special Collection Procedures, for details on capillary blood gas collection. The following supplies are needed for this procedure:

1. Heparinized capillary tube and caps or sealer
2. Metal filing and magnet
3. Container of ice
4. Warm compress (towel or washcloth)
5. Clean, dry towel
6. Sterile gauze sponge

Heel Stick

Microsamples from the heel are preferred for routine laboratory, platelet count, blood chemistry, and drug level determinations for **neonates** and infants who have not begun to stand. If an infant has compromised circulation to the extremity, is in shock, or has edema or infection at the heel, another site should be used. Avoid **heel stick** in an area that has many previous puncture sites because such a stick could cause an infection.

The lancet should be of proper pediatric size, making an incision that is less than 2.4-mm deep. Major blood vessels lie 0.3 to 1.6 mm beneath the skin at the dermal–subcutaneous junction in newborns. If an incision goes deeper, the **calcaneus** may be hit and may lead to **osteomyelitis.** [10] Commercially available heel-incision devices are designed specifically for use on infants and premature babies (see Chapter 4, Blood Collection Equipment). The standard size makes an incision 2.5 mm in length and 1.0 mm in depth. The size for premature infants incises 0.85-mm deep and 1.75-mm long.

Specific guidelines for performing a heel stick include the following:

- Do not puncture the anteromedial aspect or the posterior curve of the heel because a puncture at either site could injure the underlying calcaneus. Figure 8–3 shows the proper sites for a heel puncture.
- When holding the infant's foot, be firm but gentle. A **premature infant** in particular, has delicate tissue that may bruise easily. Holding the foot too tightly also restricts blood flow.

- Avoid excessive milking or squeezing, which causes **hemolysis** and dilutes the blood with interstitial and intracellular fluid.
- Avoid covering puncture sites with adhesive bandages because newborn skin is fragile and may macerate under the bandage.

Heel Warming. The amount of blood that can be obtained from a single heel stick is limited, so to obtain an adequate sample, prewarming the heel may be indicated. Prewarming the heel increases blood flow dramatically and arterializes the specimen. This step is essential for drawing specimens for capillary blood gas analysis.

There are several methods of warming the heel however, a surgical towel or a washcloth heated with warm water to 39 to 42°C works well. If the temperature of the towel exceeds 44°C, it may burn the infant. Wrap the warm, wet towel around the infant's foot, and encase the wrap in a plastic bag to help retain heat and to keep the patient's bed dry. Prewarming the site for 3 to 5 minutes is effective in raising the skin temperature several degrees. Chemical heel-warming packs are also available commercially for this purpose. Caution should be used if the towel is heated in a microwave oven because heating is uneven, and the towel may have hot spots. Depending on your institution's policy, you may call ahead and ask the nurse to prewarm the infant's heel, or you may apply the warm wrap, attend to another patient, then return in a few minutes to perform the heel stick.[11]

Procedure. Wash your hands, and then put on gloves. Also, if required, put on a gown and a mask. Ensure that the infant is identified properly. If the infant is not wearing an identification bracelet, have the nurse identify the infant for you. Inspect the heel area and assess for proper warmth. If it is cool or you are collecting a blood gas specimen, prewarm the foot with a warm, wet towel or a chemical heel-warming pack, according to policy. When the heel has been warmed and dried, you should disinfect the side of the heel with the alcohol swab, using firm circular motions, starting at the center of the area and working outward. Allow the alcohol to dry. Blowing on the area to hasten drying is not advised because doing so will contaminate the area. To ensure that the site is dry and free of alcohol, wipe it with a sterile cotton ball or gauze sponge.

You should use your nondominant hand to hold the infant's ankle "tennis racket" style: forefinger across the arch and thumb supporting the heel. The infant's foot should be gripped firmly but carefully to prevent bruising or injury and to avoid restricting blood flow. Using the dominant hand, hold the pediatric lancing device perpendicular to the heel. As mentioned previously, an automatic lancing device will control the incision depth, which should not exceed 2.4 mm. Next, pierce the skin with the lancet. The first drop of blood should be wiped away with the sterile gauze sponge because this drop of blood contains excess tissue fluid. As the drops form, blood is drawn into the capillary tubes and the microcollection containers, both of which should be held at a downward angle, not horizontally. Intermittent, gentle pressure with the forefinger may facilitate the blood flow. However, massaging or milking the area is not advisable because doing so causes hemolysis or dilution of the blood with tissue fluids.

If the blood flow is inadequate for collection of all required specimens, a second puncture may be needed at another heel site. In such cases, the skin is prepared as before. A puncture device should *never* be reused, and no more than two punctures should be attempted. Figure 8–4 provides a sample nursery procedure for performing a heel stick on an infant.

Care of the Heel after Collection. When collection is complete, you should evaluate the heel, place a sterile gauze sponge over the puncture site, and apply pressure until the bleeding stops. An adhesive strip should not be used because, as mentioned before, infants have delicate skin that may macerate under the Band-Aid or that may be damaged when the strip is removed.

Clean Up. Dispose of used lancing device in a sharps container. Check the infant's bed for any equipment or trash you may have left behind. Used gauze sponges, gloves, and gowns should be disposed in a biohazardous waste container. Wash your hands after removing the gloves.

Complications from Heel Stick. Some complications associated with neonatal heel sticks include cellulitis, osteomyelitis of the calcaneus, abscess formation, tissue loss, scarring of the heel, and calcified nodules. Calcified nodules occur most commonly in infants who as preemies (premature babies) or neonates received multiple heel sticks. In neonates, these nodules appear as small depressions, which progress to firm nodular lesions that appear 4 to 12 months later, migrate to the skin surface, and disappear by 18 to 20 months.[9]

Neonatal Screening

In the United States, **neonatal screening** for **phenylketonuria (PKU)** and
hypothyroidism is mandatory by law. These diseases can result in severe

242

Obtaining Blood Specimens from Infants (Heel Stick)

Principle:

To obtain blood specimens from infants with the least amount of trauma while maintaining good isolation techniques.

Procedure:

1. Locate the entrance to the nurseries (intensive care, intermediate care, and low risk). It is located on

   _____ .

2. Place blood collection tray on the table near the scrub sinks outside the nurseries.
3. Remove rings, watch, and laboratory coat.
4. Wash hands with regular soap. Control the water with foot pedals.
5. Put on a gown with ties in the back. If your clothes have long sleeves, wear a yellow paper gown. With short sleeves, wear a short-sleeved cotton gown.
6. Wear sterile gloves.
7. Pick up tray with two clean paper towels and enter nursery area.
8. Find the small metal cart and place tray on a clean diaper on the cart.
9. Discard paper towels.
10. Identify the baby by making sure that the information on the request slip is identical to that on the baby's armband.
11. After ensuring that the skin is warm, perform a heel puncture to obtain the proper blood specimens for the tests requested.
12. Hold clean cotton gauze over the puncture site until bleeding stops. Do not put adhesive strips on the baby's feet.

13. Remove all collection equipment from the crib to avoid harming the baby.
14. Before collecting blood from the next baby, wash hands at the sink inside the nursery proper and change gloves.
15. Initial the log book for all work completed.
16. Remove gown and gloves and discard in proper receptacle.
17. Wash hands.
18. When moving from one nursery area to the other, repeat the complete procedure and put on a clean gown and gloves.

Notes:

1. The baby's heel may be punctured a maximum of two times. Do not stick a baby more than twice to obtain a specimen at any given time. If a particular baby must always be punctured the maximum number of times, notify the phlebotomy supervisor and the baby's primary nurse.
2. Do not puncture a foot if bruises, abrasions, or sloughing skin is present. Call the situation to the attention of the baby's nurse.
3. To help obtain a free-flowing puncture wound from a baby who does not bleed freely, have a nurse wrap the baby's heel in a warm towel 10 to 15 minutes before the puncture is made. Prewarming the site is also necessary for collection of all specimens for capillary blood gas analysis.
4. Use only a gentle massage when obtaining blood. Excessive massaging dilutes the blood with tissue fluids and may cause hemolysis. It is sufficient to massage with your thumb and forefinger.
5. Never repuncture old puncture wounds.
6. Never remove a baby from its crib or change its position in any way without the approval of a nurse.

Figure 8–4. Sample nursery procedure for performing a heel stick on an infant.

abnormalities, including mental retardation, if not discovered and treated early. Blood spot testing for these and other diseases is performed before the newborn is 72 hours old. If blood is collected before the newborn is 24 hours of age, the screening must be repeated before the infant is 14 days old.[14]

The heel is the most frequently used site for collection of blood for screening. Appropriate collection cards are kept in the hospital laboratory or in the nursery. Circles are printed on the filter paper portion of the card; one blood drop is to be placed in each circle. It is important not to touch or contaminate the circle areas with substances other than the newborn's blood. Wash your hands and put on gloves. Then, positively identify the newborn and prepare the infant in the same manner as for a heel stick. Once the puncture is made and the blood drop appears, touch the circle area on the filter paper with the blood until the circle is filled. If the circle does not fill entirely, wipe the heel and express another, larger drop to a different circle. Do not add a second drop of blood to a previously used circle. Only one side of the filter paper should be used. Allow the paper to air dry thoroughly in the horizontal position. Direct application of blood from the heel to the card is the technique of choice; however, blood from a heparinized capillary tube may be applied if care is taken not to scratch or dent the filter paper. Make sure all the information on the screening card is completed correctly so that follow up can be done if the results are abnormal. The screening card should be placed in an envelope and sent or mailed to the laboratory within 24 hours (Fig. 8–5).

Finger Stick

A finger stick to obtain blood for routine laboratory analysis is usually preferred for children older than 1 year. Also, a finger stick may be necessary if a child has damaged veins from repeated venipuncture or if the veins are covered with bandages or casts. Do not perform a finger stick if the extremity has compromised circulation, is edematous, or is infected.

Precautions. Use a proper-sized pediatric lancet designed for the age and size of the child. An automatic lancet controls the puncture depth, which should not exceed 2.4 mm in small children. The distance from the skin surface to bone or cartilage in the middle, or third, finger is between 1.5 and 2.4 mm. Automatic incision devices are available in sizes that incise to depths of 1.75 mm, 1.25 mm, and 0.85 mm for toddlers. For a detailed description of the blood collection procedure, refer to Chapter 6, Skin Puncture Procedures.

PKU Collection Procedure

Principle:

It is a state requirement that a PKU screening be performed on all newborn patients.

Procedure:

1. Pick up completed PKU slips at nursing unit.
2. Properly identify patient.
3. Place patient's foot (limb) in dependent position.
4. Sterilize skin with alcohol; allow to *dry* and puncture with disposable lancet.
5. Allow drops to form and apply *directly* to filter paper. Apply blood to only one side of paper while viewing from other side to ensure *complete saturation* of entire circle. All five circles *must* be completely filled.
6. Allow card to dry thoroughly in a horizontal position (minimum of 3 hours). *Do not* stack wet samples.
7. Reference laboratory personnel will mail the newborn screen in an envelope provided by the State Health Department within 24 hours to the State Health Department.

Notes: Specimens may be considered unsatisfactory if

a. All circles are not completely filled.
b. All filled circles are not thoroughly saturated.
c. Uneven saturation is present because of multiple-sample application or the use of capillaries.
d. The specimens appear to be contaminated.
e. Clotted or caked blood is present on the filter paper.
f. Elution of blood from the filter paper is incomplete.
g. The filter paper is seperated from the form.
h. The specimen is received more than 5 days following the date of collection.

Figure 8–5. PKU collection procedure. (*Courtesy of Hermann Hospital Clinical Laboratories, Houston, TX, with permission.*)

Venipuncture

Venipuncture in children is used when larger quantities of blood are needed for sampling. The veins of the antecubital fossa or the forearm are most accessible and are chosen for most toddlers and children. Dorsal hand veins are preferred sites for venous access in neonates and well newborns. Other sites for venipuncture are the medial wrist, the dorsum of the foot, the scalp, and the medial ankle. If the neonate or child is receiving fluid or medication intravenously, the distal veins should be avoided for phlebotomy and preserved for IV therapy. Venipuncture is indicated for blood sampling for routine laboratory tests, sedimentation rate, blood cultures, cross-matching, coagulation studies, and drug and ammonia levels. Do not use veins in an extremity or area if there is edema or infection, or if an IV line is present. Avoid deep veins in a child with hemophilia or other bleeding disorders.

Precautions. Remove the tourniquet before withdrawing the needle. Do not use alcohol preparation pads to apply pressure because they sting and prevent hemostasis. Instead, apply pressure with the gauze sponge or a cotton ball for 3 minutes to prevent a hematoma. For neonates, use small, winged (butterfly) needles.

Equipment for Venipuncture. The equipment necessary for a pediatric venipuncture includes the following:

1. Winged infusion needle (23 or 25 gauge) or transparent hub needle (21 gauge × 1 in. or 23 gauge × ¾ in.)
2. Syringes slightly larger than the volume of blood needed
3. Large-bore or 19-gauge needle
4. Seventy percent isopropyl alcohol swab in a sterile package
5. Cotton balls or gauze sponges
6. Appropriate specimen containers
7. Tourniquet (nonlatex if child is allergic)
8. Sterile disposable gloves (nonlatex if child is allergic)
9. Blood culture:
   a. bottles, aerobic and anaerobic
   b. povidone–iodine swabs
10. Paper tape and adhesive strip
11. Marking pens
12. Biohazardous waste container

Dorsal Hand Vein Technique. The dorsal hand vein technique is appropriate for neonates and infants who are younger than 2 years old. Although the neonate will not need restraint, an older infant can be wrapped snuggly in a receiving blanket or restrained by an assistant to minimize movement. As for all procedures, positively identify the infant before beginning. Select the hand that has easily visible veins (Fig. 8–6). No tourniquet is necessary. Your middle finger and forefinger should encircle the wrist and are used to apply pressure to distend the dorsal veins (Fig. 8–7). Placing your thumb against the infant's fingers, flex the infant's wrist downward as you examine the dorsum of the infant's hand. Be careful not to bend the wrist too much or the vein may collapse. Lightly brush your finger across the back of the infant's hand as you palpate for the best vein and determine its direction. Never attempt the venipuncture if you cannot see or feel the vein. Once you have established the optimal vein, release the finger tourniquet to allow blood to recirculate. Disinfect the back of the infant's hand with the alcohol swab. Take your time and allow the area to air dry, then wipe with sterile gauze. Select the appropriate needle according to the size of the vein. Next, reposition your fingers on the infant's wrist as a tourniquet and flex the infant's hand with your thumb. Align the transparent hubbed needle bevel up, parallel to the vein. The needle should be angled about 15 degrees to the skin. The skin should be pierced 3 to 5 mm distal to the vein, then advanced slowly and carefully until the vein is punctured. As soon as blood appears in the hub, stop advancing the needle. The

Figure 8–6. The hand that is selected should have veins that are easily visible.

Figure 8–7. Positioning of health care worker's fingers for dorsal hand vein technique.

blood may flow slowly as the venous pressure is very low. Wait a few seconds, then if no blood appears, it may be necessary to gently reposition the needle. The needle need not be held because the surrounding skin will hold it in place.

As soon as the blood begins to flow, fill the microcollection tubes directly from the hub. Be careful to avoid bumping the hub and pushing the needle through the vein. Release the finger tourniquet intermittently to allow the vein to refill. If the blood flow slows or stops, gently rotating the needle without advancing it may reestablish the flow. Once the necessary tubes are filled, place a dry gauze sponge over the puncture site, and apply pressure as you quickly withdraw the needle. Continue holding pressure for 2 to 3 minutes or until the bleeding stops. An adhesive strip may be used to cover the puncture site on well babies and older infants. Do not use tape on ill neonates because their skin is fragile. Comfort the infant and offer a sucrose nipple, if permitted. Remove all used supplies, discarding them in the appropriate biohazardous containers. Discard the gloves and the gown, and wash your hands.

Dorsal hand vein venipuncture has several advantages over skin puncture: it is less stressful for the infant and the health care worker, there is less dilution of the specimen with tissue fluids and less hemolysis, and fewer punctures are required.[1,11]

Venipuncture at Other Sites. The procedure for performing venipuncture on children is similar to that for adults (see Chapter 5). The differences include the necessary preparation of the child and the parent, assistance in restraining the child, and the use of special pediatric-sized needles or winged infusion sets. After the child is securely positioned, place the tourniquet proximal to the selected vein to distend it. If necessary, the limb may be lowered, rubbed gently, or even warmed to promote dilatation of the vein. Disinfect the site thoroughly. Allow the alcohol to dry completely. Then, hold the two wings of the infusion set together in your dominant hand as your other hand pulls the skin below the puncture site taut. When inserting the needle in children, it is best to insert 3 to 5 mm below the vein. When blood appears in the tubing, release the wings of the infusion set. The skin will hold the needle in place, or you can use paper tape to secure it. Gently aspirate the syringe until the required amount of blood is withdrawn. Release the tourniquet, apply pressure over the puncture site with a gauze pad as you quickly remove the infusion set. Ask the parent or the nurse to hold pressure on the site until the bleeding stops, then apply the adhesive strip. Remove the syringe from the infusion set, attach the large-bore needle, and insert it into the collecting tubes to be filled.

Scalp Vein Venipuncture. Scalp veins may be used on infants when access to other veins is difficult or undesirable. Figure 8–8 shows the scalp veins used for peripheral vascular access.

Additional equipment required for this procedure includes a disposable razor and a large, flat rubber band. A 23- or 25-gauge winged infusion set (butterfly needle) is used for the venipuncture. The appropriate procedures should be followed: hand washing and gloving, preparing the infant, and positioning with an assistant to provide restraint. If the scalp veins are not readily visible through the hair, a disposable razor may be used to carefully shave the hair in the frontal or parietal scalp area. A prominent vein may be occluded proximally with a finger as in the dorsal hand vein technique. Feel for a pulse to prevent hitting an artery. If a vein cannot be distended with the finger, a large, flat rubber band may be placed around the upper head as a tourniquet.[14] (Placing a gauze pad under an area of the band helps in removing it after the procedure.) Disinfect the scalp with a povidone–iodine (Betadine) preparation or with alcohol, allow the scalp to dry, and then wipe it with sterile gauze. After the scalp is inspected for the desired

Figure 8–8. Scalp veins frequently used for peripheral vascular access in infants. (*From Ball J, Bindler R:* Pediatric Nursing: Caring for Children. *Norwalk, CT, Appleton & Lange, 1995, p 823, with permission.*)

vein, release the tourniquet to permit refilling of the veins. Reapply finger pressure or the rubber band. Hold the skin taut with your nondominant hand distal to the site to be punctured. Hold the infusion set with the two wings folded together and the bevel of the needle up. Position the needle at a 15-degree angle over the vein in the direction of the blood flow. Puncture the skin, and slowly advance the needle until blood begins to flow into the tubing of the needle set. Attach the syringe. Gently and slowly aspirate the blood to prevent hemolysis or occlusion by the vein wall. When sufficient blood is collected, release the finger tourniquet or rubber band. Place the sterile gauze pad over the puncture site, and apply pressure before quickly removing the needle. Apply additional pressure for several minutes to ensure that the bleeding has stopped. Fill the collecting tubes in the usual fashion. Comfort the infant by stroking him or her softly, or offering a pacifier if permitted. Be sure all used supplies are removed from the bed area.

Withdrawing Blood from IV Lines

Hospitalized children who are undergoing IV therapy, whether for total parenteral nutrition, administration of an antibiotic, or chemotherapy, often have poor veins. They may have a heparin lock or a central venous catheter when long-term access is required. Some blood tests can be performed with blood drawn from these lines; however, you must check with the nurse or the doctor and verify the policy because some hospitals limit the number of times that a line can be accessed. Also, you must confirm the amount of blood that can be drawn on the basis of the child's weight (see Table 7–1).

Equipment. The equipment required for blood withdrawal from IV lines includes the following:

1. Syringe filled with 5 mL of normal saline
2. Syringe filled with 5 mL of heparinized flush solution (1 mL for heparin lock)
3. Five-mL syringe for discard
4. Syringe for blood specimen
5. Blood collection tubes
6. Large-bore needle for transferring blood to tubes
7. Nineteen- to 25-gauge needles for gaining access to heparin lock
8. Alcohol or povidone–iodine (Betadine) swabs
9. Double stopcock for central line
10. Luer-Lok (Becton, Dickinson and Company, Franklin Lakes, NJ) catheter cap
11. Sterile 4 × 4 in. gauze sponge
12. Mask
13. Gloves

Procedure for Heparin Lock. When drawing blood from a heparin lock, disinfect the catheter cap with an alcohol or a povidone–iodine (Betadine) swab. Check patency of the line by flushing with a small amount of normal saline. Attach a needle to the discard syringe, and insert it into the cap of the heparin lock. Gently withdraw approximately 2 to 3 mL of fluid and blood, remove the syringe and needle, and discard in a sharps container. Insert another needle and syringe to collect the blood sample. When a sufficient amount of blood has been obtained, withdraw the needle and fill the collection tubes. Clean the cap of the heparin lock, then insert the syringe with the heparinized flush solution, slowly injecting the solution.

Procedure for Central Venous Catheter. Wash your hands, put on a mask and gloves, open a sterile 4 × 4 in. gauze sponge, and place it under the catheter port to serve as a sterile field. Open the sterile stopcock and attach the discard syringe to the access port closest to the child.

Attach the blood-collecting syringe to the next port and the normal saline–filled syringe to the distal port, all with sterile technique. Clean the connection site with alcohol swabs. Two or three swabs must be used to clean the site for 2 minutes. Then, allow the connection to dry. Clamp the catheter, then remove the catheter cap. Connect the pre-assembled stopcock setup, ensuring a tight seal. Unclamp the catheter, open the stopcock to the discard syringe, and withdraw 3 to 5 mL of fluid. Close that port, then open the stopcock port to the collection syringe and aspirate the required amount of blood. Close that port, and remove the syringe. An assistant can attach the large-gauge needle and fill the collection tubes. Attach the syringe with the heparinized solution to that port. Open the distal port. Gently aspirate to clear the stopcock of air, holding the syringe vertically to allow bubbles to rise. Tap the syringe to free any bubbles sticking to its side. Flush the catheter with 5 mL of saline, close that port, and then open the port to the heparinized solution and flush with 5 mL. Reclamp the catheter and remove the stopcocks. Clean the connection site of the catheter with a new alcohol preparation pad, then attach a new Luer-Lok cap.[14] Discard used items in the appropriate containers. Remove the gloves and the mask, and wash your hands.

✔ Key Terms

CALCANEUS

CHILD DEVELOPMENT

EMLA (EUTECTIC MIXTURE OF
LOCAL ANESTHETICS)

HEEL STICK

HEMOLYSIS

HYPOTHYROIDISM

LATEX ALLERGY

NEONATAL SCREENING

NEONATES

OSTEOMYELITIS

PARENTAL INVOLVEMENT

PEDIATRIC PHLEBOTOMIES

PHENYLKETONURIA (PKU)

PREMATURE INFANT

SUCROSE NIPPLE OR PACIFIER

Study Questions

1. Performing a phlebotomy on a child is challenging because
   a. a child is less emotionally mature than an adult
   b. a child is small
   c. smaller equipment must be used
   d. a child's blood clots more quickly

2. Which of the following describe the behavior of an adolescent undergoing a painful procedure?
   a. fears separation from parent
   b. embarrassed to show fear
   c. fears injury to body
   d. may not want parent present in room

3. Which of the following are important steps in preparing the child and the parent for a pediatric phlebotomy?
   a. assess their past experience with blood drawing
   b. perform the phlebotomy as quickly as possible
   c. ask the parent to leave the room
   d. use a doll or a puppet to demonstrate the procedure

4. The best location for performing a phlebotomy on a child is the
   a. bedside
   b. playroom
   c. treatment room

5. The preferred techniques for restraining a child are
   a. vertical—child sitting in parent's lap
   b. total sedation
   c. mechanical restraint
   d. supine with parent leaning over child

6. Acceptable interventions to alleviate pain include
   a. xylocaine injection
   b. sucrose nipple
   c. ice pack
   d. EMLA cream

7. The preferred site for a heel stick is
   a. anteromedial aspect
   b. medial or lateral aspect
   c. posterior curve
   d. a previous puncture site

8. The benefits of heel warming include
   a. arterializes blood
   b. dramatically increases blood flow
   c. prevents hemolysis
   d. hastens hemostasis

9. Complications of heel sticks may include
   a. osteomyelitis
   b. abscess formation
   c. paralysis of the foot
   d. calcified nodules

10. The optimal depth of a finger stick in a child is
    a. greater than 3.0 mm
    b. less than 0.5 mm
    c. less than 2.4 mm

11. The preferred techniques for obtaining blood in neonates include
    a. finger stick
    b. heel stick
    c. dorsal hand vein technique
    d. antecubital fossa venipuncture

12. Neonatal blood screening is used to identify which disease(s)?
    a. syphilis
    b. hypothyroidism
    c. cystic fibrosis
    d. PKU (phenylketonuria)

REFERENCES

1. Clagg ME: Venous sample collection from neonates using dorsal hand veins. *Lab Med* 20(4):248–250, 1989.
2. Colaizzo D, Tesler M: Children's pain: Part 4. *Nurseweek* March:14–15, 1994.

3. College of American Pathologists (CAP): *So You're Going to Collect a Blood Specimen: An Introduction to Phlebotomy,* 6th ed. Northfield, IL, CAP, 1994.
4. Jacobson PB, Manne S, Gorfinkle K, et al: Analysis of child and parent behavior during painful medical procedures. *Health Psychol* 9(5):559–576, 1990.
5. Manne S, Bakeman R: Adult–child interaction during invasive medical procedures. *Health Psychol* 11(4):241–249, 1992.
6. Marshall RE: Neonatal pain associated with caregiving procedures. *Pediatr Clin North Am* 36(4):885–903, 1989.
7. Mehne C: Cultivating a tender touch. *MT Today* September:12–16, 1992.
8. Robieux I, Eliopoulos C, Hwang P, et al: Pain perception and effectiveness of the eutectic mixture of local anesthetics in children undergoing venipuncture. *Pediatr Res* 32(5):520–523, 1992.
9. Sell EJ, Hansen MD, Struck-Pierce S: Calcified nodules on the heel: A complication of neonatal intensive care. *J Pediatr* 96(3), 1980.
10. Short BL, Avery GB: In Fletcher MA, MacDonald M (eds): *Atlas of Procedures—Neonate*. Philadelphia, J.B. Lippincott, 1993.
11. Clagg ME, Jamieson B: *Pediatric Phlebotomy*. American Society of Clinical Pathologists (ASCP) Fall Teleconference Series, No 9434, Chicago, ASCP, Sept 6, 1990.
12. Centers for Disease Control and Prevention: Anaphylactic reactions during general anesthesia among pediatric patients. *MMWR* 40(28):437–443, 1991.
13. Food and Drug Administration (FDA): Allergic reactions to latex-containing medical devices. *FDA Med Alert* Mar 29, 1991.
14. Ball J, Bindler R: *Pediatric Nursing: Caring for Children*. Norwalk, CT, Appleton & Lange, 1995.
15. Department of Health and Human Services, Centers for Disease Control and Prevention. Guidelines for isolation precautions in hospitals—Part I, Evolution of isolation practices; Part II, Recommendations for isolation precautions in hospitals. *Federal Register,* Fall 1994.
16. Kelly S. Pediatric blood collection made easy. *Lab Med* 24(4):247–248, 1993.

nine

9

ARTERIAL AND SPECIAL COLLECTION PROCEDURES

Chapter Outline

Chapter Objectives

Upon completion of Chapter 9, the learner is responsible for the following:

1. Explain the special precautions and types of equipment needed to collect capillary or arterial blood gases.

2. Describe the equipment that is used to perform the bleeding-time test.

3. Discuss the requirements for the glucose, lactose, epinephrine, and glucagon tolerance tests.

4. Differentiate cannulas from fistulas.

5. List the steps and equipment in blood culture collections.

6. List the special requirements for drawing blood through central venous catheters (CVCs).

7. Differentiate therapeutic phlebotomy from autologous transfusion.

8. Describe the special precautions needed to collect blood in therapeutic drug monitoring (TDM) procedures.

9. List the types of patient specimens that are needed for trace metal analyses.

Depending on the specific needs of individual clinical settings, health care workers may be required to perform a variety of special tests or procedures in addition to routine skin test and venipunctures. This chapter presents the basic techniques and precautions for various special tests. Extensive training sessions and supervision should accompany the student in these procedures because they can harm the patient if performed incorrectly.

ARTERIAL BLOOD GASES

✔ **Arterial blood gases (ABGs)** provide useful information about the respiratory status and the acid-base balance of patients with pulmonary (lung) disease or disorders. In addition, critically ill patients with other diseases such as diabetes mellitus benefit from ABG measurement, which is used to help manage their electrolyte and acid-base balance. Arterial blood is used rather than venous blood because arterial blood has the same composition throughout the body tissues, whereas venous blood has various compositions relative to metabolic activities in body tissues.

Arterial puncture to obtain arterial blood for blood gas evaluation requires skill and knowledge of the technique. A health care provider must undergo extensive training on arterial punctures, including demonstration of the procedure, observation, and, under the supervision of a qualified instructor, several performances on patients.

Radial Artery Puncture Site

When an ABG analysis is ordered, the experienced health care worker, nurse, medical technologist, or physician should palpate the areas of the forearm where the artery is typically close to the surface. The **radial artery,** located on the thumb side of the wrist (Fig. 9–1), is the artery most frequently used for blood collection for ABG analysis.[1] This artery has widespread collateral flow, which means that the hand area is supplied with blood from more than one artery. Arterial blood flows into the hand from both the radial and the ulnar arteries. In addition, the ra-

Figure 9–1. Technique of radial artery puncture. *(From Saunders CE, Ho MT (eds): Current Emergency Diagnosis and Treatment. Norwalk, CT, Appleton & Lange, 1992, p 922, with permission.)*

dial artery lies over ligaments and bones of the wrist and can be easily compressed to lessen the chance of a hematoma during the procedure. A drawback of using the radial artery is its small size.

To use the radial artery for blood collection for ABG analysis, the health care provider must first perform the **Allen test** to make certain

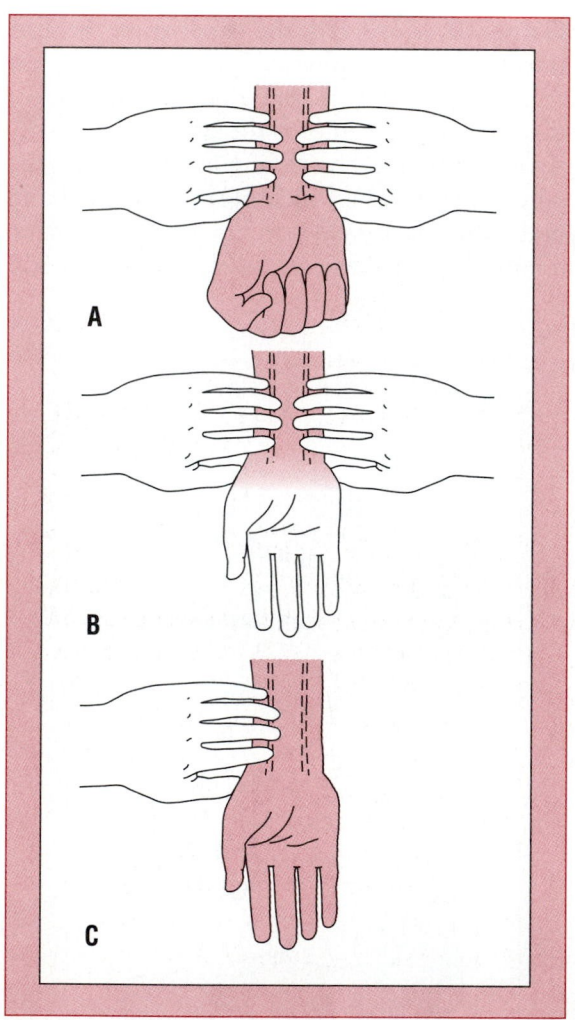

Figure 9–2. Allen test. **A.** Using the index and middle fingers, the health care worker compresses the patient's ulnar and radial arteries. The patient tightly clenches his or her fist repetitively. **B.** The patient opens the hand, and the health care worker releases the pressure. **C.** If the patients's hand refills with blood (i.e., color returns) within 5 to 10 seconds, the test is positive; if not, the test is negative.

Figure 9–3. Arteries in the arm. *(From Martini F:* Fundamentals of Anatomy and Physiology, *2nd ed. Englewood Cliffs, NJ, Prentice Hall, 1992, with permission.)*

that the ulnar and radial arteries are providing collateral circulation. The Allen test is performed as follows: (1) The health care provider compresses both arteries with the index and middle fingers, and the patient is asked to tightly clench his or her fist repetitively in order to squeeze the blood out of the hand (Fig. 9–2A). (2) The patient is then asked to open his or her hand (Fig. 9–2B), and the health care provider releases the pressure on the ulnar artery. (3) The hand should fill with blood within 5 to 10 seconds (Fig. 9–1C); if so, the Allen test is positive. If color returns to the hand after 5 to 10 seconds, the Allen test is negative. A negative Allen test indicates the inability of the ulnar artery to adequately supply blood to the hand and shows a lack of collateral circulation. Thus, the radial artery should not be used in a negative Allen test since this artery might be accidentally damaged during puncture, resulting in total lack of blood flow to the hand.

Brachial and Femoral Artery Puncture Sites

The **brachial artery** is an alternative site for blood collection for ABG analysis. The brachial artery is in the cubital fossa of the arm, as shown in Figure 9-3. Another choice, the **femoral artery,** is the largest artery used in ABG collections. It is located in the groin area of the leg, lateral to

Figure 9–4. Arteries in the leg. *(From Martini F:* Fundamentals of Anatomy and Physiology, *2nd ed. Englewood Cliffs, NJ, Prentice Hall, 1992, with permission.)*

the femur bone, as shown in Figure 9-4. Even though the brachial and femoral arteries are larger than the radial artery, they are used less frequently because they lack collateral circulation. In addition, the brachial artery lies close to the median nerve, which can be accidentally punctured. The femoral artery is a site sometimes used on patients with cardiovascular disorders. However, the possibility of releasing plaque from the inner wall of the artery in geriatric patients is a definite disadvantage of using the femoral artery as a puncture site. Usually, the femoral artery is the last choice for an arterial puncture site, and the health care provider must have expertise in obtaining blood from this artery.

Preparation of Supplies and Patient

The necessary equipment and supplies, as listed in Table 9–1, should be gathered and organized for a successful arterial puncture. The patient must be properly identified and informed of the arterial puncture procedure. It should be determined that the patient has been in a stable state for at least the previous 30 minutes (i.e., no respirator changes). The health care provider should attempt to calm the patient before drawing the specimen if the patient appears anxious. The anxiety can lead to hyperventilation, which will falsely alter the ABG levels. Before proceeding, the health care provider must also determine whether the patient is on anticoagulant therapy or is allergic to lidocaine, and the patient's temperature, oxygen concentration from the respirator (if applicable), and respiratory rate must be recorded.

Radial ABG Procedure

When an ABG analysis is ordered, the experienced phlebotomist, nurse, or physician should wash his or her hands, put on gloves, and palpate the radial artery in the radial sulcus of the forearm. The radial artery in

TABLE 9–1. EQUIPMENT AND SUPPLIES FOR AN ARTERIAL PUNCTURE

Povidone–iodine (Betadine) solution or chlorhexidine
One-half to 1 percent lidocaine to numb site
Prefilled heparinized syringe, 1 to 5 mL (especially designed plastic syringe for collections for ABG analysis)
Stopper for syringe
Needles (20 to 22 gauge, for collections for ABG analysis)
Needles (25 or 26 gauge, for lidocaine administration)
Syringe for lidocaine administration (1- or 2-mL plastic syringe)
Gauze squares to be held on site after puncture
Plastic bag or cup with crushed ice and water
Patient identification label
Laboratory requisition slip
Waterproof ink pen
Alcohol pad
Adhesive bandage strip
Oxygen measuring device to record on laboratory requisition slip the oxygen concentration on patient receiving oxygen
Thermometer to record patient's temperature on laboratory requisition slip

the patient's nondominant hand is usually the best choice. With the forefinger or first two fingers, the health care worker should press at these sites to find the artery. The thumb should never be used for palpating because there is a pulse in the thumb that may be confused for the patient's pulse. Any site that has a hematoma or that was previously used for an arterial puncture should be avoided. The patient's arm should be positioned with the wrist slightly extended and rotated. Check for adequate collateral circulation using the Allen test.

Once the radial artery site is chosen, the area should be cleaned well with povidone–iodine (Betadine) solution. No tourniquet is required because the artery has its own strong blood pressure. As in venipuncture, a syringe with a needle can be used to withdraw the sample. However, the syringe should be small (1 or 5 mL). The addition of liquid lithium heparin to coat the syringe barrel will anticoagulate the blood. Using too much liquid heparin is probably the most common preanalytical error in blood gas measurements.[2] Therefore, the amount of anticoagulant should be 0.05 mL of liquid heparin (1000 IU/mL) for each milliliter of blood. The health care worker should pull the skin taut and pierce the pulsating artery at a high angle, usually no less than 45 degrees. Little or no suction is needed because the blood flows quickly into the syringe under its own pressure. When enough sample has been drawn (usually about 1 mL), the health care worker withdraws the needle carefully to avoid introducing bubbles into the syringe, and applies gauze and direct manual pressure on the site for at least 5 minutes.

The syringe should be quickly capped, mixed with the anticoagulant, labeled, and placed in ice water *immediately* in an effort to prevent the blood gases from escaping into the atmosphere. Ideally, the specimen should be analyzed within 10 minutes of collection. Therefore, the specimen should immediately be labeled and transported to the laboratory. Before leaving the patient, the health care worker should clean the puncture site with an alcohol pad to remove the excess Betadine solution, and a pressure bandage should be left on. If bleeding from the site persists, the health care worker should apply more manual pressure and ring for assistance from the patient's primary nurse. The health care worker should never leave a patient who is bleeding, particularly after an arterial puncture. The primary nurse should be notified after an arterial puncture is performed so that the area may be checked frequently for deep or superficial bleeding.

Arterial blood results for some analytes (e.g., ammonia, glucose, lactic acid, alcohol) may differ from venous blood results because of metabolic activities. Therefore, arterial blood samples should be collected for the blood gas measurements only when specifically requested by the attending physician. In such situations, the request slip must indicate that arterial blood was collected for the analytes.

CAPILLARY BLOOD GASES

Arterial blood is the specimen of choice for testing the pH, oxygen (O_2) content, and carbon dioxide (CO_2) content of the blood. Skin puncture blood is less desirable as a specimen source because it contains blood from capillaries, venules, arterioles, and fluids from the surrounding tissue. In addition, common collection methods for capillary blood gas specimens employ an open collection system in which the specimen is temporarily exposed to room air, theoretically allowing for a brief exchange of gases (both O_2 and CO_2) before sealing the specimen from the air.

Blood for **capillary blood gas analysis** is often collected from small children and babies for whom arterial punctures can be too dangerous. They are collected from the same areas of the body as other capillary samples, such as the lateral posterior area of the heel, the great toe, or the ball of the finger. (See Chapter 8, Pediatric Phlebotomy.)

When a capillary blood gas analysis is ordered, the health care worker should choose a site and prewarm the area to ensure that good blood flow is obtained and that blood can be quickly collected, anticoagulated, and sealed from contact with room air. To prewarm the site, the health care worker must wrap a cloth or a towel that is saturated with warm water around the foot or hand for 3 to 10 minutes. Care should be taken that the warming cloth is not too hot; if the warmed cloth can be held comfortably in the hand, it is not too warm for the patient. When the health care worker is prepared to collect the blood gas specimen, the towel should be removed and the area dried. The puncture site should be cleaned and entered in the usual manner for skin punctures (as discussed in Chapter 6). A heparinized capillary tube (Fig. 9–5) with a volume of at least 100 µL should be used to collect the specimen. A metal filing may be inserted into the tube before collecting to help mix the specimen while it is entering the tube. It is extremely important that the specimen be collected with *no air bubbles,* which can distort the values obtained from the specimen. When the tube is full, the ends should be sealed with plastic caps or clay (according to individual laboratory protocol), and a magnet should be used to draw the metal filing back and forth across the length of the tube to completely mix the specimen. The tube should then be labeled and submerged in a slurry of ice water for transfer to the laboratory. The sample should be analyzed

Figure 9–5. Capillary blood gas tube.

immediately in the laboratory; however, if the specimen is stored horizontally, capped, and in the slurry of ice water, it can be kept as long as 2 hours without serious degradation. The skin puncture site should be pressed with a clean gauze sponge until the bleeding stops.

BLEEDING-TIME TEST

✔ The bleeding-time test is a useful tool for testing platelet plug formation in the capillaries. It is generally used along with other coagulation tests for diagnosing coagulopathies or problems in hemostasis, such as thrombocytopenia, qualitative platelet defects, vascular abnormalities, and von Willebrand's disease. This diagnostic tool is most frequently used as a preoperative screening test.

The test is performed by making a minor standardized incision in either the earlobe or the forearm and recording the length of time required for bleeding to cease. The duration of bleeding from a punctured capillary depends on the quantity and quality of platelets and the ability of the blood vessel wall to constrict.

Many methods have been used to measure bleeding time, the oldest dating to 1910 when Duke originally described a method in which a lancet was used to make a puncture wound in the earlobe. This test was difficult to standardize, did not allow space for repeat testing, and often caused undue apprehension in the patient. Ivy improved the bleeding-time test in 1941 by using a lancet to make puncture wounds on the forearm while maintaining a constant venous pressure with a blood pressure cuff. Both methods are difficult to reproduce because of several variables (e.g., depth of puncture, length of puncture).

Clinical research has led to the development of automated incision-making instruments for bleeding-time tests. One is called Surgicutt.[3] It is a sterile, standardized, easy-to-use, disposable instrument that makes a uniform, surgical incision. This instrument is a spring-activated surgical steel blade housed in a self-containing plastic unit from which the blade protracts and retracts automatically, eliminating the variable of blade incision. The following steps provide the procedure for the Surgicutt Bleeding Time Test.[4]

1. Prior to beginning the procedure, patients should be advised that there is an occasional scarring problem inherent in the bleeding time test. Butterfly-type bandages can reduce the potential scarring by applying one to the incision area for a 24-hour period. If there is ooze from the incision, as may be encountered in severe primary hemostatic disorders, then a pressure-type dressing should be used in conjunction with the butterfly-type bandage. If the puncture site is still bleeding beyond 15 minutes, the test should be discontinued by applying pressure to the area. A physician should be notified. The patient can also be asked if he or she has taken aspirin or other salicylates within the previous 2 weeks; these drugs interfere with the test.
2. Materials and supplies should be prepared before beginning the procedure. The following items are needed:
   - Surgicutt instrument. Each self-containing unit is sufficient for a single bleeding time determination. If package has been broken, do not use.
   - Gloves
   - Antiseptic swab
   - Blood pressure cuff (sphygmomanometer)
   - Filter paper disk (one to two Whatman's no. 1 filter paper disks per bleeding time test)
   - Butterfly-type bandage
3. Place the patient's arm on a steady support with the volar surface exposed. The incision is best performed over the lateral aspect, volar surface of the forearm, approximately 5 cm below the antecubital crease. Avoid surface veins, scars, bruises, and edematous areas. Lightly shave the area if body hair will interfere with the test.
4. Place the blood pressure cuff on the upper arm. Inflate the cuff to 40 mm Hg. The time between inflation of the cuff and the

incision should be 30 to 60 seconds. Hold at this exact pressure for the duration of the test.

5. Cleanse the area with an antiseptic swab and allow to air-dry. Remove the Surgicutt device from the package, being careful not to contaminate the instrument by touching or resting the blade-slot end on any unsterile surface.

6. Remove the safety clip. (Safety clip may be replaced if the test is momentarily delayed; however, prolonged exposure of Surgicutt to uncontrolled environmental conditions prior to use may affect its sterility.) Once safety clip is removed, DO NOT push the trigger or touch the blade slot.

7. Hold the device securely between the thumb and the middle finger. Gently rest it on the patient's forearm and apply minimal pressure so that both ends of the instrument are lightly touching the skin. A horizontal incision parallel to the antecubital crease is the most sensitive technique for the bleeding time.

8. Gently push the trigger, starting the stopwatch simultaneously. The blade will make an incision 5 mm long by 1 mm deep. Remove the device from the patient's forearm immediately after triggering. After 30 seconds, wick the flow of blood with filter paper. Bring the filter paper close to the incision, but DO NOT touch the paper directly to the incision, so as not to disturb the formation of a platelet plug.

9. Wick the blood every 30 seconds thereafter until blood no longer stains the paper. Stop the timer. Bleeding time is determined to the nearest 30 seconds. Normal ranges vary from one health care facility to another. However, most are in the approximate range of 2.0 to 8.0 minutes.

10. Remove the blood pressure cuff and cleanse the incision site with an antiseptic swab. Apply the nonallergenic butterfly-type bandage for 24 hours.

The Simplate R (Retractable) and Simplate II R are sterile, disposable devices (Fig. 9-6) used to make uniform incisions for the bleeding-time test. The spring-loaded blades are contained in a plastic housing. When triggered on the forearm, Simplate R and Simplate II R provide one and two incisions, respectively, 5-mm long by 1-mm deep. Simplate II R is used for duplicate determinations. These devices standardize bleeding-time testing by producing uniform incisions that provide reliable and reproducible results.

Possible Interfering Factors

The bleeding-time test is only a screening test, so the results of this test alone are insufficient to diagnose a specific condition. A prolonged

Figure 9–6. Simplate R (retractable) bleeding device. *(Courtesy of Organon Teknika Corp., Durham, NC.)*

bleeding time may indicate the need for further testing (e.g., platelet count). In addition, the following items should be considered:

- The ingestion of aspirin-containing products up to 7 to 10 days prior to testing may affect results.
- Other drugs (e.g., dextran, streptokinase, streptodornase, ethyl alcohol, mithramycin) may cause a prolonged bleeding time.

There are other variations of this same procedure using different devices. For reproducible results, it is important to follow the manufacturer's instructions and to teach all health care workers in the same manner.

BLOOD CULTURES

Blood cultures are often collected from patients who have fevers of unknown origin (FUO). Sometimes during the course of a bacterial infection, bacteremia may result and become the dominant clinical feature. In the case of a patient who experiences fever spikes, it is generally recommended that blood cultures be drawn before and after the spike, when bacteria may be most likely present in the peripheral circulation. It is best to draw one set of aerobic and anaerobic cultures at the time the order is given. Thirty minutes later, a second set of anaerobic and aerobic cultures should be obtained. A request for "second site" blood cultures that are obtained concurrently on opposite arms, is useful when the physician suspects bacteremia due to a local internal infection. However, a "second site" culture is *not* a very effective tool for *routine* blood culture orders and provides relatively little information that properly spaced, timed blood cultures cannot provide.[5]

Prior to beginning the procedure, the health care provider should briefly explain the test to the patient. Then, the following steps should be taken for blood culture collection:

1. Materials should be gathered and prepared next to the patient. The following items are needed: gloves, iodine scrub swab stick (10 percent povidone-iodine solution with lathering agents), acetone–alcohol swab stick, iodine prep swab stick (10 percent povidone–iodine solution), alcohol preps, two blood culture vials—one aerobic and one anaerobic, two 22- or 20-gauge needles, a syringe or evacuated tube assembly, patient identification labels, laboratory requisition slip, and pen.

2. After donning gloves, scrub the site of the venipuncture with the iodine scrub swab stick for at least 2 minutes. The excess foam should be removed with the acetone–alcohol swab stick. The phlebotomist's gloved forefinger should also be cleaned in the same manner. If the patient is known to be hypersensitive to iodine, omit the iodine scrub and clean the site twice with alcohol. A blood culture preparation kit is available commercially from Medi-Flex Hospital Products, Inc. (Overland Park, KS) (Fig. 9–7). This kit, the Blood Culture Prep Kit II, provides another method for preparing to collect blood culture specimens. It is a two-step prep system without pads or swab sticks.

3. Prep the area of the venipuncture with the iodine swab stick by beginning in the center and rubbing the swab outward in concentric circles. Do not go back over any area that has been prepped (Fig. 9–8). Allow the area to dry for 1 minute. While the area is drying, prep the tops of the blood culture vials with the iodine scrub swab stick, and prepare the needle and syringe. The syringe and needle or the evacuated tube assembly must be prepared cautiously so as not to destroy the sterility of the collection items. A second needle should be readily available.

4. The venipuncture is performed in the same manner as described in Chapter 5, and the blood is collected. Each blood culture bottle will hold 3 to 10 mL of blood. For infants and

Figure 9–7. Blood Culture Prep Kit II. *(Courtesy of Medi-Flex Hospital Products, Inc., Overland Park, KS.)*

small children, only 1 to 3 mL of blood should be collected for bacterial culture.[6] Some culture vials contain resin beads that neutralize antibiotics in the patient's blood specimen. If not neutralized, the antibiotics can inhibit bacterial growth and cause false-negative results. The iodine from the tops of the vials is replaced with an alcohol preparation. Three to 10 mL of blood is placed in the *anaerobic* vial first, then an additional 3 to 10 mL is placed in the *aerobic* vial (Fig. 9–9). If only 3 mL (or less) was obtained, placed the entire amount in the aerobic vial. Bottles such as the BBL Vacutainer vials (Becton-Dickinson Diagnostic Instrument Systems, Sparks, MD) are shaped to fit into the barrel apparatus just as an evacuated tube would, thereby eliminating one step. Also, blood can be directly inoculated into the BACTEC culture vial (Becton-Dickinson Diagnostic Instrument Systems,

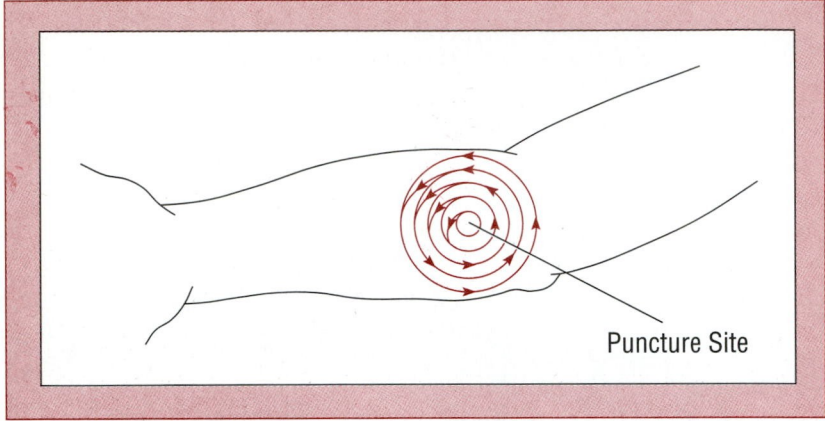

Puncture Site

Figure 9–8. Arm preparation for collection of blood culture specimens.

Sparks, MD) using a butterfly and tubing apparatus (see Fig. 9–10). Yellow-topped evacuated tubes containing **sodium polyanethole sulfonate (SPS)** may be used to collect specimens for blood culture determinations.

The blood should always be delivered gently to the vials and/or the tubes to prevent hemolysis of the cells. This is performed by directing the flow from the needle or the syringe hub along the side of the tube without foaming or extra pressure on the plunger. Evacuated tubes fill themselves, and therefore, the blood does *not* need to be forcefully ejected from the syringe. Then, invert the vials and/or tubes gently. After collecting the blood, remove the iodine from the patient's skin with an alcohol prep. The health care provider must initial the patient identification labels, indicate the time of collection on the labels, and attach a label to each vial or tube. Indicate on the request form and on the vials which culture (number) was collected if a series of blood cultures have been ordered.

Two studies have shown that the practice of changing needles after collecting blood for culture and inoculating the blood specimen into culture vials has little if any effect on the contamination of blood collected for culture.[7,8] In addition, changing needles after collecting blood for culture can lead to a needlestick injury to the phlebotomist. Careful skin cleansing was shown to be a more important factor in minimizing the specimen contamination rate than is the common practice of replacing the needle used for venipuncture with a fresh, sterile needle before inoculating the blood into culture media. If a laboratory decides to discontinue the practice of changing needles during blood culture collection, the contamination rate of blood cultures should be compared before and after the procedural change to confirm that the contamination rate has not increased.

Blood collected for culture must not be obtained through central venous catheter (CVC) lines if it cannot be obtained by venipuncture. Contamination rates may increase if the indwelling catheter is used to obtain culture specimens.[9] Also, if possible, blood should be collected below an existing intravenous (IV) line because blood above the line will be diluted with the IV fluid.

Figure 9–9. Inoculating blood culture bottles. *(Courtesy of College of American Pathologists, Northfield, IL.)*

Figure 9–10. BACTEC PLUS Aerobic/F* and PLUS Anaerobic/F* Culture Vials. *(Courtesy of Becton-Dickinson Diagnostic Instrument Systems, Sparks, MD.)*

Another source of error may involve failure to follow the sterile procedure, which results in contamination of the blood culture and misinformation for the clinician. For instance, palpating the venipuncture site after the site has been prepared without first cleaning the gloved finger can result in contamination of the culture. Likewise, failure to wipe the iodine from the tops of the vials with alcohol or using too little blood for the culture can result in a false-negative culture. Injection of air into the anaerobic bottle can cause the death of some anaerobic microorganisms and, again, result in a false-negative culture. For this reason, the anaerobic bottle must be inoculated first. Furthermore, removal of the entire metal ring on some manufacturers' bottles introduces air into the vials and could cause contamination.[5]

The Isostat system (Isolator microbial tubes) manufactured by Wampole Laboratories (Cranbury, N.J.) is a special blood culture tube system (Figs. 9–11 and 9–12). The Isolator microbial tube has (1) a stopper that fits standard blood collection vacuum holders, (2) lysing

Figure 9–11. Wampole Isolator adult microbial tube. *(Courtesy of Wampole Laboratories, Cranbury, NJ.)*

Figure 9–12. Wampole Isolator pediatric microbial tube. *(Courtesy of Wampole Laboratories, Cranbury, NJ.)*

and anticoagulating agents, (3) reagents in the tube that inactivate human immunodeficiency virus (HIV) within the normal 60-minute transport and processing time, and (4) containment adapters that help protect health care workers and laboratorians against infection due to aerosol spray or breakage during centrifugation. Using this tube affords the advantage of faster microbial test results. It also helps safeguard the laboratorian since the reagents in the Isolator tube inactivate HIV within the normal 60-minute transport and processing time. Also, the tube decreases the many procedural manipulations required during conventional blood culture collections.

GLUCOSE TOLERANCE TEST

For patients who have symptoms suggesting problems in carbohydrate metabolism, such as diabetes mellitus, the **glucose tolerance test** can be an effective diagnostic tool. The test is performed by first obtaining fasting blood and urine specimens, giving the fasting patient a standard load of glucose, and obtaining subsequent blood and urine samples at intervals, usually during a 5-hour period. Each specimen is then analyzed for its glucose content. In general, glucose levels should return to normal within 2 hours after ingestion of the glucose. With diabetic patients, the test must be carried out for 4 to 5 hours to observe how the patient metabolizes the glucose.

> **Patient Information Card Glucose Tolerance Test**
>
> **Introduction**
>
> A glucose tolerance test (GTT) has been ordered by your physician. The purpose of a GTT is to test the efficiency of your body's insulin-releasing mechanism and glucose-disposing system.
>
> You must prepare your body for the GTT by changing your eating and medication routines slightly for 3 days before the test. It is very important that you follow the instructions below in order for accurate results to be obtained.
>
> Basically, you will need to follow these three guidelines to prepare for your GTT test:
>
> 1. Your carbohydrate intake must be at least 150 g per day for 3 days prior to the GTT.
> 2. Do not eat anything for 12 hours before the GTT, but do not fast for more than 14 hours before the test.
> 3. Do not exercise for 12 hours before the GTT.
>
> **Preparation: Medication**
>
> Before proceeding with the GTT, you must tell your physician if you are currently using any of the following medications because they may interfere with test results:
>
> - Alcohol
> - Anticonvulsants (seizure medication)
> - Blood pressure medication
> - Clofibrate
> - Corticosteroids
> - Diuretics (fluid pills)

Figure 9–13. Sample patient information card. *(Courtesy of Division of Laboratory Medicine, M.D. Anderson Hospital and Tumor Institute, Houston, TX.)*

- Estrogens (birth control pills or estrogen replacement pills)
- Salicylates (aspirin, pain killers)—only if taken in high doses, such as for rheumatoid arthritis

Preparation: Diet and Exercise

Remember that for 3 days prior to your test, your diet must contain at least 150 g of carbohydrates per day. The following is a list of high carbohydrate foods:

- *Milk and milk products*—12 g of carbohydrates per serving. One serving is equal to 8 oz of milk (whole, skim, or buttermilk), 4 oz of evaporated milk, or 1 cup of plain yogurt.
- *Vegetables*—5 g of carbohydrates per serving. One serving is equal to ½ cup of any vegetable, excluding starches (e.g., potatoes, corn, or peas).
- *Fruits and fruit juices*—10 g of carbohydrates per serving. One serving is equal to ½ cup of juice, 1 small piece of fresh fruit, or ½ cup of unsweetened canned fruit, with the following exceptions:

Apple juice	⅓ cup
Grape juice	¼ cup
Raisins	2 tbsp
Watermelon	1 cup
Prunes	2 medium
Banana	½ small
Dates	2
Cantaloupe	¼ 6-in. melon
Honeydew melon	⅛ 7-in. melon

Figure 9–13. (*continued*)

- *Breads and starches*—15 g of carbohydrates per serving. One serving is equal to 1 slice of bread or 1 small roll. Other one-serving sizes are:

Bagel, English muffin	½
Tortilla	1
Cooked cereal	½ cup
Dry cereal	¾ cup
Cooked rice, noodles, pasta	½ cup
White potatoes, dried beans and peas	½ cup
Yams	¼ cup
Corn	⅓ cup
Crackers	5–6

- *Meats, cheeses, and fats*—These foods contain few or no carbohydrates.
- *Miscellaneous*

Ice cream	½ cup	15 g of carbohydrates
Sherbet	½ cup	30 g of carbohydrates
Gelatin	½ cup	30 g of carbohydrates
Jams, jellies	1 tbsp	15 g of carbohydrates
Sugar	1 tsp	4 g of carbohydrates
Carbonated beverage	6 oz	20 g of carbohydrates
Hard candy	2 pcs	10 g of carbohydrates
Fruit pie	⅙	60 g of carbohydrates
Cream pie	⅙	50 g of carbohydrates

Figure 9–13. (*continued*)

| Plain cake | ¹⁄₁₀ | 30 g of carbohydrates |
| Frosted cake | ¹⁄₁₀ | 38 g of carbohydrates |

Preparation: General Health

The following physical conditions should be reported to your doctor because they too may affect the results of your test:

- Acute pancreatitis
- Adrenal insufficiency
- Diabetes mellitus
- Hyperinsulinism (excess insulin secretion, resulting in hypoglycemia)
- Hyperthyroidism
- Hypopituitarism (decreased function of pituitary gland)
- Pregnancy
- Stress

If you have any difficulty making the necessary alterations in your diet or medication schedule, please inform your doctor. For accurate test results, the instructions on this card must be followed.

Figure 9–13. (*continued*)

When a glucose tolerance test is to be performed, the patient should be given complete instructions about the procedure so that his or her cooperation can be ensured (Fig. 9–13). For best results, the patient should eat normal, balanced meals for at least 3 days prior to the test. Twelve hours prior to the beginning of the test, the patient should fast completely. Water intake is strongly encouraged because frequent urine specimens are required throughout the procedure. Other beverages, including unsweetened tea or coffee, are not allowed. Smoking, tobacco chewing, and gum chewing (including sugarless gum) should be discouraged until the completion of the test because they may stimulate digestion and interfere with the interpretation of the results. If a patient is chewing gum prior to or during the test, note this on the requisition slip.[10]

During the test, the patient drinks a standard dose of glucose, usually 75 or 100 g for adults or approximately 1 g/kg of body weight for children and small adults. A dose of 100 g is recommended for diagnosis of gestational diabetes.[10] Commercial preparations are available as flavored drinks to make the glucose more palatable. The patient must start and finish the drink within 5 minutes. Water intake is encouraged throughout the procedure. If the patient should vomit at any point in the procedure, the physician should be notified immediately to decide whether the test should be continued or stopped.[10]

When the patient finishes drinking the solution, the time is noted, and 30-, 60-, 120-, and 180-minute blood and urine specimens are obtained. Thus, if the glucose is administered to the patient at 7:30 AM, at 8:00 AM the 30-minute blood and urine specimens are obtained from the patient. This collection is followed by collections of blood and urine specimens at 8:30 AM (60 minutes), 9:30 AM (120 minutes), and 10:30 AM (180 minutes) (Fig. 9–14). The tubes should be labeled with the time, as well as "30 minutes," "1st hour," and so on. If blood is obtained initially by venipuncture, all succeeding specimens must also be venous blood. Similarly, if capillary blood is used, all specimens should be collected by microtechnique because the values and methods of analysis may vary between the two types of samples. If serum samples are used instead of plasma samples with a preservative, the tubes should be centrifuged immediately after collection, then the serum should be separated from the blood cells and placed in the refrigerator to inhibit glucose utilization by the blood cells.

POSTPRANDIAL GLUCOSE TEST

The 2-hour **postprandial glucose test** can be used to screen patients for diabetes because glucose levels in serum specimens drawn 2 hours after

Figure 9–14. Graph of glucose tolerance test results.

a meal are rarely elevated in normal patients. In contrast, diabetic patients usually have increased values 2 hours after a meal.

For this test, the patient should be placed on a high carbohydrate diet 2 to 3 days before the test. The day of the test, the patient should eat a breakfast of orange juice, cereal with sugar, toast, and milk to provide an approximate equivalent of 100 g of glucose. A blood specimen is taken 2 hours after the patient finishes eating breakfast. The glucose level of this specimen is then determined, and the physician can decide whether further carbohydrate metabolism tests (such as a glucose tolerance test) are needed.

EPINEPHRINE AND GLUCAGON TOLERANCE TESTS

Epinephrine increases blood sugar by accelerating glycogenolysis (the breakdown of glycogen). The **epinephrine tolerance test** is used to determine the availability and the quantity of liver glycogen by stimulating an increase in blood sugar by epinephrine injection.

First, a fasting blood sugar (glucose level) is obtained. Then, the physician or another qualified professional injects 10 minims of a

1 : 1000 solution of epinephrine hydrochloride intravenously. Thirty minutes after the injection, another blood sample is taken for glucose level determination. The blood sugar should rise at least 30 mg/dL higher in the 30-minute sample and should return to the fasting level in about 2 hours. If the patient's blood sugar level does not respond or rises only slightly, several disease states may be responsible. If glycogen storage is depleted, the epinephrine has little effect, and the blood sugar may increase only slightly. Such conditions exist in patients with hepatocellular damage, such as patients who have cirrhosis or a fatty liver. If glycogen stores are present but not readily available, although they may be present, the epinephrine has little effect on blood sugar. Von Gierke's disease can interfere with the availability of glycogen for conversion to sugar.

Because a low response to an epinephrine injection can be attributed to several disease states and other factors, this test is not considered a diagnostic tool. Rather, it is used along with other carbohydrate metabolism studies.

The **glucagon tolerance test** is conducted like the epinephrine tolerance test, except glucagon is injected instead. In fact, often the two stimulants may be given in combination to test liver glycogen stores. The amount of the stimulants given should be determined by the ordering physician and administered by a qualified professional or physician. Various health care workers may be involved in drawing the blood samples for glucose determinations and may be responsible for labeling and delivering the specimens to the laboratory.

LACTOSE TOLERANCE TEST

Some otherwise healthy adults experience difficulty in digesting lactose, a milk sugar. They appear to lack a mucosal lactase enzyme that breaks down the lactose into the simple sugars glucose and galactose. Instead, gastrointestinal discomfort may result, followed by diarrhea. These patients usually show no further symptoms if milk is removed from their diet.

To determine if a patient suffers from lactose intolerance, a physician may order a **lactose tolerance test.** A 3-hour glucose tolerance test should be performed 1 day in advance to determine the patient's normal glucose curve. A lactose tolerance test should be performed the next day in the same manner as the glucose tolerance, substituting the same amount of lactose for the glucose given the previous day. Fasting, 1-hour, 2-hour, and 3-hour blood samples are drawn and tested for glucose. When the results are graphed, the curve should be similar to that obtained from the glucose tolerance test, if the patient has the mucosal lactase enzyme and digests the sugar properly. If the patient is intolerant to lactose, his or her blood glucose level will increase by no more than 20 mg/dL from the fasting sample level.

The health care worker should be sure that a bathroom is located near the patient testing area because patients who are lactose intolerant may experience severe discomfort during the testing.

False-positive lactose tolerance test results have been known to occur in 25 to 33 percent of the patients tested who had normal lactase activity in small intestine biopsy specimens. Such results have been attributed to slow gastric emptying, not to the absence of the lactase enzyme.

THERAPEUTIC DRUG MONITORING (TDM)

Laboratory drug monitoring of therapeutic agents is a complex endeavor that requires much coordination among laboratory, nursing, and pharmacy personnel. A basic understanding of the variables, information needed, and definitions of terms is important to obtain accurate laboratory results.

To adequately evaluate the appropriate dosage levels of many drugs, the collection and evaluation of specimens for trough and peak levels is necessary. The trough level is the lowest concentration in the patient's serum; that is, the specimen should be collected immediately prior to administration of the drug. The peak level is the highest concentration of a drug in the patient's serum. The time required to reach the highest concentration varies with the mode of administration (intramuscular injection v. IV infusion) and the rate at which the drug is infused. In addition, random levels may be appropriate for monitoring the drug dosage if the drug is administered by continuous infusion and if enough time has elapsed for the drug to reach equilibrium. The time of collection is much more critical for drugs with shorter half-lives (e.g., gentamicin, tobramycin, and procainamide) than for those with longer half-lives (e.g., phenobarbital and digoxin). Specimens for therapeutic drug monitoring (TDM) should *not* be collected immediately following dosing.[11,12]

As a result of all these factors, laboratory personnel must acquire and document additional information when performing these tests. A health care worker may be asked to acquire the following information: patient's name; patient's identification number; patient's location; test ordered; requesting physician; collection time and date; whether the order is for a peak level, a trough level, or a continuous-infusion random level determination; time and date of last dose; time and date of next dose; and a nurse's verification that the dose was administered. Specific specimen guidelines for each drug should be established by pharmacy and laboratory staff and strictly adhered to.

Evacuated blood collection tubes without the plasticizer tris(butoxyethyl)phosphate (TBEP) on the tube top are suitable for most collections used to monitor drugs.[13] However, to prevent the possibility that the blood may come into contact with an interfering stopper, blood specimens should be maintained in an upright position after collection. In addition, because falsely low levels of lidocaine, phenytoin, and pentobarbital occur with the use of gel serum separator tubes, this type of evacuated blood collection tube should be avoided in TDM unless the gel serum separator tube has been evaluated and determined not to cause interferences.[14]

Most TDM assays should be performed on clotted blood. The National Committee for Clinical Laboratory Standards (NCCLS) has devised toxicology and drug-monitoring requirements for blood collection containers; these requirements can be helpful to the pharmacy and laboratory personnel who are responsible for establishing specific specimen guidelines for each drug.

COLLECTION FOR TRACE METALS (ELEMENTS)

Testing for trace metals involves the use of specially prepared trace metal evacuated blood collection tubes. Also, special acid-washed plastic syringes are usually suitable for trace metal testing. For aluminum level determinations, a needle that is free of aluminum must be used. For lead level determinations, lead-free heparinized evacuated blood tubes equipped with sterilized stainless steel needles should be used for blood collection.[15] Specific specimen collection guidelines should be established as part of the clinical laboratory's technical procedures for trace metal testing.

VASCULAR ACCESS DEVICES (VADs)

Drawing blood specimens through CVC lines requires special techniques, training, and experience. A CVC, also called a central venous line, is one of numerous vascular access devices (VADs). The CVC is usually inserted into the subclavian vein, which is in the chest area below the clavicle. A dressing covers the tubing that extends above the skin. Another type of VAD is a peripherally inserted central catheter (PICC), which is inserted into the peripheral venous system with a lead into the central venous system. A PICC is usually placed in the arm, in the basilic or cephalic vein. The PICC should not be used for blood collection because it may collapse during aspiration. An **implanted port** is another VAD that is a small chamber attached to an indwelling line. This port is surgically implanted beneath the skin.

A **heparin lock,** a device that can be inserted into a VAD, is used for medication administration and blood collection. This device is flushed with a heparin solution (Fig. 9–15) on a scheduled basis to prevent blood clots from developing in the line. Because a heparin solution is used in this device, coagulation specimens must not be collected from it, otherwise, the solution will falsely alter coagulation test results.

Usually, managers of health care facilities require nursing or laboratory personnel to take specialized training courses prior to allowing them to collect blood from a VAD. The IV line is a direct pathway into the patient's bloodstream. Each time the IV system is entered, the possibility of contamination and infection exists. However, if aseptic technique is strictly adhered to, this procedure can provide a relatively safe means of access to the VAD and can save the patient some of the trauma of undergoing frequent venipunctures for laboratory studies. In regard to the CVC line, its use should be limited to once daily unless other instructions are received from a physician. Specific criteria must be established at each health care facility for obtaining blood through a VAD.

Figure 9–15. Heparin lock flush solution.

Drawing Blood Through a CVC

To draw blood through a CVC, a 20-mL syringe is the largest syringe recommended for use with a soft-wall catheter because larger sizes may collapse the catheter wall. The patient should be positioned with the catheter hub at or below the level of the patient's heart to prevent possible air emboli when the CVC is entered. Nursing or medical staff should be consulted before opening the CVC line to avoid interrupting medication, which is extremely vital to the maintenance of the patient's care. When drawing blood from multilumen catheters, the lumen(s) not being drawn should be clamped during the procedure to prevent dilution of the blood sample being drawn.

The following equipment and supplies should be prepared prior to the procedure: laboratory requisition forms, tubes, and labels for the specimen; sterile gloves; two or three 20-mL disposable syringes; one 10-mL disposable syringe; one 10-mL syringe filled with injectable normal saline, used for flushing the catheter; two or three sterile needles; a 4 × 4-in. piece of sterile gauze; a linen protector to provide a clean work area; a plastic or paper container for wastes or soiled items; adhesive tape; a sterile heparin cap; alcohol wipes; and 100 U/mL heparin (optional).

The procedure may involve the following steps but is subject to differences among hospitals and must be performed by *authorized personnel only.*[16]

1. Check patient's chart for physician's order to draw blood through CVC.
2. Obtain laboratory requisitions and labels that reflect patient location and tests for which blood is needed.
3. Check labels against slips and patient's identification bracelet as described in Chapter 5.
4. Determine amount of blood to be drawn so that correct size syringe(s) can be used.
5. Assemble equipment, wash hands, and put sterile gloves on.
6. Aseptically draw up to 10-mL injectable normal saline and cap with sterile needle cover to maintain sterility. Take all supplies to bedside in a tray or other enclosed container to avoid a needle stick.
   Note: Take *only* tubes for the patient, no others.
7. Identify patient by armband ID, noting full name and hospital number. Check against preprinted labels
8. Explain procedure to patient.
9. Provide adequate room and light for procedure.
10. Position patient by elevating the bed to a comfortable working

level and making the bed flat, and have catheter hub at or below the level of the patient's heart.

11. After placing linen protector on bed, place tray of supplies on protector. Place sterile 4 × 4 in. gauze under connection site.

12. If IV is infusing, clamp off mainline IV tubing. Close slide clamp on short microbore tubing.

13. Loosen IV tubing connection or heparin cap. Aseptically disconnect IV tubing or injection cap from short microbore tubing, holding short microbore tubing and IV tubing "up" to avoid contamination.

14. Cap IV tubing with sterile needle and needle cover, and aseptically insert 10-mL syringe in short microbore tubing.

15. Unclamp short microbore tubing. Aspirate (slowly and steadily) 5 to 10 mL blood. Remove syringe with blood and place in tray in order to discard later.

16. Aseptically insert syringe of correct size for needed blood specimen into short microbore tubing.

17. Open the slide clamp on short microbore tubing and slowly aspirate blood in the quantity needed.

18. Close slide clamp on short microbore tubing. Remove syringe and place sterile needle on syringe.

19. Quickly and aseptically insert the 10-mL syringe with normal saline into the short microbore tubing. Open slide clamp on short microbore tubing.

20. Gently irrigate catheter with 5 mL normal saline.

21. Close slide clamp on short microbore tubing; temporarily leave syringe with 5 mL normal saline in place.

22. Place blood into blood collection tubes as previously described.

23. Open slide clamp on short microbore tubing. Complete irrigation of catheter with remaining 5 mL normal saline. Close slide clamp on short microbore tubing.

24. Aseptically reconnect IV tubing to short microbore tubing. Open clamp on IV tubing and slide clamp on short microbore tubing.

25. Determine that IV fluids are infusing properly at rate set by unit nurse.
    Note: If pump is being used, make certain pump is ON and alarm is ON. If the rate of IV flow appears altered, the nurse should be notified *immediately.* Retape connection between short microbore tubing and IV tubing.

26. Make sure the patient is in a safe and comfortable position with the bed down, siderails up, and bedside table and call light accessible to patient. Place used equipment and supplies in

appropriate discard containers. The needles should NOT be recapped before discarding.

27. Write the date, time, and initial labels on blood specimens and place tubes of blood with the correct lab requisitions. Dispatch to laboratory in usual manner.

28. Document completion of procedure and any problems in the patient's medical record.

    Note: The uncapped used needles should NOT be placed on the patient's bed, but rather in an appropriate container until they can be properly discarded.

CANNULAS AND FISTULAS

A **cannula** is a tubular instrument that is used in kidney patients to gain access to venous blood for dialysis or blood collection. Blood should be drawn from the cannula of a kidney patient only by specially trained personnel because the procedure requires special techniques and experience.

A **fistula** is an artificial shunt in which the vein and artery have been fused through surgery. It is a permanent connection tube located in the arm of the kidney dialysis patient. The health care worker should use extreme caution when collecting a blood specimen from a kidney dialysis patient and avoid using the arm with the fistula as the site for venipuncture. If no other location can be found for the venipuncture site, the patient's arm must be cleaned *thoroughly* prior to blood collection. If the venipuncture site in this arm becomes infected, the inflammation in the blood vessels of the arm may shut down all the veins, requiring surgery to place a new shunt in the kidney dialysis patient.

DONOR ROOM COLLECTIONS

Properly trained health care providers may be employed in a regional blood center or a hospital blood donor center to screen and collect blood from donors. This section summarizes the procedure outlined by the American Association of Blood Banks (AABB).[17] Only an experienced, properly trained health care worker or technologist should be considered for this function because a physical, emotional, or traumatic experience may keep a donor from volunteering in the future.

Donor Interview and Selection

Not everyone who wants to donate blood is eligible, so the interviewer must determine the eligibility of each potential donor. Carefully determining donor eligibility not only helps prevent the spread of disease to blood product recipients, but also prevents untoward effects on the potential donor.

The following information should be kept on file on every donor indefinitely and initially obtained from every prospective donor, regardless of his or her ultimate acceptability:[17]

1. Date of donation.
2. Name: last, first, and middle initial.
3. Address.
4. Telephone number.
5. Gender.
6. Age and birth date. (Donors should be at least 17 years of age; however, minors may be accepted if written consent is obtained in accordance with applicable state law. Elderly prospective donors may be accepted at the discretion of the blood bank physician.)
7. Written consent form signed by the donor: (1) allowing the donor to defer from being a donor if he or she has risk factors for HIV, the causative agent of acquired immunodeficiency syndrome (AIDS), or (2) authorizing the blood bank to take and use his or her blood.
8. A record of reasons for deferrals, if any.
9. Social security number or driver's license number (may be used for additional identification but is not mandatory).
10. Name of patient or group to be credited, if a credit system is used.
11. Race [not mandatory, but this information can be useful in screening patients for a specific phenotype (chromosomal makeup)].
12. Unique characteristics about a donor's blood. (Blood from donors that is negative for cytomegalovirus or that is Rh-negative group O blood is used for neonatal patients.)

To help minimize the incidence of dizziness, fainting, or other reactions to blood loss, donors are encouraged to eat within 4 to 6 hours of donating blood. Eating a light snack just before the phlebotomy may help prevent these reactions, but a donor should not be required to eat if he or she does not want to do so.

Blood bank records must link each component of a donor unit [red blood cells (RBCs), white blood cells (WBCs), platelets, etc.] to its disposition. If the donation is a "replacement for credit" for a particular patient, the donor must supply the patient's name or the group name that is to be credited.

A brief physical examination is required to determine whether the donor is in general good condition on the day that he or she is to donate blood. The physical examination entails a few simple procedures easily mastered by the health care worker:

1. *Weight.* Donors must weigh at least 110 lb (50 kg); if the weight is less, the volume of blood donated must be carefully monitored and care taken that not too much blood is drawn. Also, the anticoagulant in the bag must be modified for the lesser donation. Most blood banks will not routinely accept donors who weigh less than 110 lb.

2. *Temperature.* The donor's oral temperature must not exceed 37.5°C (99.6°F).

3. *Pulse.* The donor's pulse should be regular and strong, between 50 and 100 beats per minute. The pulse should be taken for at least 30 seconds.

4. *Blood pressure.* The systolic blood pressure should measure 90 to 180 mm Hg, and the diastolic blood pressure should be between 50 and 100 mm Hg. People with blood pressure outside these limits should be deferred as donors and referred to their physicians for evaluation of a possible health problem.

5. *Skin lesions.* Both arms should be examined for signs of drug abuse, such as needle marks or sclerotic veins. The presence of mild skin disorders such as psoriasis, acne, or a poison ivy rash does not necessarily prohibit an individual from donating unless the lesions are in the antecubital area or the rash is particularly extensive. Donors with purulent skin lesions, wounds, or severe skin infections should be deferred, as should anyone with purplish-red or hemorrhagic nodules suggestive of Kaposi's sarcoma (an HIV-associated clinical sign). The skin at the site of the venipuncture must be free of lesions.

6. *General appearance.* If the donor looks ill, excessively nervous, or under the influence of alcohol or drugs, he or she should be deferred.

7. *Hematocrit or hemoglobin values.* The hematocrit value must be no less than 38 percent for donors. The hemoglobin value must be no less than 12.5 g/dL. A finger stick is commonly used to draw blood for such determinations. The health care worker may either collect blood in a hematocrit tube for centrifuging and reading or use the copper sulfate method, in which the hemoglobin is qualitatively determined. (For further details on the copper sulfate method, please refer to the AABB technical manual.)[17]

An extensive medical history must be taken on all potential donors, regardless of the number of previous donations on record. Most blood bank donor rooms have a simple card listing all the questions to be asked and "yes" or "no" columns that are used to indicate the donor's responses. The health care provider should refer to the protocol of the donor room at the institution's blood bank or the AABB technical manual, which sets guidelines for donor screening and acceptance.

Collection of Donor's Blood

The health care worker in a donor room must operate under the supervision of a qualified, licensed physician. Blood should be collected by using aseptic technique; a sterile, closed system; and a single venipuncture. If a second venipuncture is needed, an entirely new, sterile donor set is necessary; the first is discarded according to the contaminated material disposal protocol of the institution.

A donor should never be left alone either during or immediately after blood collection. The health care worker should be well versed in donor reactions, equipment safety precautions, first-aid techniques, and location of first-aid equipment in case it is needed in the course of donation.

The health care worker should prepare the antecubital portion of the donor's arm in the same manner as for collection of a blood culture specimen (Fig. 9–16). The blood-collecting bag should be placed conveniently, and the tubing should be extended to ensure that it has no kinks that would prevent a free flow. After the arm is properly prepared, the tourniquet should be replaced and the donor given instructions to open and close the hand during the course of the phlebotomy (Fig. 9–17). A 15-gauge regular or 17–gauge thin-walled needle is used most often. The 17-gauge thin-walled needle is preferable because it has the internal diameter of a 15-gauge needle and the outside diameter of a 17-gauge needle; that is, it has the large-bore size of a 15-gauge needle, but the smaller total size of the 17-gauge needle. The sterile needle is uncapped, and with a quick, sure motion, the needle is slipped under the skin and into the vein. As the draw begins, the needle and tubing should be taped in place and a dry, sterile gauze sponge laid on top. The health care worker should encourage the donor to continue to slowly open and close the hand and to report any discomfort or dizziness that occurs.

The health care worker should make sure that the blood in the bag mixes the anticoagulant during the collection, either manually or by placing it on a mechanical agitator. If the collection process takes more than 8 minutes to complete, platelet concentrates or antihemophilic factor preparations may not be possible. However, as long as the flow is constant and the bag contents continue to be mixed well, no time constraints are necessary.

Once the proper amount of blood is collected (405 to 495 mL), the phlebotomy should be stopped, the tubing clamped off with a hemostat or some other temporary clamp, the tourniquet or blood pressure cuff

Venipuncture Site Preparation

1 Purpose

To provide the phlebotomist with instructions on how to correctly perform an arm scrub that will ensure that the venipuncture site is free of bacteria

2 Scope

To be performed by the phlebotomist prior to any venipuncture collection procedure

3 Procedure

Materials Needed:
Iodophor [polyvinylpyrrolidone, (PVP), titratable iodine, 0.75 to 1 percent]
Iodophor (titratable iodine, 1 percent)
Cliniswab tincture of green soap (Clinipad Corp., Greenwich, CT)
Sterile gauze
Tourniquet or blood pressure cuff

3.1 Inspect both arms of the donor as well as other exposed skin areas for the presence of skin disease or a rash, a recent tattoo, or scars suggestive of intravenous drug use.

    3.1.1 If any abnormal findings are detected, defer the donor.

    3.1.2 If no abnormal findings are detected, select a large, firm vein in an area free of skin lesions or rash.

    3.1.3 Use either a tourniquet or an inflated blood pressure cuff to make the veins more prominent. Ask the donor to open and close his or her hand a few times.

3.2 Apply the blood pressure cuff or the tourniquet, and determine the site for venipuncture.

    3.2.1 The point at which you intend to insert the needle will be the focal point of the scrub.

    3.2.2 Preparing a completely aseptic site for venipuncture is impossible; however, a state of surgical cleanliness can be achieved to provide maximum assurance of a sterile product.

3.3 Before performing the scrub procedure, ask the donor if he or she is allergic to iodine.

3.4 If the donor is allergic to iodine, use the following scrub procedure:

Figure 9–16. Venipuncture site preparation. *(Courtesy of Gulf Coast Regional Blood Center, Houston, TX.)*

3.4.1 Using a sterile, disposable Cliniswab tincture of green soap swab stick, thoroughly scrub a 3-in. area (minimum) around the venipuncture site for at least 2 minutes.

3.4.2 From the center point of the venipuncture site, using a sterile, disposable Cliniswab, apply acetone–alcohol solution, working outward in concentric circles over the scrub area for a 3-in. minimum diameter.

3.4.3 Cover the area with dry, sterile gauze. Let the acetone–alcohol solution soak for 1 minute or until dry.

3.5 If the donor is not allergic to iodine, use the following scrub procedure:

3.5.1 Using a sterile, disposable swab of iodophor (PVP of 0.75 to 1 percent titratable iodine), vigorously scrub an area 3 in. minimum in diameter around the venipuncture site for at least 30 seconds to clean away body oils, dirt, and so forth.

3.5.1.1 Excess foam must be removed, but the arm need not be dry before you proceed to the next step.

3.5.2 From the center point of the venipuncture site and using a sterile, disposable iodine scrub, apply iodophor (PVP titratable iodine, 1 percent solution).

3.5.2.1 Work the swab outward in concentric circles over the scrub area for a 3-in. minimum diameter and let stand. The solution need not be completely dry before the venipuncture is performed.

3.5.2.2 Cover the area with dry, sterile gauze.

3.5.2.3 *Do not wipe the iodine off the scrub site before venipuncture.*

4 Procedural Notes

4.1 The venipuncture site must be in the center of the 3-in. preparation area.

4.2 Do not wipe off the solution prior to performing the venipuncture.

4.3 Failure to properly prepare the venipuncture site may allow contaminants to reach the donor or the patient receiving components drawn from the donor's blood.

Figure 9–16. (*continued*)

---

5 References

5.1 American Association of Blood Banks; 11th ed., Bethesda, MD, 1993.

5.2 Klein HG: Standards for blood banks and transfusion services, 16th ed.

5.3 Food and Drug Administration, 21 CFR 640.

Figure 9–16. (*continued*)

released, the needle removed, and pressure placed over the site for several minutes. It is advisable that the donor be instructed to raise his or her arm over the head while holding the gauze with pressure over the puncture site. This method minimizes bleeding into the site and surrounding tissues, but also helps restore the integrity of the vascular tissue. The donor should not be allowed to bend the arm until the bleeding stops; otherwise, the tissue may be further traumatized by bleeding into the area below the skin, as well as encouraging the vascular tissue to overlap and form scar tissue on the site during the healing process. A pressure bandage may be placed over the site once the bleeding stops. The blood in the bag and tubing should be mixed well, properly labeled, and stored in accordance with blood bank standards.

If the donor complains of dizziness or other discomfort, he or she should be encouraged to remain seated or prostrate for 10 to 15 minutes or longer. If the donor appears to be well, he or she should be encouraged not only to drink more fluids than usual to replace the volume loss, but also to refrain from strenuous exercise or work until after a full meal. Refreshments should be offered to the donor as a courtesy and as an opportunity for the donor to restore some of the lost body fluids. Any adverse reactions experienced by the donor should be recorded on the donor card. If the donor leaves before staff members recommend that he or she does so, this fact should also be noted on the donor's medical record.

THERAPEUTIC PHLEBOTOMY

Therapeutic phlebotomy is used in the treatment of some myeloprolif- erative diseases, such as polycythemia, or other conditions in which the removal of blood benefits the patient. Records in the blood bank should

Venipuncture

1 Purpose

To provide instructions for performing the venipuncture collection procedure

2 Scope

To be performed by the phlebotomist for every whole blood collection

3 Procedure

Materials Needed:
Tourniquet or blood pressure cuff
Blood bag pack
Tape
Gauze

3.1 Reapply the tourniquet or inflate the blood pressure cuff.
3.2 Ask the donor to open and close his or her hand until the previously selected vein is again prominent.
    3.2.1 *Do not touch the scrubbed area.* This precaution prevents possible contamination of the unit and/or harm to the donor.
    3.2.2 If you are unable to locate the vein, remove the iodine or other solution, choose the venipuncture site, and prepare the site again.
3.3 Clamp tubing.
    3.3.1 With a plastic hemostat, clamp the in-line tubing of the primary bag at approximately the fifth segment.
        3.3.1.1 Fold the tubing so that it is double-clamped. This step will prevent anticoagulant from running out of the in-line tubing into the bag and will prevent air contamination of the unit when the needle cap is removed.
3.4 Perform the venipuncture:
    3.4.1 Uncover a sterile needle by removing its cap.
        3.4.1.1 Twist the needle cover to remove the cap.
    3.4.2 Perform the venipuncture immediately.
        3.4.2.1 Do not pinch the tubing to remove anticoagulant from the needle tip because doing so will allow air to enter the tubing.

Figure 9–17. Venipuncture. *(Courtesy of Gulf Coast Regional Blood Center, Houston, TX.)*

3.4.3 Release the clamp.

3.4.4 Tape the tubing to the donor's arm.

3.4.5 Turn on the shaker if an electric shaker is being used.

3.4.6 Instruct the donor to open and close his or her hand slowly and continuously during the collection. This maneuver helps the movement of blood into the container.

3.4.7 Position dry, sterile gauze over the venipuncture site so that the gauze will be in the proper position when the needle is removed.

4 Procedural Notes

4.1 Mix the blood and anticoagulant frequently during collection. Such mixing can be done without removing the blood bag from the scale. Take care not to squeeze the bag, but lift the bottom end and rock it in a back-and-forth motion similar to that of a shaker. This mixing should be done frequently, immediately after completing the venipuncture. *When the primary container is almost filled, take care when mixing the blood with the anticoagulant to prevent premature tripping of the scale.*

5 References

5.1 American Association of Blood Banks, 11th ed., Bethesda, MD, 1993.

5.2 Klein HG: Standards for blood banks and transfusion services, 16th ed.

5.3 Food and Drug Administration, 21 CFR 640.

Figure 9–17. (*continued*)

indicate the patient's diagnosis, the physician's request for the phlebotomy, and the amount of blood to be taken. The medical director of the blood bank must decide whether the patient is to be bled in the donor room or in a private section of the blood bank. Some patients are visibly ill and weak, and their presence may have an adverse psychological effect on the healthy donors in the donor room. When a patient is obviously ill, his or her physician or the medical director of the blood bank should be present during the phlebotomy. Generally, the patient should be bled more slowly than a healthy donor, and the resting period should be extended.

The blood obtained through therapeutic bleeding may be used for homologous transfusion if the unit is deemed suitable by the director of the blood bank. If it is to be used, the recipient's physician must agree to use the blood for his or her patient, and a record of the agreement should be kept. The unit is then labeled and processed in the usual manner. The label must indicate that the blood is the result of a therapeutic bleed and must include the patient's diagnosis. If the unit is unsuitable for transfusion, the entire unit is disposed of in the usual manner for contaminated wastes.

AUTOLOGOUS TRANSFUSION

✔ A practice that is frequently used now is **autologous transfusion:** the patient donates his or her own blood before anticipated surgery. The reason for this type of transfusion is that the safest blood a recipient can receive is his or her own blood. The autologous transfusion prevents transfusion-transmitted infectious diseases (e.g., HIV, hepatitis) and eliminates the formation of antibodies in the transfused patient.

THE EMERGENCY CENTER

The atmosphere in an emergency center differs from that in any other area of the hospital. Most emergency rooms are chronically filled with people in pain whose medical problems range from ralatively minor injuries or illnesses to major, traumatic injuries. In addition to those who come to the emergency center for immediate treatment of acute injuries or illnesses, some patients have no regular physician and use the local emergency center for treatment of chronic illnesses such as coughs and colds. Family members often accompany the patients and may be highly emotional and vocal about their concern for their loved ones.

This range of patients and families with varying needs who demand attention from the limited staff can create a highly charged atmosphere. In most emergency centers, the patients are prioritized in a central reception area, often referred to as a *triage area,* as they arrive. Those who need immediate attention are seen first, and those whose conditions are more stable are seen later. However, even when the patients are prioritized according to their illnesses, the routine can be upset if a trauma patient arrives by ambulance and requires immediate life-saving measures. Although personnel at the triage desk may attempt to maintain a stable and orderly work flow in the emergency center, medical emergencies and critically ill or injured patients are unavoidable and must be handled professionally. The emergency center is an unpredictable setting; even though guidelines are placed on the flow of patients, the unexpected can occur at any moment.

Recognizing that the emergency center setting is stressful, the health care provider has two important responsibilities. First, he or she must be completely familiar with all the equipment and well versed in all blood-collecting procedures. If called on to collect stat (immediate) blood specimens from a critically injured person about to go to surgery, the health care worker must respond quickly and must successfully obtain the correct specimen in the right volume. He or she may not have enough time to collect another specimen if the first one is unsuitable. Consequently, only experienced health care workers should accept positions in the emergency center, where skills must be well mastered and automatic. The second responsibility is to follow directions quickly and correctly. In a critical situation, the health care worker must be able to follow the orders exactly and not require extensive, time-consuming directions. Only an experienced, confident, mature health care worker is suited to the unpredictable emergency environment.

Another factor present in the emergency center, which may cause a great deal of stress in some persons, is the sight and sound of traumatically injured patients in pain. Profuse bleeding, disfigurement, moaning, and groaning are common occurrences in this setting. Health care workers should be aware of their own reactions to critically injured patients. If they find the setting too stressful, they should opt for work on the general floors of the hospital or in a clinic where the sights and sounds are more predictable and controlled. The health care worker who chooses to work in an emergency center must learn to do his or her job with single-mindedness and to ignore anything that may distract from obtaining high-quality samples with speed and accuracy.

Obviously, in such a stress-charged atmosphere, tension runs high and minor personality conflicts occur more readily than in other more routine surroundings. All emergency center personnel must learn to resolve and quickly dismiss irritations and losses of temper that may otherwise interfere with the delivery of good emergency medical care. Only a mature, responsible person can cope well with the emergency center environment.

A career in emergency medicine is not for everyone; some people can work in the stressful setting for only a limited amount of time, whereas others would work nowhere else. The excitement of being part of a team of professionals who routinely provide life-saving treatment to critically injured patients has an attraction that cannot be easily duplicated in any other area of patient care. Health care workers must choose the environment that is best suited to their temperament and where they can best deliver quality patient care.

✔ *Key Terms*

ALLEN TEST

ARTERIAL BLOOD GASES (ABGs)

AUTOLOGOUS TRANSFUSION

BLEEDING-TIME TEST

BLOOD CULTURES

BRACHIAL ARTERY

CANNULA

CAPILLARY BLOOD GAS ANALYSIS

CENTRAL VENOUS CATHETER (CVC)

CENTRAL VENOUS LINE

EPINEPHRINE TOLERANCE TEST

FEMORAL ARTERY

FISTULA

GLUCAGON TOLERANCE TEST

GLUCOSE TOLERANCE TEST

HEPARIN LOCK

IMPLANTED PORT

LACTOSE TOLERANCE TEST

PERIPHERALLY INSERTED CENTRAL CATHETER (PICC)

POSTPRANDIAL GLUCOSE TEST

RADIAL ARTERY

SODIUM POLYANETHOLE SULFONATE (SPS)

THERAPEUTIC PHLEBOTOMY

TRACE METALS

VASCULAR ACCESS DEVICES (VADs)

Study Questions

For the following, choose the ONE best answer:

1. A cannula is
   a. the fusion of a vein and an artery
   b. a good source of arterial blood
   c. a tubular instrument used to gain access to venous blood
   d. an artificial shunt that provides access to arterial blood

2. A milk sugar that sometimes cannot be digested by healthy individuals is
   a. glucose
   b. glucagon
   c. lactose
   d. lactate

3. Which of the following is the preferred site for blood collection for ABG analysis?

   a. subclavian artery   c. ulnar artery
   b. femoral artery   d. radial artery

4. Which of the following supplies is *not* needed during an arterial puncture for an ABG determination?

   a. tourniquet   c. lidocaine
   b. heparin   d. syringe

5. What is the reason for performing the Allen test?

   a. to obtain the oxygen concentration of the patient
   b. to determine whether the patient's blood pressure is elevated
   c. to test for the possibility of a hematoma
   d. to determine that the ulnar and radial arteries are providing collateral circulation

6. When blood is drawn from the radial artery for an ABG determination, the needle should be inserted at an angle of no less than

   a. 20 degrees   c. 45 degrees
   b. 30 degrees   d. 65 degrees

7. Which of the following evacuated tubes is preferred for the collection of a blood culture specimen?

   a. yellow-topped evacuated tube
   b. green-topped evacuated tube
   c. light blue–topped evacuated tube
   d. red-topped evacuated tube

8. During a glucose tolerance test

   a. a standard amount of glucose drink is given to the patient, then a fasting blood collection is performed
   b. the patient should be encouraged to drink water throughout the procedure
   c. the patient is allowed to chew sugarless gum
   d. all the patient's specimens are timed from the fasting collection

9. The bleeding-time test is used to

   a. check for vascular abnormalities
   b. diagnose diabetes mellitus
   c. determine whether the patient's blood pressure is low
   d. assess liver glycogen stores

10. One purpose for autologous transfusion is to prevent the possibility that

    a. the transfused patient will develop diabetes mellitus
    b. antibodies will form in the transfused patient
    c. antigens will form in the transfused patient
    d. polycythemia will develop in the transfused patient

REFERENCES

1. National Committee for Clinical Laboratory Standards (NCCLS): *Percutaneous Collection of Arterial Blood for Laboratory Analysis.* NCCLS Document H11-A2, Villanova, PA, NCCLS, Vol 12, no 8, 1992.
2. National Committee for Clinical Laboratory Standards (NCCLS): *Blood Gas Preanalytical Considerations: Specimen Collection, Calibration, and Controls.* NCCLS Document C27-A, Villanova, PA, NCCLS, 1993.
3. Smith C: Surgicutt: A device for modified template bleeding times. *J Med Technol* 3(4): 1986.
4. International Technidyne Corporation: *Surgicutt: Package Insert of Procedure.* Edison, NJ, International Technidyne Corporation.
5. Balows A (ed): *Manual of Clinical Microbiology,* 5th ed. Washington, DC, American Society for Microbiology, 1991.
6. Campos JM: Detection of bloodstream infections in children. *Eur J Clin Microbiol Infect Dis* 8:815, 1989.
7. Isaacman DJ, Karasic RB: Lack of effect of changing needles on contamination of blood cultures. *Pediatr Infect Dis J* 9:274, 1990.
8. Krumholz HM, Cummings S, York M: Blood culture phlebotomy: Switching needles does not prevent contamination. *Ann Intern Med* 13:290, 1990.
9. Baron EJ, Peterson LR, Finegold SM (eds): *Bailey & Scott's Diagnostic Microbiology.* St. Louis, Mosby, 1994.
10. National Diabetes Data Group: Classification and diagnosis of diabetes mellitus and other categories of glucose intolerance. *Diabetes* 28:1039, 1979.
11. College of American Pathologists (CAP): *Clinical Laboratory Handbook for Patient Preparation and Specimen Handling: Fascicle IV—Therapeutic Drug Monitoring and Toxicology.* Skokie, IL, CAP, 1985.
12. Bittikofer J: Toxicology (Chap 27). In Bishop M, Duben-Engelkirk J, Fody E (eds): *Clinical Chemistry: Principles, Procedures, Correlations.* Philadelphia, J. B. Lippincott, 1992.
13. Janknegt R, Lohman J, Hooymans PM, et al: Do evacuated blood collection tubes interfere with therapeutic drug monitoring? *Phar Weekbl (Sci)* 5:287–291, 1983.
14. Quattrocchi F, Karnes H, Robinson J, et al: Effect of serum separator blood collection tubes on drug concentration. *Ther Drug Monit* 5:359–362, 1983.
15. Meranger J, Hollebone B, Blanchette G: The effects of storage times, temperature and container types on the accuracy of atomic absorption

determination of Cd, Cu, Hg, Pb and Zn in whole heparinized blood. *J Anal Toxicol* 5:33–41, 1981.

16. Woodard E: *Laboratory Liaison Technician Manual.* Houston, TX, Division of Laboratory Medicine, M.D. Anderson Hospital and Tumor Institute, 1988.

17. Walker RH (ed): *Technical Manual of the American Association of Blood Banks,* 11th ed. Arlington, VA, 1993.

ten

10

HOME, HOSPITAL BEDSIDE, AND NURSING HOME COLLECTIONS

Chapter Outline

Chapter Objectives
Glucose Monitoring
Blood Gas and Electrolyte
   Analysis
Blood Coagulation Monitoring
Hematocrit and Hemoglobin

Cholesterol Screening
Future Trends
Self Study
   Key Terms
   Study Questions

Chapter Objectives

Upon completion of Chapter 10, the learner is responsible for the following:

1. List two other terms that are synonymous with *point-of-care testing*.

2. Identify four analytes whose levels can be determined through point-of-care testing.

3. Describe the most widely used application of point-of-care testing.

4. Given the abnormal and normal control values for glucose from a daily run, plot the control values on the appropriate quality control charts.

With new emerging technology, laboratory testing services and results delivery have expanded beyond the laboratory to the hospital bedside, the home, the nursing home, and any other direct-contact patient setting.[1] The terms used for these direct laboratory services include *decentralized laboratory testing, on-site testing, alternate-site testing, near-patient testing,* **patient-focused testing, point-of-care testing,** and *bedside testing.* As innovations in point-of-care instrumentation continue to evolve, nurses, laboratorians, and other health care providers will increasingly perform additional on-site laboratory testing to obtain various types of laboratory test results. The demand for point-of-care testing is increasing because rapid turnaround of laboratory test results is necessary for prompt medical decision making.

GLUCOSE MONITORING

One of the most widely used applications of point-of-care testing is blood glucose monitoring, in which commercially available instruments, such as the one shown in Figure 10–1, are used to determine blood glu-

Figure 10–1. HemoCue β-Glucose Analyzer. *(Courtesy of HemoCue, Inc., Mission Viejo, CA).*

TABLE 10–1. BLOOD GLUCOSE MONITORS

Instrument (Manufacturer)	Features
Glucometer Encore (Miles Diagnostics Division, Elkhart, IN)	Quality control (QC) management capability Memory function includes date and time; thus, no timing Above-average accuracy No wiping required Easy to operate
Accu-Chek easy (Boehringer Mannheim Corp., Mannheim, Federal Republic of Germany)	QC and patient data management capability with AccuData GTS Memory function includes date, time, and patient identification number Above-average accuracy
One Touch II Hospital (Life Scan, Mountain View, CA)	QC data management capability Automated QC features Available for use in three languages Memory function includes date and time Above-average accuracy Easy to use
β-Glucose analyzer (HemoCue, Inc., Mission Viejo, CA)	Refrigerated temperature required for test cuvettes Above-average accuracy Memory capability is available Easy to operate

cose levels. Such determinations allow the physician to choose appropriate treatment regimens for patients with **diabetes mellitus,** a chronic disease in which the pancreas cannot produce enough **insulin** or cannot use the insulin that it does produce. Insulin is a chemical that is released into the bloodstream by the pancreas when glucose levels in the blood increase after meals. Insulin causes the glucose to be absorbed from the blood into the body tissues, where it is used for energy. Because of the lack of insulin in patients with diabetes mellitus, glucose is not properly absorbed by the tissues, and the glucose levels within the blood increase. If the blood glucose levels become too elevated, the diabetic patient can enter a state of metabolic acidosis, which can result in shock and then death. Because research has shown that strict glucose control in patients with diabetes mellitus is necessary to prevent serious complications, pocket-size glucose reflectance meters are used in point-of-care testing to help these patients monitor and maintain glucose levels within the acceptable range. During the past decade, small glucose-monitoring instruments such as those described in Table 10–1 became commonplace in the home, in the nursing home, and at the hospital bedside.

These "rapid" methods require whole blood samples collected by skin puncture from the finger, heel (for infants), or a flushed heparin line. As for any blood collection procedure, appropriate safety protocols must be followed (e.g., wearing gloves), and disposal of potentially contaminated waste must be part of the quality control and safety guidelines. These bedside procedures are handy for quick screening in a hospital or outpatient setting. However, *extreme caution* must be taken to provide a rigid, up-to-date, quality control and training program for personnel before they begin to implement such procedures. Variance in methodology and lack of quality control on reagents and equipment can lead to serious medical consequences for patients being tested.[2,3] Therefore, careful adherence to manufacturers' instructions, a thorough evaluation of the monitoring devices, and strict adherence to daily quality control procedures will ensure a more accurate and precise screening tool. In addition, careful recording of the results must include the date, time, and health care worker identification, as well as verification that the results are from the bedside (or patient's home) rather than the clinical laboratory. In some health care facilities, bedside test results are recorded on special bedside testing forms or in a separate section of the patient's medical record.

To perform the blood glucose determinations, health care providers must be aware of the total quality assurance procedures that are required to obtain accurate and precise results. A skin puncture is customarily performed to obtain the blood for these bedside glucose assays. The patient's finger should be cleansed with alcohol and allowed to dry. A microcollection lancet is used to puncture the finger. The first drop of blood is wiped away with a dry, sterile gauze pad, and the next drop is allowed to fall from the finger onto the reagent strip or pad. After the specified time indicated on the instrument's instruction sheet elapses, the blood drop is removed by blotting or by washing, and the strip is placed in the instrument to obtain a glucose reading. The timing of the reaction is critical, and most of these instruments call the time to the attention of the operator by buzzing or by sounding an alarm.

The HemoCue β-Glucose Analyzer (HemoCue, Inc., Mission Viejo, CA) (Fig. 10–1) is an instrument used for bedside glucose testing. This instrument differs from others since it obtains test results from capillary, venous, or arterial whole blood. It uses a microcuvette rather than a test strip and does not require blotting.

Some glucose-monitoring instruments should be calibrated with glucose standards (calibrators). The glucose values must be monitored daily with **quality control material,** and whenever a battery is changed, or the meter is cleaned. This control material should be similar to the patient's specimen in order to determine if the analytic system is working properly. For example, the glucose control material should be based on the use of whole blood because this type of body fluid is used for measurements with bedside glucose-monitoring instruments.

Each day, the glucose assay is performed on patients' blood specimens, control material must be analyzed. The control value obtained each day is plotted on a chart under the appropriate date, and the daily plots are joined with a straight line (Fig. 10–2). Interpretation of this chart is based on the fact that for a normal distribution, 95 percent of

Figure 10–2. Quality control record.

the values about the mean, or average ($\bar{x}$), should be within ± 2 standard deviations (SD) of the mean (average), and the fact that 99 percent of the values are within ± 3 SD of the mean. Tolerance limits are determined by pooling the data obtained during a 20-day test period and referring to the mean $\pm$ 2 SD. If a daily control value exceeds the tolerance limits, corrective action must occur according to the manufacturer's directions and be documented for future reference.

Another quality control measure that can be taken when bedside glucose-monitoring instruments are used is purchasing the reagent strips and controls in quantities that enable health care workers to use constant pools of the same lot number. This leads to reproducibility of the glucose results. Required preventive maintenance of each meter is critical for accurate results.

Some point-of-care glucose-testing instruments can store and download calibrators, controls, and patients' results and can thus provide a complete instrument log for quality assurance interpretation. Table 10–2 provides a list that will help lead to quality results through *avoidance* of these problems.

BLOOD GAS AND ELECTROLYTE ANALYSIS

Blood gas analysis for critical patient care needs can also be accomplished through patient-focused testing (Fig. 10–3). **Blood gas analysis** involves measurement of the partial pressure of oxygen (Po_2), the par-

TABLE 10–2. PROBLEMS TO AVOID IN BEDSIDE GLUCOSE TESTING

Specimen is inappropriately stored.
Wrong volume of specimen is collected.
Specimen is collected at wrong time.
Instrument blotting/wiping technique is not performed according to manufacturer's directions.
Reagents are outdated.
Timing of the analytical procedure is incorrect.
Reagents are not stored at proper temperature, leading them to deterioration.
Patient has not dieted properly for procedure.
Patient's result/time/date/etc., are mislabeled.
Recording of result is incorrect.
Battery for instrument is weak or dead.
Calibrators and/or controls are not properly used.
Results are not sent to appropriate individuals in timely manner.

Figure 10–3. i-STAT system for point-of-care testing. *(Courtesy of i-STAT Corporation, Princeton, NJ.)*

tial pressure of carbon dioxide (P_{CO_2}), and pH. The P_{O_2} and P_{CO_2} are analyzed whenever a patient has a heart or lung disorder. The blood pH determines whether the blood is too acidic or too alkaline. All these analytes must be closely monitored in emergency care situations, critical care units, cardiac intensive care units, and other units requiring immediate patient diagnosis and treatment.

In addition to monitoring blood gases, patient-focused testing instruments such as those shown in Figures 10–3 and 10–4 can measure blood electrolyte levels—sodium (Na^+), potassium (K^+), chloride (Cl^-), and bicarbonate (HCO^-_3) levels. These electrolyte measurements, as well as blood gas analysis, are needed immediately in critical care situations.

These instruments require preventive maintenance and quality control similar to the glucose-monitoring instruments. However, these instruments measure more than one analyte and thus have more complex

Figure 10–4. Nova Biomedical stat profile analyzer. *(Courtesy of Nova Biomedical, Waltham, MA.)*

operational, quality control, and maintenance needs than the glucose monitors. Consequently, as a health care professional involved in collecting blood and determining the analytes' results with these instruments, it is extremely important to be thoroughly trained in the use of the instruments prior to actually testing patients' blood.

BLOOD COAGULATION MONITORING

Similar to glucose monitoring, monitoring blood coagulation through point-of-care testing provides immediate results that can be used in controlling bleeding or clotting disorders in patients.[4] A blood coagulation instrument such as the CIBA Corning Biotrack 512 coagulation monitor (CIBA Corning Diagnostics Corp., Medfield, MA) is a handheld instrument that can measure prothrombin time (PT) and activated partial thromboplastin time (APTT) from an unmeasured drop of whole blood, providing results in 3 minutes. Again, the health care provider using this instrument must be trained appropriately in the preventive maintenance and quality control parameters in order to obtain accurate results.

**The University of Texas–Houston Health Science Center (UTHHSC)
Medical Mobile Van**

Technical Procedure   Hematocrit, or Packed Cell Volume (PCV)

Principle of the Test

The hematocrit represents the volume of circulating blood that is occupied by erythrocytes and is expressed as a percentage. The method used for the determination is centrifugation with the StatSpin centrifuge (Norfolk Scientific, Inc., Norwood, MA) procedure. The hematocrit test helps the physician to identify patients at risk of developing anemia and to manage patients who have anemia. Anemia is a less than normal number of erythrocytes in the volume of packed cells. The most common cause of anemia throughout the world is iron deficiency. A decrease in the hematocrit value results in lack of energy, reduced resistance to infections, and an increased risk of abnormality in pregnancy. An increased hematocrit value can result from polycythemia, hemoconcentration, and/or cardiac disease.

The reference intervals based on Texas Department of Health (TDH) values are as follows:

40–54% (males)
38–47% (females)
44–64% (newborns)
35–49% (14–90 days)
30–40% (6 months–1 year)
31–43% (1 year–10 years)

The critical limits are based on TDH levels:

<34% or >54% (male)—counsel
<31% or >47% (female)—counsel

If levels are in critical range, rerun. If the same, Nurse Practitioner refers to rural health clinic.

Materials and Reagents Required

Heparin-coated microcapillary tubes
Gloves
Microcentrifuge
Controls
Laboratory tissues

Figure 10–5. Technical procedure for hematocrit, or packed cell volume (PCV), determinations. *(Courtesy of The University of Texas–Houston Health Science Center, Houston, TX.)*

Specimen Collection

The technical procedure for finger puncture should be followed for blood collection. It is extremely important to wear gloves and a protective laboratory coat during the collection and testing procedures. Microcapillary tubes treated with ammonium heparin (color-coded red) should be used for the capillary blood collection. These tubes should be stored in a cool, dry place.

To perform the microcollection, hold the microcapillary tube by the end that has the color-coded band. Fill to the color-coded band. After filling, tilt the banded end downward until the blood moves halfway between the band and the end of the tube. Hold the tube in a horizontal position and push the *dry* (banded) end of the tube fully into the vertically held sealing compound. Twist and remove. Using a laboratory tissue, wipe off any blood that is forced from the other end.

Precautions

- Do not squeeze, or "milk," the finger before or during the procedure; doing so can result in an abnormally low reading.
- Do not collect blood in the microcapillary tube while the patient's finger is still wet with alcohol, or a low reading will result. Allow the finger to air dry before collection.

Test Procedure

1. Put the microcapillary tube (sealed end toward the outer rim) in any of the 12 positions on the hematocrit microcentrifuge. This rotor need not be balanced. Screw the cover in place.
2. Holding the rotor by the black "cover knob," attach the rotor to the rotor holder. (*Important:* Always hold the hematocrit rotor by the black knob on the rotor cover when pressing it firmly in a downward motion onto the rotor holder and when removing the rotor from the centrifuge. Pressing on the outer edges of the hematocrit rotor may result in damage to the rotor.)
3. Centrifuge the hematocrit rotor.
4. After the rotor stops, remove the rotor. To read the hematocrit value, place the rotor in the middle of the illuminated magnifying reader. Follow the directions on it as follows:
   Position the reader so that the base of the red blood cell column intersects the 0 (zero) line and the 100 percent line intersects the top of the plasma. Read the height of the red

Figure 10–5. (*continued*)

blood cell column directly from the scale. Interpolate between the markings to 1 percent.

Quality Control

- Use the controls daily purchased for the microhematocrit procedure.
- To verify the adequacy of cell packing, on a daily basis select one or more tubes (preferably with a hematocrit value of more than 50 percent, if available), centrifuge, and read. Spin these tubes a second time. The difference between the initial reading and the second reading should be 1 percent or less.

Preventive Maintenance of Microcentrifuge

- The timer should be calibrated with a stopwatch every 2 weeks.
- Speed can be checked by using the cell-packing procedure described under Quality Control.

References

StatSpin Procedure.
National Committee for Clinical Laboratory Standards (NCCLS): *Physician's Office Laboratory Guidelines,* 2nd ed. Document POL1-T2, Villanova, PA, June 1992.
Becan-McBride K, Ross D: *Essentials for the Small Laboratory and Physician's Office.* St. Louis, Mosby-Year Book, 1988.

Figure 10–5. (*continued*)

HEMATOCRIT AND HEMOGLOBIN

The hematocrit [Hct, packed cell volume (PCV), Crit] represents the volume of circulating blood that is occupied by red blood cells (RBCs). It is expressed as a percentage; thus, a hematocrit value of 38 percent indicates that 38 mL of each 100 mL of peripheral blood is composed of RBCs. Hematocrit values are obtained to aid in the diagnosis and evaluation of anemia, a less than normal number of erythrocytes, and may be used to evaluate blood volume and total RBC mass. Shown in Figure 10–5 (see pages 313–315) is a technical procedure for hematocrit. For accurate test results, remember not to squeeze the tissue to obtain capillary blood because doing so will dilute the sample with tissue fluid.

Determining a patient's hemoglobin level is another test to aid in the diagnosis and evaluation of anemia and other blood abnormalities.

Figure 10–6. HemoCue β-Hemoglobin Analyzer. *(Courtesy of HemoCue, Inc., Mission Viejo, CA.)*

The hemoglobin test has been determined by the American Medical Association (AMA) to be more accurate than the hematocrit test in diagnosis and treatment. A point-of-care analyzer that can be used to measure hemoglobin is the HemoCue β-Hemoglobin System (HemoCue, Inc., Mission Viejo, CA) (Fig. 10–6). A patient's venous, capillary or arterial whole blood sample placed in the microcuvette and inserted into this instrument provides the patient's hemoglobin value.

CHOLESTEROL SCREENING

Another laboratory testing procedure that health care providers are performing through point-of-care testing is cholesterol screening. Total blood cholesterol values can be monitored with a disposable, one-step, quantitative procedure by using the AccuMeter (ChemTrak, Inc., Sunnyvale, CA).[5] Its measurement is from finger stick whole blood or venous heparinized whole blood. This analytic system is somewhat different from other patient-focused testing systems in that it uses no instrumentation. Thus, preventive maintenance, calibration, and function checks are not necessary. However, after blood application, a visual evaluation of the colored bar height of the cholesterol reaction must occur in good lighting for accurate results. Also, it is imperative to have a sufficient sample size of 40 μL or more to obtain accurate cholesterol results.

FUTURE TRENDS

More point-of-care testing procedures are evolving that will inevitably involve phlebotomists, nurses, patient care technicians, and others who are providing care at the hospital bedside, nursing home, and/or home. For each new procedure, the health care worker must make a point of learning in detail the preventive maintenance, quality control, and calibration requirements in order to provide accurate test results.

✔ *Key Terms* ——————————————————

BLOOD GAS ANALYSIS   PATIENT-FOCUSED TESTING

DIABETES MELLITUS   POINT-OF-CARE TESTING

INSULIN   QUALITY CONTROL MATERIAL

Study Questions ——————————————————

For the following, choose the ONE best answer:

1. Insulin is released into the bloodstream when
   - a. blood cholesterol levels decrease
   - b. blood glucose levels decrease
   - c. blood glucose levels increase
   - d. blood cholesterol levels increase

2. Diabetes mellitus is caused by the inability of the pancreas to make or to use
   - a. glucose
   - b. cholesterol
   - c. sodium
   - d. insulin

3. In which of the following organs is insulin produced?
   - a. gall bladder
   - b. pancreas
   - c. liver
   - d. kidney

4. After the skin is punctured to obtain blood for glucose monitoring
   - a. use the first drop of blood for the glucose test
   - b. use an alcohol pad to remove the first drop of blood
   - c. use a dry, sterile gauze pad to remove the first drop of blood
   - d. squeeze the patient's finger to make a big first drop of blood for the monitor

5. Prior to using reagent strips and/or controls in point-of-care testing, the blood collector should
   - a. check the date when the bottle was opened
   - b. check the expiration date
   - c. verify that they were stored at the appropriate temperature
   - d. all of the above

6. To increase the blood flow from the skin puncture site for patient-focused testing,

   a. squeeze the punctured finger
   b. massage the area
   c. puncture another site adjacent to the first puncture site
   d. none of the above

7. Blood gas analysis measures

   a. Na^+ and K^+
   b. Pco_2, Po_2, and pH
   c. Cl^- and HCO_3^-
   d. Pco_2, Na^+, and Cl^-

8. Blood coagulation monitoring through point-of-care testing measures

   a. PT and APTT
   b. PT and Pco_2
   c. Po_2 and Pco_2
   d. PT, APTT, and pH

9. Which of the following is a blood glucose monitor?

   a. One Touch II Hospital (Life Scan, Mountain View, CA)
   b. i-STAT (i-STAT Corporation, Princeton, NJ)
   c. AccuMeter
   d. AccuMonitor

10. Electrolyte monitoring through point-of-care testing measures

    a. Na^+, K^+, PT, and APTT
    b. Pco_2, Po_2, and Na^+
    c. Na^+, K^+, Cl^-, and HCO_3^-
    d. Pco_2, Cl^-, HCO_3^-, and Po_2

REFERENCES

1. Tsai WW, Nash DB, Last JV: Point-of-care testing: Barriers and facilitators to implementation. *Clin Lab News* October:14, 1994.
2. National Committee for Clinical Laboratory Standards (NCCLS): *Ancillary (Bedside) Blood Glucose Testing in Acute and Chronic Care Facilities (Tentative Guidelines)*. NCCLS Document C30-T, Villanova, PA, NCCLS, Vol 11, no 8, June 1991.
3. Joint Commission for Accreditation of Healthcare Organizations (JCAHO): *Accreditation Manual for Pathology and Clinical Laboratory Services*. Oakbrook Terrace, IL, JCAHO, 1993.
4. Despotis GJ, Sontoro SA, Spritznagel E, et al: Prospective evaluation and clinical utility of on-site monitoring of coagulation in patients undergoing cardiac operation. *J Thorac Cardiovasc Surg* 107(1):271–279, 1994.
5. Allen MP, DeLizza A, Ramel U, et al: A noninstrumental quantitative test system and its application for determining cholesterol concentration in whole blood. *Clin Chem* 36:1591–1597, 1990.

eleven

11

URINALYSIS AND BODY FLUID COLLECTIONS

Chapter Outline

Chapter Objectives
Urine Collection
  Pregnancy Test
  Single-Specimen Collection
  Timed Collections
Cerebrospinal Fluid
Fecal Specimens
Seminal Fluid
Amniotic Fluid
Other Body Fluids
Culture Specimens

Other Nonblood Procedures
  Throat and Nasopharyngeal
    Culture Collections
  Skin Tests
  Gastric Analysis and Hollander
    Test
  Sweat Chloride by Iontophoresis
Self Study
  Key Terms
  Study Questions

Chapter Objectives

Upon completion of Chapter 11, the learner is responsible for the following:

1. Identify the types of body fluid specimens, other than blood, that are analyzed in the clinical laboratory, and the correct procedures for collecting and/or transporting these specimens to the laboratory.

2. Identify the various types of specimens collected for microbiological, throat, and nasopharyngeal cultures and the protocol that health care workers must follow when transporting these specimens.

3. List the types of patient specimens that are needed for gastric and sweat chloride analyses.

4. List three types of urine specimen collections and differentiate the uses of the urine specimens obtained from these collections.

In addition to collecting and transporting blood specimens, health care workers usually are involved in the collection and/or transportation of urine and other body fluid specimens. The health care worker should be careful when transporting body fluids because they are difficult to obtain and because the quality of the clinical laboratory test result is only as good as the specimen that is collected and transported to the testing site as quickly as possible under appropriate environmental conditions. Also, because such specimens may be biohazardous, the health care worker must adhere to universal precautions (see Chapter 12, Infection Control, and Chapter 13, Safety and First Aid) during collection and transportation of these specimens. Just as for blood collections, the laboratory request slip must accompany the specimen, which must be properly labeled with the patient's name, the patient's identification number, the date, the time of collection, the type of specimen, and the attending physician's name.

URINE COLLECTION

Routine urinalysis (UA) is one of the most frequently requested laboratory procedures because it can provide a useful indication of body health. It can be performed on a "first morning" or "random" urine specimen. Various diseases and disorders such as those listed in Table 11–1 can be detected through a routine UA. Some of the more common types of urine specimen collections and their uses are provided in Table 11–2.

The routine UA includes a physical, a chemical, and sometimes a microscopic analysis of the urine sample. The physical properties include the following: color, transparency v. cloudiness, odor, and concentration as detected through a specific gravity measurement. The chemical analysis for abnormal constituents is determined by using plastic strips impregnated with color-reacting substances that test for the presence of glucose, protein, blood [red blood cells (RBCs) and hemoglobin], white blood cells (WBCs), bacteria, bilirubin, and other constituents. The plastic strip, which has a separate reagent pad for each chemical test, is dipped into the urine briefly. The color of each reagent pad is compared to a color chart usually shown on the outer label of the reagent strip container. The results are reported according to the reagent label specifications (e.g., trace, 1+, 2+, and so on for a positive result,

TABLE 11–1. ABNORMAL URINE TEST RESULTS AND ASSOCIATED CONDITIONS

Abnormal Urine Test Result	Associated Condition
Presence of protein in urine (proteinuria)	Kidney disease Prolonged exercise Chemical poisoning
Presence of hemoglobin in urine (indicates blood destruction)	Kidney disease Malaria Severe burns Chemical poisoning
Presence of bilirubin in urine	Liver disease Obstructive jaundice
Presence of glucose in urine (glycosuria)	Diabetes mellitus
Presence of leukocytes in urine (white blood cells)	Infection of the kidney Infection of the urinary bladder Infection of the urethra
Presence of ketone bodies in urine (ketosis)	Diabetes mellitus Starvation

or negative when no reaction occurs). The strip is discarded after it is used one time. The urine may also be viewed microscopically for the presence of blood cells, bacteria and other pathogenic microorganisms, crystals, and casts.

Some other tests that can be performed on urine specimens are the pregnancy, myoglobin, and porphyrin tests. Urine is also the specimen of choice for drug abuse testing. Other laboratory procedures associated with the urinary system include the **creatinine clearance test** to determine the ability of the kidneys to remove creatinine from the blood, and the **blood urea nitrogen (BUN) test** to measure the amount of urea in the blood.

TABLE 11–2. TYPES OF URINE SPECIMEN COLLECTIONS AND THEIR USES

Specimen Type	Reason for Collection	Use
Random	This type of specimen is most convenient to obtain.	Routine urinalysis (UA)
First urine of the morning	This urine excretion is the most concentrated.	Protein, nitrite, microscopic analysis Routine urinalysis (UA)
Fasting	Metabolic abnormalities are suspected.	Glucose level determinations for diabetes mellitus testing
Clean-catch midstream	The specimen is free of contamination.	Culture for bacteria and/or microscopic analysis
Timed (e.g., 2 hour, 4 hour, 24 hour)	The excretion rate of the analyte can be determined.	Creatinine clearance test, urobilinogen determinations, hormone studies

Pregnancy Test

Human chorionic gonadotropin (HCG) is the first detectable analyte produced in pregnancy. Thus, its determination in the urine or serum is the basis of pregnancy tests. HCG is a hormone produced by the placental cells beginning approximately 10 days after conception (implantation of the ovum).

The urinary excretion of HCG peaks during the first trimester of pregnancy at approximately 10 weeks. Several types of assays are used to determine urinary HCG levels. An example of a frequently used enzyme immunoassay for HCG is the Hybritech Icon II HCG urine assay (Hybritech, Inc., San Diego, CA). The procedure for this assay follows:

✔
1. Obtain a **random urine sample** from the patient.
2. Drop five drops of patient's urine onto the center of the Icon II HCG membrane, allowing each drop to absorb into the membrane before adding the next.
3. Drop three drops of the antibody–enzyme conjugate reagent (bottle A) in rapid sequence onto the Icon II membrane so that the reagent covers the entire surface.
4. Wait 1 minute.
5. Dispense wash solution (buffer in kit) by directing flow toward the inner wall of the test cylinder. Fill the cylinder to the fill line and wait for drainage of the wash solution before proceeding.
6. Dispense three drops of the substrate reagent (bottle B) in rapid sequence onto the membrane so that the reagent covers the entire surface of the membrane.
7. Wait 2 minutes.
8. Stop the reaction by filling the cylinder to the fill line with wash solution.
9. With the indicator mark facing the user, observe the color development at the test zone and the positive reference zone. Formation of a circular blue dot in the test area confirms the presence of HCG. A built-in negative control indicates when a test result is invalid because of interfering substances.

Pregnancy tests are performed not only because of inquiry regarding pregnancy, but also for other medical reasons. Some of these reasons include the following:

- Certain surgical and diagnostic procedures (e.g., x-rays, colon surgery) are postponed or reconsidered if the patient is pregnant.
- Genetic counseling and/or plans to investigate, through cytogenetic and genetic studies, the possibility of familial defects in the infant may occur if the pregnancy test is positive.

- The HCG level is elevated in the urine of persons having various types of neoplasms and tumors (e.g., lung carcinoma).

Single-Specimen Collection

The preferred urine specimen for most analyses is the first voided urine of the morning, when urine is the most concentrated. The urine collection containers must be clean and dry prior to the collection process. For routine UA procedures, appropriate containers include plastic disposable cups or bags (for infants) with a capacity of 50 mL. The containers must be properly labeled, free of interfering chemicals, able to be tightly capped, and leakproof. The specimen should be transported to the UA section promptly for analysis within 2 hours after the patient voids. If transportation or analysis cannot occur within this time period, the urine should be refrigerated.

Another type of single-specimen urine test is the urine culture and sensitivity (C&S). This specimen requires a clean-catch midstream urine collection. The patient is instructed to void approximately one half of the urine into the toilet, a portion is collected in a readily available sterile container (Fig. 11–1), and the rest is allowed to pass into the toilet.[1]

If asked, "What is a *clean-catch urine specimen?*," the procedure should be described, stating that this type of specimen is used to detect the presence or absence of infecting organisms. The specimen must be free of contaminating matter that may be present on the external genital areas. Thus, the following steps should be explained to a female patient who is to obtain a clean-catch midstream urine specimen:

1. The woman should separate the skin folds around the urinary opening and clean this area with mild antiseptic soap and water.
2. Holding the skin folds apart with one hand and after urinating into the toilet, the patient should urinate into a sterile container. The container should not touch the genital area.
3. The health care worker or sometimes patient will label the container with her name and the time of collection and deliver it to the requested location.
4. Health care personnel should refrigerate the urine specimen immediately.

For a male patient, the following procedure should be adhered to for obtaining a clean-catch midstream urine specimen:[2]

1. The man should wash the end of his penis with soapy water and then let dry.
2. After allowing some urine to pass into the toilet, the patient should collect the urine in the sterile container. The container

Figure 11–1. Midstream urine collection catch kits. *(Courtesy of Evergreen Scientific, Los Angeles, CA.)*

should not touch the penis. Steps 3 and 4 are the same as those for a woman.

The urine specimen must be transported to the microbiology section promptly. If it cannot be taken to the area for microbiological culturing within 1 hour of collection, the specimen should be refrigerated to prevent an overgrowth of contaminate bacteria.

Timed Collections

For some laboratory assays, such as the creatinine clearance test, urobilinogen determinations, and hormone studies, 24-hour (or other timed period) urine specimens must be obtained. Incorrect collection and improper preservation of this type of specimen are two frequent errors affecting timed collections. Thus, the health care worker should be aware of the protocol for collecting a 24-hour urine specimen so that he or she can assist other health care professionals and the patient in preventing collection errors. The following steps should be followed for a 24-hour urine collection:[3]

1. The patient should be given a chemically clean, wide-mouthed, 3- to 4-L container with a tight-fitting lid. The laboratory personnel should add any required preservatives to the container prior to giving it to the patient. Patients should not be allowed to submit urine specimens in their own jars because the jars might not be chemically clean and would not contain the required preservatives. The preservative and any associated precautions should be written on the collection container label. The label should be placed on the container, not on the lid. Other information on the label should include the following:

- Patient's name
- Patient's identification number
- Starting collection date and time
- Ending collection date and time
- Name of the requested laboratory test

Other information that may be required by the facility includes

- Physician's name
- Patient's location (e.g., hospital room, outpatient)

2. The patient should be instructed verbally that the collection of the 24-hour urine specimen begins with emptying the bladder and discarding the first urine passed. This first step in the collection process should start between 6 and 8 AM, and the exact time should be written on the container label.

3. Except for the first urine discarded, all urine should be collected during the next 24-hour period. The patient should be reminded to urinate at the end of the collection period and to include this urine in the 24-hour collection. The patient should be told to urinate before having a bowel movement because fecal material in the urine specimen will make the specimen unacceptable for collection.

4. Because urine is an ideal culture medium for microorganisms that decompose chemical constituents, the patient should be instructed to refrigerate the entire specimen after adding each collection during the 24-hour period.

5. Some preservatives for 24-hour urine collection are corrosive if accidentally spilled or if the patient comes in contact with them during collection. Thus, the patient should be warned of any preservatives in the container.

6. The patient should be informed not to add anything except urine to the container and not to discard any urine during the collection period.

7. A normal intake of fluids during the collection period is desirable unless otherwise indicated by the physician.
8. Some laboratory assays require special dietary restrictions; these instructions should be given to the patient.
9. If possible, medications should be discontinued for 48 to 72 hours preceding the urine collection as a precaution against interference in the laboratory assays.
10. The 24-hour urine specimen should be transported to the clinical laboratory as soon as possible. The specimen should be placed in an insulated bag or a portable cooler to maintain the cool temperature.
11. Following the verbal instructions for the 24-hour urine collection, the patient should be provided with written instructions (non–English speaking patients should receive instructions in their native language) as a reminder.

CEREBROSPINAL FLUID

✔ **Cerebrospinal fluid (CSF)** is obtained by a physician through a spinal tap, or lumbar puncture. The fluid is usually collected in three sterile containers numbered in the order in which they were collected. The first tube is usually contaminated with blood. Thus, the second and third tubes are usually used for analysis. Tests commonly performed on CSF include total protein level, glucose level, cell count, microbiological, chloride level, and cryptococcal antigen determinations. CSF must be transported immediately to the clinical laboratory for stat analysis.

FECAL SPECIMENS

✔ Stool (fecal) specimens are commonly collected in order to detect parasites [e.g., **ova and parasites (O&P)**], enteric disease organisms (e.g., *Salmonella, Shigella, Staphylococcus aureus*), and viruses. The specimen is collected in a wide-mouthed plastic or waxed cardboard container with a tight fitting lid. If the patient is to collect the stool specimen at home, he or she should be given a collecting container and instructed to avoid urinating in the container because urine can kill the microorganisms in the collected stool specimen. For children, the container can be placed under the toilet seat so that the child can sit on the toilet. The patient should be instructed to wash the outside of the specimen container after collection and to wash his or her hands thoroughly. The specimen container must be properly sealed to prevent leakage and contamination because fecal material from patients with infectious intestinal diseases is extremely hazardous. The specimen must be transported to the laboratory immediately and maintained at body temperature (37°C) for detection of parasitic infections.

In addition to the collection of stool specimens for microorganism detection, feces are collected to detect invisible (occult) quantities of blood that do not alter the appearance of the stool. Laboratory determination of **occult blood** assists in the confirmation of the presence of blood in black stools and can be helpful in detecting gastrointestinal (GI) tract lesions and colorectal cancer. Feces for occult blood tests are often collected by the patient using special test cards such as Hematest (Miles Laboratories, Inc., Elkhart, IN). The cards can be mailed or brought to the health care facility after collection. Manufacturers have also developed occult blood tests that can be performed at home without collecting a stool specimen. A chemically impregnated pad is dropped into the toilet by the patient after he or she has a bowel movement. The patient watches for a color change that he or she reports to the physician via a special test result card supplied with each patient kit. The health care workers involved in specimen collection and transportation should be aware of the procedural steps for these occult blood tests to instruct the patient for proper collections.[4]

SEMINAL FLUID

Semen is examined in the clinical laboratory to: 1) determine the effectiveness of vasectomy; 2) investigate the possibility of sexual criminal charges, and 3) assess fertility. Before collection of a semen specimen, the patient should be given clear instructions for proper specimen collection. Semen must be collected in containers that are clean and free of trace detergents. Condoms can be used but must be washed free of spermicidal substances prior to use. Specimens must not be exposed to extremes of temperature or light prior to being submitted to the clinical laboratory and should be transported within 2 hours of collection.

AMNIOTIC FLUID

Fluid that bathes the fetus within the amniotic sac is called **amniotic fluid.** It may be collected by a physician when the pregnant patient is at approximately 16 weeks' gestation so that fetal abnormalities can be detected through chromosomal analysis and chemical tests such as the alpha-fetoprotein (AFP) assay. Occasionally, amniotic fluid is obtained in the last trimester of pregnancy to determine the lung maturity of the fetus. When transporting amniotic fluid to the laboratory, the specimen must be protected from light and transported immediately.

OTHER BODY FLUIDS

In addition to the fluids just discussed, other types of body fluids that sometimes must be transported to the laboratory include synovial fluid, which is extracted aseptically from joint cavities, and fluid aspirated from body cavities (e.g., pleural fluid obtained from the lung cavity, pericardial fluid from the heart cavity, peritoneal fluid from the abdominal cavity).

Upon receiving any type of body fluid for transportation, it is important to verify that the container is properly labeled with the patient's name, the patient's identification number, the date, the time of collection, and the type of body fluid collected.[4]

CULTURE SPECIMENS

Other specimens that the health care worker may be requested to transport to the clinical laboratory include sputum (fluid from the lungs, containing pus), throat and sinus drainage cultures, wound cultures, ear or eye cultures, and skin cultures. The health care worker should be extremely careful while transporting each type of specimen because the specimens can easily become contaminated and may be biohazardous. For safety, the health care worker needs to wear gloves when handling and transporting these specimens in their containers.

OTHER NONBLOOD PROCEDURES

Throat and Nasopharyngeal Culture Collections

Nasopharyngeal cultures are often performed to detect carrier states of *Neisseria meningitidis, Corynebacterium diphtheriae, Streptococcus pyogenes, Haemophilus influenzae,* and *Staphylococcus aureus.* For infants and children, from whom significant sputum cultures are difficult to obtain, nasopharyngeal cultures may be used to diagnose whooping cough, croup, and pneumonia. Throat cultures are most commonly obtained to determine the presence of streptococcal infections. Because coughing may force organisms from the lower respiratory tract into the nasopharynx, it may be best to perform a throat culture on a child or an infant and stimulate coughing in order to obtain a more significant nasopharyngeal culture. Health care workers should be thoroughly taught the correct procedures before they are allowed to acquire specimens from patients.

When a throat culture is ordered, the patient should be instructed to open the mouth wide, as if to yawn. A light source should be directed into the mouth and throat so that areas of inflammation, ulceration, exudation, or capsule formation can be readily seen. A tongue blade or spoon is used to depress the tongue and to prevent contamination with organisms from the oral cavity. A sterile cotton swab should be used to brush both tonsillar areas, the posterior pharynx, and all other areas of possible infection.[5]

The swab can then be placed in a special transport medium or the fluid on the swab can be inoculated directly onto agar in a Petri dish by rolling the swab across a small area of the medium. The specimen can then be transported to the laboratory, where it may be spread out, or "streaked," for distribution of the microorganisms. A Gram-stained smear is often useful to provide preliminary indications of infection and should be made with the swab by rolling it across a sterile slide before placing it in a transport medium or inoculating plate agar. The slide, the swab, and any inoculating media should be taken to the laboratory and processed as soon as possible after collection. The culture should be placed under optimal growth conditions for suspected pathogens (i.e., the culture should be incubated). Timely processing of the specimen helps prevent overgrowth of normal flora, which can inhibit or mask any pathogenic organisms present.

Nasopharyngeal specimens should be obtained with a Dacron- or cotton-tipped flexible wire that can be easily sterilized prior to use. Commercially packaged sterilized swabs are also available. The swab is passed gently through the nose and into the nasopharynx, where it is rotated. Then, the swab is carefully removed and placed in a transport medium or the fluid on the swab is inoculated onto a medium for isolation. Again, the timely processing of all specimens is crucial for best results.

Skin Tests

On occasion, a nurse or other health care worker may be asked to perform a **skin test.** The health care worker should check the policies of the health care facility prior to performing the procedure. Skin tests are simple and relatively inexpensive. They determine whether a patient has ever had contact with a particular antigen and has produced antibodies to that antigen. A wide range of disease states stimulate antibody responses in individuals. Tests range from detection of ragweed and milk allergies in hypersensitive individuals, to detection of tuberculosis and fungal infections in persons who have had contact with these organisms.

The skin test is administered by pulling 0.1 mL of diluted antigen into a tuberculin syringe. All air bubbles should be expelled by holding the syringe vertically and tapping the sides of the barrel. The volar surface of the patient's forearm should be cleaned with alcohol and prepared in the same manner as for a venipuncture (see Chapter 5). The area should be devoid of scars, skin eruptions, and excessive hair. Holding the syringe at a slight angle (approximately 20 degrees), the needle should be slipped just under the skin. The plunger should be pulled back to ensure that a blood vessel has not been entered. The fluid may be slowly expelled into the site. The needle should be promptly removed, and only slight pressure applied, with gauze, over the site. Care should be taken that the fluid does not leak onto the gauze or run out of the injection site. The patient should hold the arm in an extended position until the site has time to close and retain the fluid. A bandage should not be used over the site because it may absorb some of the fluid and distort the results of the skin test by causing skin irritation from the adhesive.

The patient should report any reaction, no matter how slight, to the physician. Also, a return visit for proper interpretation of the skin reaction should be scheduled with the physician. At some health care agencies, the patient is asked to note the exact size of the reaction site and to indicate this size on a prelabeled card that can be mailed back to the institution. When this is the case, patients should be fully informed about how to read these reactions.

Gastric Analysis and Hollander Test

✔ **Gastric analysis** and the **Hollander test** both involve gastric (stomach) fluid to determine gastric function in terms of stomach acid production. The gastric analysis measures gastric acid secretion in response to stimulation from histamine or pentagastrin, whereas the Hollander test uses insulin to stimulate gastric secretions. Both tests involve passing a tube through the patient's nose and into the stomach. Both tests also require intravenous (IV) administration of the stimulant. Therefore, although the health care worker may be asked to assist and to draw specimens as required, the responsibility for properly intubating the patient (using fluoroscopic examination) and administering the stimulant intravenously should rest with the physician or the nurse. The health care worker can be present to assist in patient care and to draw any required blood specimens, but under *no* circumstances should be expected to carry out the procedure. Improper placement of the tube poses a high risk to the patient and could result in a punctured lung if the tube enters the bronchial system instead of the esophagus. The health care worker can and should be responsible for proper labeling of gastric and blood samples when he or she is present and assisting during the procedure.

Sweat Chloride by Iontophoresis

The sweat chloride test is used in the diagnosis of cystic fibrosis.[6] Cystic fibrosis is a disorder of the exocrine glands, generally thought to be enzymatic in nature, that causes changes in mucus-producing glands in the body. Primarily affected are the lungs, upper respiratory tract, liver, and pancreas. Patients with cystic fibrosis produce chloride in their sweat at two to five times the level produced by healthy individuals.

For the laboratory evaluation, pilocarpine hydrochloric acid (HCl) is iontophoresed into the skin of the patient to stimulate sweat production. The sweat is absorbed onto preweighed gauze pads, then the weight of the sweat is determined. The pad is then diluted with deionized water, and the chloride is generally read by titration with a chloridometer.

When a health care provider receives an order to perform a sweat chloride test on a patient, he or she should properly prepare for the procedure under the supervision of a medical technologist. Four cups and lids should be preweighed with two 2-in.-square gauze pads in each cup. Only two cups are normally used, but the other two can be used as backups, if needed.

Choosing a site with the largest surface area (in children and infants, the leg is best suited), the health care worker should wipe the surface of the skin with a gauze pad soaked in deionized water. Next, the area is wiped dry. Another 2-in.-square, eight-ply gauze pad is soaked in 0.07 moles/liter sodium bicarbonate and placed on the cleaned area. The negative electrode is placed on the gauze and taped securely to the skin. The electrode should not come into direct contact with the skin at any time when the current is on.

Another gauze square is soaked in 0.33 percent pilocarpine HCl and placed on the skin next to the sodium bicarbonate square, but not touching it. The positive electrode should be placed on this piece of gauze and taped securely in place. Again, care should be taken that the electrode does not come into direct contact with the skin at any time during the procedure. Before the current is turned on, the area between and around the secured gauze squares should be wiped dry.

Next, the current is turned on and very slowly increased to 1 mA. The current must be incremented slowly because a sudden increase may electrically shock the patient. After 10 minutes, the current is decreased to zero. The switch is turned off and the electrodes and gauze squares are removed and discarded. Reagent-grade water is used to wipe off the pilocarpine HCl area, which is then wiped dry.

A 2×2-in. square of thin waxed film, such as Parafilm, should be cut out and handled with clean forceps. Using the forceps, the film can be placed against the cleaned area and tape it securely onto the skin on adjacent sides. Still using the forceps, two gauze pads from a preweighed cup are removed and placed between the Parafilm and the skin. The remaining side can be taped securely. Tape may also be applied across the top of the Parafilm to prevent it from tearing. A timer should be started for 1 hour. During that period, the procedure should be repeated on the other arm or leg.

After 1 hour, the tape should be carefully removed and the gauze sponges removed with forceps and returned to the original cup. The lid must be placed tightly on the cup and the cup weighed again. After weighing, 200 µL of deionized water should be added to the cup. The lid should be replaced and wrapped securely with Parafilm. The gauze sponges should equilibrate 2 to 3 hours or overnight. The cups and a record of the weights measured during the procedure should be taken to the laboratory, where a clinical laboratory scientist will measure the chloride with the chloridometer and calculate the results.

✔ Key Terms

AMNIOTIC FLUID	OVA AND PARASITES (O&P)
BLOOD UREA NITROGEN (BUN)	PERICARDIAL FLUID
CEREBROSPINAL FLUID (CSF)	PERITONEAL FLUID
CLEAN-CATCH MIDSTREAM	PLEURAL FLUID
CREATININE CLEARANCE	RANDOM URINE SAMPLE
CULTURE AND SENSITIVITY (C&S)	SKIN TEST
GASTRIC ANALYSIS	SPUTUM
HOLLANDER TEST	SWEAT CHLORIDE TEST
OCCULT BLOOD	SYNOVIAL FLUID

Study Questions

For the following, choose the ONE best answer:

1. What type of urine specimen is needed to detect an infection?
   a. random
   b. clean catch
   c. routine
   d. 24 hour

2. Which of the following types of specimens is most frequently collected for analysis?
   a. amniotic fluid
   b. urine
   c. CSF
   d. pericardial fluid

3. Which of the following body fluids is extracted from joint cavities?
   a. pleural fluid
   b. peritoneal fluid
   c. synovial fluid
   d. pericardial fluid

4. The O&P analysis is requested on what type of specimen?
   a. CSF
   b. amniotic fluid
   c. fecal
   d. synovial fluid

5. Fetal abnormalities are detected through analysis of
   a. pleural fluid
   b. peritoneal fluid
   c. amniotic fluid
   d. CSF

6. The occult blood analysis is frequently requested on what type of specimen?

   a. CSF
   b. fecal
   c. throat culture
   d. seminal fluid

7. Ketosis is frequently detected with which of the following conditions?

   a. liver disease
   b. diabetes mellitus
   c. chemical poisoning
   d. infection

8. Which of the following body fluids is obtained from the abdominal cavity?

   a. synovial fluid
   b. pericardial fluid
   c. peritoneal fluid
   d. CSF

9. Which of the following can be used in children and infants to diagnose whooping cough?

   a. CSF culture
   b. nasopharyngeal culture
   c. amniotic fluid culture
   d. pericardial fluid culture

10. What is the specimen of choice for drug abuse testing?

   a. CSF
   b. urine
   c. synovial fluid
   d. gastric fluid

REFERENCES

1. Garza D: Urine collection and preservation, in Ross DL, Neely AE (eds): *Textbook of Urinalysis and Body Fluids*. New York, Appleton-Century-Crofts, 1983, p 61.
2. Free AH, Free HM: *Urinalysis in Clinical Laboratory Practice*. Cleveland, CRC Press, 1975.
3. National Committee for Clinical Laboratory Standards (NCCLS): *Routine Urinalysis and Collection, Transportation, and Preservation of Urine Specimens*. NCCLS Document GP16-T, Villanova, PA, NCCLS, December 1992.
4. Henry J (ed): *Clinical Diagnosis and Management by Laboratory Methods*. Philadelphia, W.B. Saunders, 1991.
5. Becan-McBride K, Ross D: *Essentials for the Small Laboratory and Physician's Office*. Chicago, Mosby-Year Book, 1988.
6. National Committee for Clinical Laboratory Standards (NCCLS): *Sweat Testing: Sample Collection and Quantitative Analysis*. NCCLS Document C34-P, Villanova, PA, NCCLS, March 1993.

BEDSIDE GLUCOSE TESTING

A 59-year-old Hispanic woman having non–insulin dependent diabetes mellitus tested her glucose level at home on March 14, 1995, and obtained a glucose reading of 320 mg/dL using a test strip. Because she was having symptoms of sweating, feeling bad, and feeling lightheaded, the woman went to her physician the next day. Her physician immediately hospitalized her for treatment of uncontrolled diabetes. During the hospitalization, the following glucose meter v. clinical laboratory comparisons were performed:

DATE	GLUCOSE METER RESULTS (mg/dL)	LABORATORY TEST RESULTS (mg/dL)
3/15/95	151	198
3/16/95	192	238
3/17/95 (AM)	96	267
3/17/95 (PM)	120	246

From product performance specifications, hospital personnel determined that the comparisons for March 15 and March 16 were within the acceptable product performance variation range. However, the last two comparisons fell outside the acceptable range. The patient indicated that she followed the preventive maintenance schedule described in the documentation packaged with the glucose meter. The calibration was checked weekly, and the last calibrator reading, which was performed on March 17, was in range. A control run on March 16 resulted in a reading of 129 mg/dL, with confidence limits of 90 to 120 mg/dL.

Questions:

1. What is the problem in this case study?
2. What troubleshooting technique(s) should have been implemented to resolve this problem?

SAFETY PROCEDURES

IV

*P*art IV provides a more detailed look at regulatory factors that affect the health care professional in practicing phlebotomy and associated procedures. The chapters cover methods for protecting patients and providers from the risks of infections and hazardous situations, ways to document information about phlebotomy practices, and procedures for proper transportation of specimens.

Chapter 12, Infection Control, describes the essentials of infection control, which include surveillance, knowledge of the chain of infection, and isolation protocol. Detailed procedures are presented that are designed to protect the patient from infections and to protect the employee from being exposed. Infection control programs designed for various hospital units are also described.

Chapter 13, Safety and First Aid, provides basic procedures for safe handling of specimens, equipment, and reagents in the work setting. Topics covered include fire, electrical, radiation, mechanical, and chemical safety procedures, as well as emergency care procedures.

Chapter 14, Documentation and Transportation, provides the essentials of documentation and the clinical or medical record. Special components that relate to phlebotomy practice are highlighted, such as specimen requisition forms, labels, and reports. Specimen transportation and delivery procedures are also described.

twelve

12

INFECTION CONTROL

Chapter Outline

Chapter Objectives

Upon completion of Chapter 12, the learner is responsible for the following:

1. Define the term *nosocomial infection.*

2. Identify the basic programs for infection control.

3. Explain the proper techniques for hand washing, gowning, gloving, masking, double bagging, and entering and exiting the various isolation areas.

4. Identify the potential routes of infection and methods for preventing transmission of microorganisms through these routes.

5. Describe the various isolation procedures and reasons for their use.

The condition in which the body is invaded with pathogenic bacteria, fungi, viruses, or parasites is called *infection.* **Nosocomial infections** are those that are acquired after admission to a health care facility, such as a hospital, a clinic, a nursing home, or a psychiatric institution. Approximately 5 percent of all hospitalized patients in the United States acquire nosocomial infections.[1] These infections are often harmful to the patient and costly to both patients and insurers; each year, millions of dollars are spent on nosocomial infections. In an attempt to control them, **infection control programs** have been developed. Using guidelines established by the Centers for Disease Control and Prevention (CDC), the Joint Commission for Accreditation of Healthcare Organizations (JCAHO), and state regulatory agencies, managers of each health care institution are responsible for developing and implementing an infection control program. These programs usually address the issues of **surveillance,** reporting, **isolation procedures,** education, and investigation of epidemics within the health care institution. An infection control nurse or practitioner usually works closely with or in the clinical microbiology laboratory and communicates with personnel in the health care facility to make the necessary assessments.

SURVEILLANCE

In most health care institutions, the infection control program involves monitoring and collecting data on several specific populations such as (1) patients at a high risk of infection; (2) patients with previously acquired infections; (3) personnel or patients accidentally exposed to a communicable disease, contaminated equipment, or hazardous reagents; and (4) patients in certain areas of the hospital or in certain rooms. The health care worker should be aware of these special circumstances for two reasons. First, the health care worker can take the necessary precautions to prevent infecting him- or herself or the patient. Second, the health care worker can mentally prepare to deal with these special patients in a professional and humanistic manner. Because each health care facility has its own infection control program and policy manual, the health care worker should read and be familiar with both.

Infection control surveillance also involves classification of infections according to prevalence rates. The prevalence rates of commonly identified nosocomial infections are represented in Figure 12–1. Each of the infections cited in this figure can be transmitted in a variety of ways,

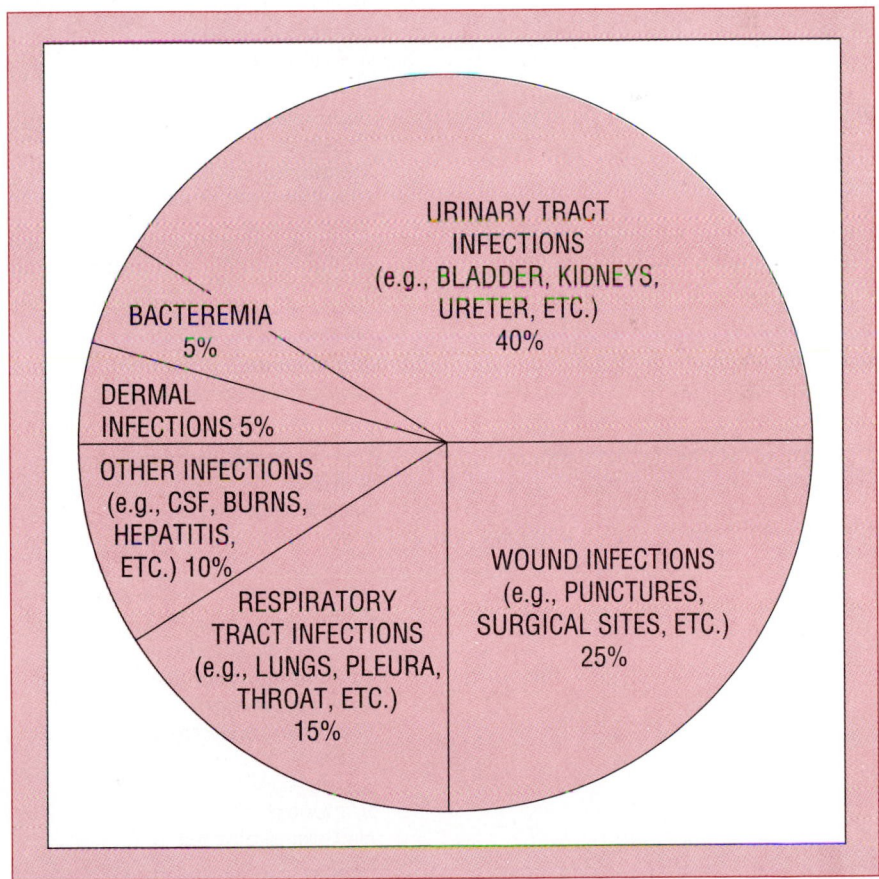

Figure 12–1. Prevalence of nosocomial infections. CSF, cerebrospinal fluid. *(From Castle M, Ajemian E: Hospital Infection Control. New York, John Wiley & Sons, 1987, with permission.)*

TABLE 12–1. PATHOGENIC AGENTS CAUSING NOSOCOMIAL INFECTIONS

Body Areas or Hospital Areas	Commonly Identified Pathogenic Agents
Blood and cerebrospinal fluid	Any microorganisms
Burn unit	All Gram-negative bacilli Gram-positive rods Fungi
Dialysis unit	Hepatitis and other viruses Bacteria Fungi
Ear	*Pseudomonas aeruginosa* *Streptococcus pneumoniae* Gram-negative bacilli
Eye	*Staphylococcus aureus* *Neisseria gonorrhoeae* Gram-negative bacilli *Moraxella lacunata* *Haemophilus influenzae* *S. pneumoniae* *P. aeruginosa*
Gastrointestinal tract	*Salmonella* sp. *Shigella* sp. *Yersinia enterocolitica* Enteropathogenic *Escherichia coli* *Vibrio cholerae* *Campylobacter* sp. Parasitic protozoans *Candida albicans* Some viruses
Genital tract	*N. gonorrhoeae* *Haemophilus vaginalis* *C. albicans* (yeast)
Intensive care or postoperative care unit	Any microorganisms
Nursery unit	*S. aureus* Group B *Streptococcus* *E. coli* *S. pneumoniae* Other Gram-negative bacilli Viruses
Respiratory tract	*Streptococcus pyogenes* *Corynebacterium diphtheriae* *Bordatella pertussis* *Staphylococcus epidermidis* *S. aureus* *S. pneumoniae* *H. influenzae* Any Gram-negative bacilli Fungi Certain viruses

(continued)

TABLE 12–1. *(Continued)*

Body Area or Hospital Areas	Commonly Identified Pathogenic Agents
Skin	*S. aureus*
	S. pyogenes
	C. albicans
	Smallpox
	Herpes virus
	Enterovirus
	Measles
Urinary tract	Any microorganism in sufficient numbers
Wounds and abscesses	Any microorganisms

and each health care worker should realize that he or she can be a potential recipient or transmitter of infectious agents. Table 12–1 lists causative agents for nosocomial infections.

Infection control programs also monitor employee health programs. The primary objective is to minimize the risk of infection or hazardous circumstances for employees and patients. Most employees are screened for the following diseases prior to employment: measles, mumps, tuberculosis, hepatitis, diarrheal disease, syphilis, and skin diseases. Immunization for a variety of diseases is often made available initially and throughout employment, free of charge. Often, the hospital stipulates policies for employees with specific infections or employees who have been exposed to certain infections, such as those listed in Table 12-2.

For the employee's protection, many types of warning labels are used. Among these are color-coded isolation signs and radiation hazard signs. Radiation signs may be posted on the hospital doors of patients treated with radioactive isotopes. In general, a short period of contact with these patients is not significant; however, the National Committee for Clinical Laboratory Standards (NCCLS) recommends that pregnant employees avoid contact with these patients.[2]

CHAIN OF INFECTION

Nosocomial infections result when the **chain of infection** is complete. The three components that make up the chain are **source, mode of transmission,** and **susceptible host.**[3]

Source

In a normal environment, relatively few things are sterile; therefore, potential sources of infection cover a wide range. Inanimate objects, as

TABLE 12–2. EMPLOYEE INFECTIONS OR SPECIAL CIRCUMSTANCES[a]

Disease	Work Status	Duration of Work or Work Limitations
AIDS	May work with restriction	Evaluated by Employee Health Physician
Draining abscess, boils, and so forth	Off	Until drainage stops, if employee has patient contact
Chicken pox (varicella)	Off	For 7 days after eruption first appears in normal host, provided lesions are dry and crusted when they return

Diarrhea
  Shigella
  Salmonella
	Variable	Individual, depending on extent of symptoms, cultures, and evaluation by Personnel Health Service

Gonorrhea	May work	
Hepatitis A	Off	Must bring note from private physician upon return
Hepatitis B	Off	Must bring note from private physician upon return
Herpes simplex	May work	Evaluation by Personnel Health Service, depending on work area
Herpes zoster	No patient contact	If able to work, may do so
Influenza and URI	Variable	Evaluation by Personnel Health Service, depending on work area
Impetigo	Off	No patient contact until crusts are gone
German measles (rubella)	Off	Until rash clears (minimum of 5 days)
Measles	Off	Until rash clears (minimum of 4 days)
Mononucleosis	Off	At discretion of private physician
Positive PPD conversion	May work	Evaluation and follow-up by Personnel Health Service
Pregnancy (first or second trimester)	May work	Avoid contact with patients having viral or rickettsial infections or those being treated with radioactive material
Pregnancy (third trimester)	May work	Avoid contact with patients in any type of isolation
Active TB	Off	Until under treatment and smears are negative for 2 weeks
Scabies	Off until treated	
Strep throat (group A)	Off	May work 24 hours after being placed on appropriate antibiotic therapy and symptom free

Abbreviations: PPD, purified protein derivative; TB, tuberculosis; URI, upper respiratory tract infection.
[a] Sample guideline for employees with infection; their work status and when they can return to work.
Adapted from Castle M. Ajemian E: Hospital Infection Control. New York, John Wiley & Sons, 1987, with permission.

well as people, are colonized with various microorganisms, many of which help carry out normal body functions. Some of these microorganisms, however, are more pathogenic than others. For example, relatively few *Shigella* organisms need to be ingested before a diarrheal infection occurs. However, with *Salmonella*, large numbers of the organisms must be ingested before symptoms appear. Conversely, numerous anaerobic and aerobic bacteria must be present in the gastrointestinal (GI) tract for normal metabolism to occur.

Regarding the sources of nosocomial infections, infection control practitioners must consider the amount of contamination, viability of the infectious agent, virulence of the agent, length of time from contamination to contact, and the manner in which the agent is transmitted from the source. Sources of nosocomial infection are numerous in the health care environment (Table 12–3). For instance, human hands provide a warm, moist environment for microorganisms. Therefore, a physician, phlebotomist, or nurse can transmit organisms from themselves or an infected patient to another potential host. Uniforms or other clothing that comes in contact with infectious agents and is then worn around other patients is another potential source of infection. Likewise, medical instruments that come into contact with open wounds, mucous membranes, or organs can transmit microorganisms. For example, an instrument such as a fiber-optic bronchoscope may be used repeatedly only if thoroughly decontaminated after each use. Otherwise, it may be implicated in transmitting bacterial pneumonia. Although many other pieces of invasive equipment are also potential transmitters unless adequately sterilized, some pieces of equipment that can become contaminated with bacteria are less likely to cause infection. As an example, tourniquets come in contact with intact skin but are less likely sources of infection. However, they should also be decontaminated after use.

TABLE 12–3. CONSIDERATIONS FOR SOURCES OF NOSOCOMIAL INFECTIONS

Health care personnel (e.g., lack of hand washing between patients)

Visitors

Medical instruments [e.g., contaminated needles, intravenous (IV) catheters, Foley catheters, bronchoscopes, respiratory therapy equipment]

Medical reagents (e.g., IV fluid)

Other patients (e.g.,those having severe wound drainage)

Mode of Transmission

The second link in the chain of infection involves transmission from the source to the next host. **Pathogenic agents** may be transmitted by five modes: (1) direct contact, (2) air, (3) medical instruments, (4) other objects, and (5) other vectors. Direct contact involves close or intimate contact with an infected person. For example, some patients acquire staphylococcal infections, chicken pox, hepatitis, or diarrhea after touching other infected individuals. During contact, the infective microorganism rubs off one person onto another. Hand washing is the best means of preventing infections transmitted by this route.

Microscopic airborne droplets may carry infectious agents, such as the causative agent of tuberculosis and Legionnaire's disease. Droplets may become airborne in the following instances: when an individual coughs or sneezes, when linens are shaken, when dust is stirred by sweeping, or when ventilation is inadequate. Preventive measures include wearing a mask, isolating specific patients, and ensuring good ventilation.

As mentioned previously, invasive medical instruments may expose a susceptible patient to pathogenic agents. To prevent instrument-induced infections, health care personnel should change or decontaminate instruments such as tourniquets and catheters after each use. Needles should be used only once, then disposed of in appropriate containers.

Other inanimate objects, such as toys in the pediatric areas, common toilets and sinks, linens, and water fountains are all potential modes of transmission. Objects that can adhere to infectious agents and transmit infection are called **fomites.** Common health care facility fomites are listed in Table 12–4. Preventing transmission by fomites can be accomplished by following isolation techniques, using **sterile technique** for injections or venipuncture, wearing gloves during equipment handling, and restricting the use of common toys or facilities.

Many insects (mosquitoes, ticks, fleas, mites) and rodents act as vectors in transmitting infectious diseases such as plaque, rabies, and malaria. Patients may be exposed to these vectors in unsanitary conditions or in areas where the diseases are prevalent.

Susceptible Host

The third link in the chain of infection is the susceptible host. Factors that affect a host's susceptibility are age, drug use, the degree and nature of the illness, and the status of the immune system. The patient's progress in the hospital significantly affects his or her chances of ac-

TABLE 12–4. FOMITES COMMONLY FOUND IN HEATLH CARE FACILITIES

Computer keyboards
Door knobs
Telephones
Countertops
Scrub suits
Phlebotomy trays
Eyeglasses
Pens and pencils
Water-faucet handles
Laboratory coats
Manuals and books
Phlebotomy supplies and equipment
IV equipment

quiring an infection. Underlying diseases, such as diabetes, acquired immune deficiency syndrome (AIDS), and cancer, as well as therapeutic measures (chemotherapy, radiation therapy, antibiotics), all change the status of the body and make it a potential host for infection.

Breaking the Chain

Infection control programs aim at breaking the infection chain at one or more links, as shown in Figure 12–2. Hand-washing procedures for sterile technique, proper waste disposal, appropriate laundry services, and housekeeping are ways of controlling the sources. Isolation techniques, control of insects and rodents, and use of disposable equipment and supplies help interrupt the modes of transmission. Host susceptibility is controlled by speeding the patient's recovery. Immunizations, transfusions, proper nutrition, medication, and adequate exercise all help the patient to regain health.

ISOLATION PROCEDURES

Isolation procedures, methods of removing diseased individuals from society, date to antiquity. Although the supplies for and methods of isolation have been updated, the fear of being contaminated and the stigma associated with a patient in isolation are still present. The psychological effects of being a patient in isolation are profound. Therefore, the health care provider should make an effort to reduce these patients' anxiety by communicating in a calm, professional, and reassuring manner.

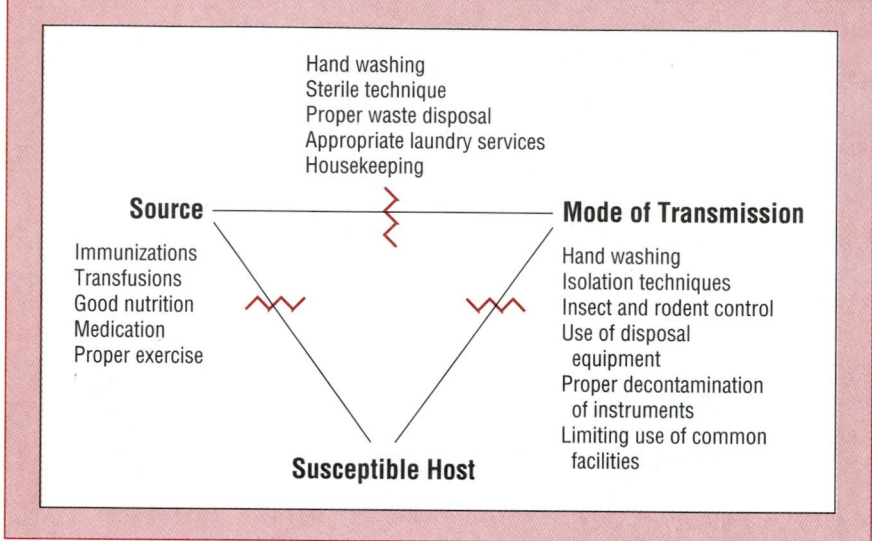

Hand washing
Sterile technique
Proper waste disposal
Appropriate laundry services
Housekeeping

Source ——————————————→ **Mode of Transmission**

Immunizations
Transfusions
Good nutrition
Medication
Proper exercise

Hand washing
Isolation techniques
Insect and rodent control
Use of disposal
  equipment
Proper decontamination
  of instruments
Limiting use of common
facilities

Susceptible Host

Figure 12–2. The chain of nosocomial infection can be interrupted by infection control procedures.

New CDC Isolation Guideline

In the past, isolation procedures were established in varying degrees. They ranged from sterile rooms or wards to isolation procedures for one disease only. Isolation techniques were formally divided into two types by the CDC: category-specific precautions and disease-specific precautions.[3] The new federal guideline on hospital isolation precautions may clarify the instances in which specific infection control actions should be taken.[4] The change should avoid the inconsistent use of universal precautions and **body substance isolation (BSI)** practices (both described later in this chapter) among health care facilities.

Under the new guideline: (1) **standard precautions** are combined with isolation practices for moist and potentially infectious body substances (BSI practices) into a single set of safeguards, which are to be used for the care of all patients; (2) the old categories of isolation and disease-specific precautions have been collapsed into three sets of precautions based on the route of transmission: airborne, droplet, and contact; and (3) specific syndromes in both adult and pediatric patients that are highly suggestive of infection are listed.

Hospitals have the option to continue with alternative isolation procedures; therefore, they may continue with previously used procedures. The most common types of procedures in use have been the category-specific isolation precautions, shown in Figure 12–3 and discussed later in this chapter and in Figure 12–4.

Standard Precautions

Standard precautions are a combination of the universal precautions and the BSI practices. These precautions apply to blood, *all* body fluids, nonintact skin, and mucous membranes. Standard precautions are designed to reduce the risk of transmission of microorganisms from both recognized and unrecognized sources of infection in health care facilities. All the steps of the universal precautions apply to the standard precautions for health care workers involved in blood collection.

Category-Specific Isolation Precautions

Strict or Complete Isolation. **Strict (complete) isolation** has been required for patients with contagious diseases—that is, diseases that may be transmitted by direct contact and by air. Examples include anthrax, rabies, smallpox, measles, chicken pox, plague, diphtheria, and streptococcal and staphylococcal pneumonia. The patients are housed in private rooms with closed doors, and all articles in the room should be handled as if they are contaminated. Patients are usually restricted to their rooms. If they must be moved, they should be covered appropriately. Personnel entering these rooms must wear gowns, masks, and gloves. Hand washing is critically important. All items taken into the room must be left there in the appropriate location (Fig. 12–4).

Figure 12–3. Isolation signs and warning signs.

Isolation Technique for Laboratory Personnel

Principle:

Laboratory personnel must practice isolation techniques when collecting specimens from infectious patients. Doing so helps prevent transmission of the disease to the laboratorian and to other patients by means of the technologist.

Procedure:

1. Check the sign posted on the door of an isolation room. It will tell you the type of isolation and to what extent the isolation procedures must be followed. The types of isolation are as follows:
   a. *Complete (strict):* anthrax, rabies, smallpox, measles, chicken pox
   b. *Respiratory:* whooping cough, meningococcal meningitis, mumps, rubeola
   c. *Protective (reverse):* immuno-suppressed or burn patient
   d. *Drainage/secretion:* postoperative, skin infections
   e. *Enteric: Salmonella, shigella,* typhoid fever, hepatitis A
   f. *Contact:* group A strep, pneumonia, rubella
   g. *Tuberculosis (or AFB):* tuberculosis
2. Check with the nursing station to find out the patient's diagnosis. Female personnel who are pregnant or think they might be should avoid all patients isolated for viral or rickettsial infections. Pregnant women in their last trimester should not go into *any* isolation rooms.
3. Except for protective isolation, any equipment taken into the room must be left there. Make sure that a needle–tube assembly, a tourniquet, and a pen are in the room before entering. Protective isolation rooms should have the needle–tube assembly and a tourniquet already in the room. Isolation rooms will have either an anteroom in which isolation equipment is kept or a cart outside the door for the same purpose.
4. Put on a sterile gown, touching only the inside. Make sure that your back is completely covered, and tie the belt. Pull the sleeves all the way down.
5. Place a mask over your nose and mouth. Tie both ties comfortably around your head. For AFB isolation, a fitted high-efficiency particulate air (HEPA) respirator must be worn.

Figure 12–4. Isolation technique for laboratory personnel. *(From Hermann Hospital Clinical Laboratories, Houston, TX, with permission.)*

6. Put on disposable gloves, trying not to touch the palms with your hands. When entering a protective isolation room, wash your hands thoroughly before you put on *sterile* disposable gloves. Pull the gloves up over the sleeves of the gown.

7. Invert the isolation bag halfway inside out and leave it near the door outside the room. Take only the equipment that you will need into the room. Leave the requisition slip on the cart outside the room.

8. Check the patient's armband and collect your specimen. Label the specimen with the information on the patient's armband, leaving the pen in the room.

9. Dispose of the needle in the sharps biohazardous box in the room. Throw the cotton swab and any gauze flats into the biohazardous container in the room.

10. Before placing the tubes in the isolation bag, wipe the outside of the tubes with a paper towel moistened with cold water to remove any blood that may be on the outside of the tubes. Touching only the inside of the biohazardous bag, place the tubes inside the bag, standing in the doorway of the room. Touch only the inside of the bag; avoid touching other items or areas outside the room with gloved hands.

11. Wash your gloved hands in the patient's room. Dry your hands and turn off the faucet with a paper towel.

12. Remove your gown by breaking the paper tie and touching only the inside. Fold it with the contaminated side on the inside and discard it.

13. Remove the first glove.

14. Remove your other glove by sliding the index finger of the opposite hand between the glove and your hand. Discard the gloves.

15. Wash your hands again, using a paper towel to turn off the faucet.

16. Leave the unit: Place a clean paper towel over the door knob and open the door. Hold the door open with one foot and discard the paper towel in the wasetbasket beside the door. Place the tubes of blood in the isolation container for return to the laboratory.

17. Check the labeled tubes against the requisition slip to be sure that the patient from whom blood was collected was the patient for whom the tests were ordered.

Figure 12–4. (*continued*)

> 18. Wash your hands at the nursing station before going to the next patient's room.
>
> *Quality Control:*
>
> The only means of quality control is strict adherence to the procedure.

Figure 12–4. (*continued*)

✔ *Respiratory Isolation.* **Respiratory isolation** has been required for patients with infections that may be transmitted over short distances through the air (droplet transmission). Examples include whooping cough, meningococcal meningitis, mumps, and measles. Patients are housed in private rooms with closed doors. Anyone entering the room must wear a mask, as should the patient if he or she is moved. All contaminated supplies should be disposed of in the patient's room.

✔ *Enteric Isolation.* **Enteric isolation** has been required for patients with infections that are transmitted by ingestion of the pathogen. Examples include diarrheal diseases—such as *Salmonella, Shigella, Escherichia coli, Yersinia, Staphylococcus, Campylobacter, Vibrio,* and amebic dysentery—and other parasitic infections. Ideally, patients should be housed in private rooms. Their bathroom facilities should *not* be used by hospital personnel, other patients, or visitors. People entering these rooms should wear gowns and gloves. All contaminated materials should be disposed of in the patient's room.

✔ *Drainage/Secretion Isolation.* **Drainage/secretion isolation** has been required after surgery or if a patient is admitted with a skin infection. Postoperative wounds, catheters, and intravenous (IV) apparatuses may become infected, and microorganisms can be transmitted to other patients by direct or indirect contact. Patients are generally restricted to their rooms, and all entering people should wear gowns and gloves. When these patients are moved, procedures to prevent transmission should be implemented (e.g., covering the infected site).

✔ *Contact Isolation.* **Contact isolation** was designed to prevent the spread of highly transmissible infections that do not warrant strict isolation but are conveyed primarily by direct contact. This type of isolation is necessary for pediatric patients having acute respiratory infections (e.g., influenza, pneumonia), patients with major skin infections that are draining severely, and patients with antibiotic-resistant microorganisms. Masks are required for health care workers who must go near the patient. Gowns are indicated if soiling is likely, and gloves are always indicated for performing the phlebotomy. Hands must be washed before and after the use of gloves. The gown, mask, and gloves must be discarded or bagged and labeled before they are sent for decontamination and reprocessing.

Tuberculosis Isolation. **Tuberculosis isolation** has been indicated for patients with infectious tuberculosis. This type of isolation is sometimes referred to as *AFB* (acid-fast bacilli) to protect the patient's confidentiality. Because multiple cases of drug-resistant tuberculosis have been reported, new guidelines were developed for health care workers who come in contact with these patients. The new guidelines emphasize the importance of and necessity for wearing an appropriate mask when the health care worker must share air space with the patient having infectious tuberculosis. A mask must be appropriately fitted to *each* health care worker who cares for patients with active tuberculosis. On October 10, 1993, the **Occupational Safety and Health Administration (OSHA)** implemented a policy that requires the use of National Institute for Occupational Safety and Health (NIOSH)–approved high-efficiency particulate air (HEPA) respirators as a minimum level of respiratory protection when health care workers enter AFB isolation rooms.[5]

Disease-Specific Isolation Precautions

Another type of isolation precautions has been designed to prevent the transmission of most of the common infectious diseases in the United States. This type of isolation protocol has been used less often than the category-specific precautions because **disease-specific isolation** precautions include specific procedures for dealing with more than 150 diseases. These diseases are listed in the older version of the CDC isolation guideline.[6]

BSI Practices

Body substance isolation (BSI) is a newer, alternative isolation system. This type of isolation focuses on the isolation of potentially infectious moist body substances (blood, urine, saliva, feces, sputum, wound drainage, and other body fluids).[7] This isolation technique is based on the presumption that all body substances may carry infectious agents and thus precautions should be used whenever health care personnel are working with any of these substances.

The BSI technique focuses on isolation of moist body substances through the use of barrier precautions, primarily gloves, and diagnosis of patients who have some of the diseases that are transmitted by air. A stop-sign alert (Fig. 12–5) must be placed on the door of any room inhabited by a patient with one of these diseases. Before entering a room with a stop-sign alert, the health care worker must consult the floor nurse who will determine whether he or she should wear a mask to collect the blood specimens.

Body substance isolation includes the following:[7]

1. Gloves must be worn for contact with blood, body fluids, secretions, mucous membranes, nonintact skin, and all moist substances from the body. Gloves *must* be changed between patients. Hand washing must also occur after and before each patient's blood collection. If running water is not available (e.g., home health care setting), the health care provider should use the decontaminating rinses or foams available through various vendors for hand washing.
2. A fluid-resistant gown, a mask, and goggles should be worn when secretions, blood, or body fluids are likely to spill or splash onto the clothing of the health care worker.
3. Soiled articles must be placed in a biohazardous container or bag. If the container or bag is contaminated on the outside, it

**REPORT TO FLOOR NURSE
BEFORE ENTERING**

STOP

**FAVOR DE ANUNCIARSE A LA ENFERMERA DE PISO
ANTES DE ENTRAR AL CUARTO**

Figure 12–5. Stop-sign alert for body substance isolation.

should be placed in a double bag, as discussed subsequently in this chapter.

4. Needles should never be recapped. They, and other sharp items (e.g., lancets), should be placed in rigid, puncture-resistant, biohazardous containers that display the required labels. Before going to off-site settings (e.g., home health care visits), the health care worker must remember to take a biohazardous container along for sharps disposal.

5. Private rooms and additional precautions are necessary for patients with certain diseases (e.g., pulmonary tuberculosis, contagious diseases requiring strict isolation, cancer patients requiring reverse isolation).

6. Health care workers must be immunized against infectious agents transmitted by airborne or droplet routes (e.g., measles, mumps, rubella) before entering the rooms of patients with these infections.

UNIVERSAL PRECAUTIONS FOR HEPATITIS AND HIV

Patients who are infected with blood-borne pathogens such as hepatitis or HIV cannot always be readily detected. Therefore, the CDC states that "under universal precautions, all patients should be assumed to be infectious for HIV and other blood-borne pathogens."[8] These universal precautions eliminate the need for a separate isolation category of "blood and body-fluid precautions." However, other categories of isolation precautions should be retained if conditions are appropriate. The following six points summarize the necessary precautions for preventing the transmission of blood-borne pathogens.[8,9]

1. All health care workers should routinely use appropriate barrier precautions to prevent skin and mucous membrane exposure when contact with blood or other body fluids of any patient is anticipated. Barriers (e.g., gloves, facial masks, respirators, gowns, shields) are also referred to as *personal protective equipment (PPE)*. Gloves should be worn (a) for touching blood and body fluids, mucous membranes, or nonintact skin of all patients; (b) for handling items or surfaces soiled with blood or body fluids; and (c) for performing venipunctures and other vascular access procedures. Gloves should be changed after contact with each patient. Masks and protective eyewear or face shields should be worn to prevent exposure of mucous membranes of the mouth, nose, and eyes during procedures that are likely to generate droplets of blood or other body fluids. Fluid-resistant gowns or aprons should be worn during procedures

that are likely to generate splashes of blood or other body fluids. As explained in the section of this chapter entitled "Tuberculosis Isolation," a personal respirator should be used if the risk of aerosolized *Mycobacterium tuberculosis* is present.

2. Hands and other skin surfaces should be washed immediately and thoroughly if contaminated with blood or other body fluids. Hands should be washed immediately after gloves are removed.

3. All health care workers should take precautions to prevent injuries caused by needles, scalpels, and other sharp instruments or devices (a) during procedures, (b) when cleaning used instruments, (c) during disposal of used needles, and (d) when handling sharp instruments after procedures. To prevent needle-stick injuries, health care workers should not recap needles, purposely bend or break them by hand, remove them from disposable syringes, or otherwise manipulate them by hand. After they are used, disposable syringes and needles, scalpel blades, and other sharp items should be placed in puncture-resistant containers for transport to the reprocessing area.

4. Although saliva has not been implicated in HIV transmission, to minimize the need for emergency mouth-to-mouth resuscitation, health care workers should ensure that mouthpieces, resuscitation bags, or other ventilation devices are available for use in areas in which the need for resuscitation is predictable.

5. Health care workers who have exudation lesions or weeping dermatitis should refrain from all direct patient care and from handling patient care equipment until the condition resolves.

6. Pregnant health care workers are not known to be at greater risk of contracting HIV infection than health care workers who are not pregnant; however, if a health care worker develops HIV infection during pregnancy, the infant is at risk of infection resulting from perinatal transmission. Because of this risk, pregnant health care workers should be especially familiar with and strictly adhere to precautions to minimize the risk of HIV transmission.

OSHA STANDARDS FOR OCCUPATIONAL EXPOSURE TO BLOOD-BORNE PATHOGENS

OSHA, an agency of the US Department of Labor, requires employers to provide measures that will protect workers exposed to biological hazards. On December 6, 1991, OSHA standards for occupational exposure to blood-borne pathogens, based mainly on the use of the hepatitis B vaccine and the previously described CDC recommendations regarding universal precautions, were published.[9] These standards require the employer to provide the following:

1. An implementation and compliance program requiring all employers and employees to observe universal precautions.
2. PPE devices to minimize the risk of infection from blood-borne pathogens (e.g., fluid-resistant gowns, goggles, respirators).
3. Engineering practice controls that isolate or remove the blood-borne pathogen hazard from the health care facility (e.g., sharps disposal containers, self-sheathing needles).
4. Work practice controls that change the manner in which a blood collection task is performed to reduce the likelihood of exposure (e.g., prohibiting needle recapping; prohibiting eating, drinking, or smoking in the clinical laboratory).
5. Appropriate cleaning methods in blood and other body fluid collection areas to prevent exposure to infectious agents (e.g., use of 10 percent solution of household bleach as a disinfectant for the area).
6. The hepatitis B virus (HBV) vaccine available at no cost to employees. The HBV vaccine protects against HBV, as well as delta hepatitis. The hepatitis virus is the most frequently occurring laboratory-associated infectious agent. It attacks the liver and is a life-threatening blood-borne pathogen. Currently, it is the most infectious occupational health hazard in health care facilities.
7. Postexposure follow-up for employees exposed to HBV and HIV. The follow-up must involve an immediate confidential medical evaluation of the employee. The employee's medical record must include the employee's name, social security number, and HBV vaccination dates. Health care workers are concerned about HIV because it is a blood-borne pathogen that leads to a poor prognosis (i.e., development of AIDS) if workers are exposed by needle stick or another method. Although the incidence of HIV infections occurring as a result of on-the-job exposure is relatively low, caution must be used because no vaccine is available for protection.
8. Training and educational information on blood-borne pathogens (e.g., HIV and HBV) available for employees at no cost and accessible during the employees' working hours. These training sessions must occur at the beginning of task assignment involving occupational exposure to blood-borne pathogens. Each employee must have annual training on this

topic, and each employer must maintain an accessible copy of OSHA's blood-borne pathogen standards with statements that relate these standards to the specific health care facility's environment.

9. Labels and signs that warn of biological hazards and contaminated waste. These labels and signs must be affixed to appropriate refrigerators, freezers, waste containers, and storage cabinets containing infectious materials. The labels must be fluorescent orange or orange-red, bearing the word *biohazard* in English and other predominant languages spoken in the region (e.g., *peligro biologico* in Spanish). In addition, the biohazard symbol shown in Chapter 13, Figure 13–4 should be on the label. Alternatively, red or orange bags may be substituted for labels.

Blood-Borne Exposure Procedures

OSHA requires managers at health care facilities to provide a confidential medical evaluation, treatment, and follow-up for any employee who has had a blood-borne exposure incident (e.g., needle stick).

Immediately after an exposure incident, the employee must (1) decontaminate the needle-stick site with an appropriate antiseptic (e.g., iodine) for 30 seconds or (2) flush the exposed mucous membrane site (e.g., eyes) with water for 10 minutes. Then, he or she should report the incident to his or her supervisor, who will direct the employee to the appropriate clinic for medical evaluation, treatment, and counseling.

The medical evaluation involves the following five steps:[8]

1. The exposed health care worker's blood is tested for HIV in an accredited laboratory.
2. The source individual is identified and tested for HIV and HBV, if the person gives permission.
3. If the source individual tests positive for HIV, the exposed health care worker is given counseling and evaluated for HIV infection immediately, 6 weeks, 12 weeks, and 6 months later. Also, azidothymidine (AZT) therapy is provided to the exposed employee as soon as possible, preferably within 1 hour of exposure.
4. If the source individual does not consent to testing and is in a high-risk category, the exposed health care worker is given immune globulin or an HBV vaccination.
5. The exposed health care worker is counseled to be alert for acute viral symptoms within 12 weeks of exposure.

This entire medical evaluation must be completely confidential.

ISOLATION FOR HOSPITAL OUTBREAKS

Occasionally, outbreaks of particular infections occur in one or more hospital areas. For example, infection control surveillance may reveal that the nursery unit is having an excessive number of cases of staphylococcal infection. To control the outbreak, the infection control staff may dictate the need for special precautions, isolation procedures, or employee screening for staphylococcal carriers. Any health care worker entering or exiting these areas should be made aware of the special circumstances.

PROTECTIVE, OR REVERSE, ISOLATION

Many patients are put in isolation not because they have an infection, but because they are highly susceptible to infection and need to be protected from the external environment. Therefore, this type of isolation is referred to as **protective (reverse) isolation.** In general, keeping the patient in a private room and using good hand-washing techniques are sufficient precautions for health care workers caring for patients in protective isolation, but additional precautions such as gowns, gloves, and masks may also be used. Articles may be removed from the room and do not need to be double bagged because these patients do not have infections. However, articles *entering* the room must be sterile or carefully decontaminated.

A few hospitals in the United States have large protective isolation facilities for patients with combined immunodeficiencies who must live in an environment that is completely sterile. All food and articles are sterilized before they are taken into the patient's room. Some patients must live their entire lives in such a protected environment.

INFECTION CONTROL IN HOSPITAL UNITS

Other areas where patients are at a high risk of infection are the nursery, the burn unit, the postoperative care unit, or intensive care unit (ICU), and the dialysis unit. The clinical laboratory plays an important role in infection control in these hospital units and is also subject to specific infection control procedures.

Infection Control in a Nursery Unit

Newborns are easy targets for infections of all sorts because their immune systems are not fully developed at birth. Neonates may pick up pathogens from their mothers, other babies, or hospital personnel. The best way to minimize infection is to use gloves and an antiseptic for hand washing. Special clothing may be worn by nursery personnel, changed daily, and limited to the unit. Bibs should be used and discarded after contact with only one baby. Often, a baby is assigned a single nurse to limit the possible sources of infection transmission. Babies whose mothers have genital herpes must be isolated from other infants. Mothers with genital herpes must also be isolated. All individuals having contact with either the mothers or the children must be gowned and gloved, and double-bagging procedures must be used for disposal of contaminated articles in the patient's room.

Infection Control in a Burn Unit

Patients with burns are also highly susceptible to infection. In some institutions, infection rates for burn patients are lower because of the availability of a completely isolated environment for each patient. Each bed is surrounded by a plastic curtain with sleeves. Hospital personnel use these sleeves when having contact with the patient. All supplies and equipment are kept outside the curtain.[1]

In hospitals lacking these facilities, burn patients are housed in private rooms. Gowning, gloving, **double bagging** (as described later in this chapter), and strict hand-washing procedures should be used. All articles in the room, as well as the room itself, should be disinfected or sterilized frequently.

Infection Control in an ICU or a Postoperative Care Unit

Patients in ICUs are more critically ill and, by nature, more susceptible to infections. In most hospitals, ICUs are open areas, with numerous patients in one large room so as to be more easily monitored. Patients with known infections should be isolated according to the types of infections they have, and strict hand-washing and gloving policies are necessary in all ICUs.

Postoperative patients are susceptible to infection because surgical wounds or drains enable bacteria to gain easy access to deeper tissues. Again, each patient who becomes infected should be isolated and dealt with according to the type of infection acquired.

Infection Control in a Dialysis Unit

Patients needing dialysis are most often immunosuppressed, which makes them a high-risk group for contracting infection, especially hepatitis. Protective gowns and gloves may be worn in the unit, and strict hand-washing and gloving techniques should be adhered to.

Infection Control in the Clinical Laboratory

The clinical laboratory contributes to infection control programs in the following manner:

1. Maintaining laboratory records for surveillance purposes
2. Reporting on infectious agents, drug-resistant microorganisms, and outbreaks
3. Evaluating the effectiveness of sterilization or decontamination procedures

Laboratory personnel must be cautious because they often handle specimens with infectious agents. Laboratorians have a higher incidence of hepatitis antigen, tuberculosis, tularemia, and Rocky Mountain spotted fever than that of other hospital personnel.[1] Many of these infections are acquired by aerosol spray, needle sticks, spills, mouth pipetting, and eating, drinking, or smoking in the laboratory. Such danger can easily be prevented or minimized by adhering to policies that prohibit mouth pipetting, eating, drinking, and smoking in the laboratory. Other useful procedures include hand washing; gloving; wearing protective clothing such as laboratory coats, scrubs, and face shields, if appropriate; surface decontamination; and careful disposal of needles.

The health care worker should remember that the quality of laboratory test results is only as good as the specimen collected. If the specimen is contaminated or improperly collected, laboratory test results reflect this fact and may be misleading. If sloppy techniques are used, the potential for mistakes and infection is greater. Table 12–5 details the infection control policies that health care workers must follow during blood collection.

TABLE 12–5. INFECTION CONTROL RESPONSIBILITIES REQUIRED IN BLOOD COLLECTION

Maintaining good personal hygiene, including wearing clean clothes, keeping hair clean and tied back if necessary, keeping fingernails clean, and washing hands frequently

Maintaining good health by eating balanced meals in the designated areas, getting enough sleep, and getting enough exercise

Reporting personal illnesses to supervisors

Becoming familiar with and observing *all* isolation policies

Learning about the job-related aspects of infection control and sharing this information with others

Cautioning all personnel working with known hazardous material (this can be done with proper warning labels)

Reporting violations of the policies

Reporting potential candidates for infection control (e.g., patients who are jaundiced)

SPECIFIC ISOLATION TECHNIQUES

In most hospitals, all supplies required for isolation procedures are located in an area or on a cart just outside the patient's room. After washing their hands, health care personnel may put on the appropriate PPE just prior to entering the room.

Hand Washing

Hand washing is the most important procedure in the prevention of disease transmission in hospitals. It should be the first and last step of any isolation procedure (Fig. 12–6A–C). Scrubbing for surgery requires a different procedure than washing hands for general patient care. For general purposes, hand washing usually removes potential pathogens but does not necessarily sterilize the hands. Good technique involves soap, warm running water, and friction.[1] Soap removes oils that may hold bacteria to the skin. Many varieties of soap are available for gen-

A.

Figure 12–6. Specific isolation techniques: hand washing, gowning, masking, gloving, and double bagging. **A.** Hand-washing techniques should involve soap lather, friction between hands, and thorough washing between fingers. **B.** Washing should include the wrist areas. **C.** Lather should be rinsed. Rinsing should continue until all soap is removed. If the water must be turned off by hand, a clean paper towel should be used to grab the faucet. **D.** Gowns should be large enough to cover all clothing. Sleeves should be pulled down and the back covered. **E.** The mask should be tied in two places and should fit comfortably. **F.** Gloves should be pulled over the ends of gown sleeves. **G–I.** After specimen collection, the gown should be removed from inside out. **J.** Double bagging involves two individuals, one inside the room and one outside.

B.

C.

D.

E.

Figure 12–6. (*continued*)

Figure 12–6. (*continued*)

eral purposes. However, health care personnel who purchase supplies should choose soaps that are mild, easy to use, and form a good lather. Warm running water washes away loosened debris and lathers the soap. Friction from rubbing the hands together loosens and removes dead skin, oil, and microorganisms. The health care worker should thoroughly rub both sides of each hand and between each finger. Hands should be rinsed in a downward position. After rinsing, the faucet should be turned off by grasping the handles with paper towels to prevent reinoculation of microorganisms onto the hands.

Gowning

After hand washing, a sterile gown should be put on by touching only its inside surface. It should have long sleeves and be large and long enough to cover all clothing (Fig. 12–6D). Gowns are generally made of cloth or paper. The health care worker's back must be completely covered, the belt tied, and the sleeves pulled all the way to the wrists.

Masking

After gowning, a mask (if necessary) may be put over the nose and mouth (Fig. 12–6E). Often, a small metal band on the mask can be shaped to fit the nose. Two ties are usually made, the first around the upper portion of the head and the second around the upper portion of the neck. Most masks become ineffective after prolonged use (20 minutes).[1]

Gloving

Chemically clean disposable gloves may be used for most isolation procedures. The exception is protective isolation procedures, for which *sterile* disposable gloves should be used. Gloves should be pulled over the ends of gown sleeves (Fig. 12–6F). Rings and other pieces of jewelry should not be worn because they may puncture a glove during patient contact.

Entering and Exiting the Room

Isolation bags for transporting specimens are often available. The bag may be turned halfway inside out and left near the door outside the room, or someone may be available to hold the bag outside the door. Only the needed supplies should be taken into the room. Phlebotomy requisitions may be left outside the room on the isolation cart. If drawing a blood specimen, the health care provider may use a tourniquet in the room or leave the one brought in. The specimen should be labeled at the bedside and the pen left in the room. Used needles, swabs, and so forth should be put in appropriate containers inside the room. Any blood on the outside of the specimen container should be removed with a paper towel. While standing in the doorway, and touching only the inside of the isolation bag, the health care worker should place the specimen inside the bag. Gloved hands should be washed in the room. The faucet may be turned off with a paper towel.

The mask, if used, can be removed by carefully untying the lower tie first, then the upper one. Only the ends of the ties should be held. The mask should then be properly disposed of inside the room. In some cases, a special container for masks is placed just outside the room to prevent exposure of hospital personnel to airborne diseases while inside.

The gown is removed by first breaking the paper tie or untying the sash. It should be removed and folded with the contaminated side turned inside and with care taken not to touch the uniform (Fig. 12–6G–I). One glove may be removed, and the second one can be slipped off by sliding the index finger of the ungloved hand between the glove and the hand.

Just before leaving the room, however, hands must be washed again and a paper towel used to turn off the faucet. A clean paper towel should be used to open the door. The door should be held open with one foot and the used paper towels discarded in the wastebasket directly inside the patient's room.

Once outside the room, the requisition forms may be checked again, placed carefully in the isolation bag, and sealed. Care must be taken to avoid touching the inside of the bag holding the specimen. Personnel should wash their hands again before proceeding with other duties.

Disposing of Contaminated Items

Trash, linens, and other articles in an isolation room may be removed by using one sturdy biohazardous bag or the double-bagging procedure. Double bagging involves putting contaminated material in one bag and sealing it inside the room. A different person should stand outside the doorway with another opened, clean, impermeable bag (Fig. 12–6J). The person standing outside the room should have the ends of the bag folded over the hands to shield them from possible contamination. The sealed bag from the room may then be placed inside the clean bag. The person outside the room can then fold over the edges, expel the air, and seal the outer bag. The bag must be labeled with biohazard warnings.

PREVENTION OF LABORATORY-ACQUIRED INFECTIONS

As mentioned previously, health care workers must be extremely cautious with biohazardous specimens. Policies and procedures for handling such specimens should be defined in the laboratory policy manual and should be reviewed periodically by health care workers who collect and transport specimens. Infections from these specimens may be spread during collection and handling by means of several routes. The actual occurrence of an infection from a biohazardous specimen depends on the virulence of the infecting agent and the host's susceptibility. The following are possible routes of infection from collected specimens and therefore should be considered when health care personnel must collect or process specimens for laboratory assays:

1. *Skin contact.* Virulent organisms can enter through skin abrasions and cuts or through the conjunctiva of the eye. Thus, scratches from needles and broken glass must be avoided. If the health care worker has a cut or an abrasion, he or she should always wear a laboratory coat, gloves, and protective adhesive tape over the cut or abrasion to prevent possible inoculation from infectious specimens. He or she must also avoid rubbing the eyes.

2. *Ingestion.* Failure to wash contaminated hands and subsequent handling of cigarettes, gum, food, or drinks can result in an infection from a biohazardous specimen. Each employee must comply with the safety rules of the laboratory to prevent transmission of infections.

3. *Airborne.* As discussed in other sections, aerosol spray created from patient's specimens by careless splashing or centrifugation must be prevented. Dangerous, infectious aerosol spray can be caused from popping stoppers off blood specimen vacuum tubes and centrifugating the blood specimens. To protect against blood exposure during this hazardous step, manufacturers recently developed different types of items that minimize airborne transmissions (see Chapter 4, Blood Collection Equipment). Prior to centrifugation, vacuum tubes should be inspected for cracks and tubes with wet rims should be wiped dry. The centrifuge brake should not be applied to save time because braking can cause infectious aerosol formation. Centrifuged infectious specimens must not be poured because of the potential hazards from aerosol formation. Instead, the contents should be transferred by using a disposable pipette with a rubber bulb or its equivalent and gently transferring the contents down the wall of the aliquot tube or tubes.

STERILE TECHNIQUE FOR HEALTH CARE WORKERS

All health care personnel should realize that bacteria and other microorganisms can be found everywhere. For example, human skin is covered with bacteria. Because of this fact, all health care personnel should be responsible for cleanliness and maintaining sterility when handling instruments, catheters, IV supplies, or other devices that come into contact with patients.

The health care worker is responsible for using sterile supplies for skin punctures and venipunctures and antiseptics for patient preparation. Alcohol pads are often used to cleanse skin sites for venipuncture. Although rubbing with alcohol pads destroys most of the bacteria, it does not destroy all microorganisms. A special decontamination procedure is required to obtain a sterile site. Venipuncture for blood cultures requires this type of preparation, as discussed thoroughly in Chapter 9.

New needles and most blood collection tubes are sterilized by the manufacturers. Once the covering of a needle or a lancet is removed, the needle or lancet should not touch anything until it punctures the skin. If it accidentally touches *anything* prior to contact with the skin site, it must be discarded appropriately and replaced with a new one. If a nee-

TABLE 12–6. COMMON ANTISEPTICS AND DISINFECTANTS FOR THE HEALTH CARE SETTING

Compound	Uses and Restrictions
Alcohols	
Ethyl (70%)	Antiseptic for skin
Isopropyl (70%)	Antiseptic for skin
Chlorine	
Chloramine	Disinfectant for wounds
Hypochlorite solutions	Disinfectant
Ethylene oxide	Disinfectant (toxic)
Formaldehyde	Disinfectant (noxious fumes)
Glutaraldehyde	Disinfectant (toxic)
Hydrogen peroxide	Antiseptic for skin
Iodine	
Tincture	Antiseptic for skin (can be irritating)
Iodophors	Antiseptic for skin (less stable)
Phenolic compounds	
1–2% Phenols	Disinfectant
Chlorophenol	Disinfectant (toxic)
Hexachlorophene	Antiseptic for skin (used in surgery)
Chlorhexidine	Antiseptic for skin
Hexylresorcinol	Antiseptic for skin
Quaternary ammonium compounds	Antiseptic for skin (ingredient in many soaps)

dle is used for an unsuccessful venipuncture, it too *must* be discarded and replaced with a new one before another puncture is attempted.

Sterile technique and isolation procedures may require sterile gloves. If this is the case, the health care worker must make sure that the package of gloves indicates that they are sterile. Some manufacturers produce gloves that are *chemically clean* but not necessarily *sterile*. Most sterile gloves are available in various hand sizes. If the gloves do not fit properly, they may interfere with the procedure.

Disinfectants and Antiseptics

Disinfectants are chemical compounds used to remove or kill pathogenic microorganisms.[10] Chemical disinfectants are regulated by the Environmental Protection Agency (EPA). Antiseptics are chemicals used to inhibit the growth and development of microorganisms but do not necessarily kill them. Antiseptics may be used on human skin, whereas disinfectants are generally used on surfaces and instruments because they are too corrosive for direct use on skin. An intermediate-level disinfectant with a product label claiming that the disinfectant is HIVcidal or tuberculocidal, or a disinfectant having a chlorine bleach dilution of 1 : 10, should be used to disinfect tourniquets and items contaminated with blood or other body fluids. A more diluted solution of chlorine bleach (1 : 32) is used for routine cleaning of surfaces.[11] Table 12–6 lists some of the more common hospital disinfectants and antiseptics used.

✔ Key Terms

Antiseptics

Body Substance Isolation (BSI)

Chain of Infection

Contact Isolation

Disease-Specific Isolation

Disinfectants

Double Bagging

Drainage/Secretion Isolation

Enteric Isolation

Fomites

Infection Control Programs

Isolation Procedures

Mode of Transmission

Nosocomial Infections

Occupational Safety and Health Administration (OSHA)

Pathogenic Agents

Protective (Reverse) Isolation

Respiratory Isolation

Source

Standard Precautions

Sterile Technique

Strict (Complete) Isolation

Surveillance

Susceptible Host

Tuberculosis Isolation

Study Questions

The following may have one or more answers:

1. Which of the following types of nosocomial infections are most prevalent?
   a. dermal infections
   b. wound infections
   c. respiratory tract infections
   d. urinary tract infections

2. Name the links in the chain of infection.
   a. poor isolation technique
   b. susceptible host
   c. source
   d. mode of transmission

3. What is/are the primary function(s) of isolation procedures?
   a. keep the hospital clean
   b. prevent transmission of communicable diseases
   c. protect the general public from disease
   d. provide protective environments

4. Nurses, physicians, and other health care workers are responsible for knowing the procedures of which type(s) of isolation?

   a. strict
   b. drainage/secretion
   c. enteric
   d. protective, or reverse
   e. respiratory
   f. universal precautions

5. Which of the following precautions prevents infectious aerosol spray?

   a. popping the cap on a vacuum collection tube rather than twisting it
   b. inspecting vacuum tubes for cracks prior to centrifugation
   c. applying the centrifuge brake to save time during centrifugation of specimens
   d. pouring the specimens into the required aliquot tubes

6. Protective isolation is generally used for

   a. an adult patient with active tuberculosis
   b. a pediatric patient who has an immunodeficiency
   c. an adult patient with meningitis
   d. a pediatric patient who has whooping cough

7. Which of the following laboratory-acquired infections is most prevalent?

   a. HIV infection
   b. Rocky Mountain spotted fever
   c. HBV infection
   d. tuberculosis

8. Enteric isolation may be required for patients with infections such as

   a. tuberculosis
   b. whooping cough
   c. *Salmonella*
   d. Rocky Mountain spotted fever

9. According to the OSHA standards for occupational exposure to blood-borne pathogens, which of the following is a PPE?

   a. 10 percent household bleach
   b. fluid-resistant gown
   c. goggles
   d. respirator

10. In Spanish, *peligro biologico* refers to the English term

    a. hepatitis
    b. biohazardous
    c. blood-borne pathogen
    d. *Salmonella*

REFERENCES

1. Bennett JV, Brachman PS (eds): *Hospital Infections,* 3rd ed. Boston, Little, Brown & Co, 1992.

2. National Committee for Clinical Laboratory Standards (NCCLS): *Protection of Laboratory Workers from Infectious Disease Transmitted by Blood, Body Fluids and Tissues*. NCCLS Document M29-T2, Villanova, PA, NCCLS, 1991.
3. Castle M, Ajemian E: *Hospital Infection Control*. New York, John Wiley & Sons, 1987.
4. Department of Health and Human Services—Centers for Disease Control and Prevention (CDC): Guideline for isolation precautions in hospitals: Part I. Evolution of isolation practices and Part II. Recommendations for isolation precautions in hospitals. *Federal Register* Fall 1995.
5. Decker M: OSHA enforcement policy for occupational exposure to TB. Special report. *Infect Control Hosp Epidemiol* 4(12):689–693, 1993.
6. Garner JS, Simmons BP: CDC guideline for isolation precautions in hospitals. *Am J Infect Control* 12:103, 1984.
7. Lynch P, Jackson MM, Cummings MJ, et al: Rethinking the role of isolation precautions in the prevention of nosocomial infections. *Ann Intern Med* 107:243, 1987.
8. Guidelines for prevention of transmission of human immunodeficiency virus and hepatitis B virus to health-care and public-safety workers. *MMWR* 38(S-6):1989.
9. US Department of Labor and Occupational Safety and Health Administration (OSHA): Occupational exposure to bloodborne pathogens; final rule (29 CFR 1910.1030). *Federal Register* Dec 6:64004–64182, 1991.
10. Luebbert P: Choosing the appropriate disinfectant. *Lab Med* 23(2):126, 1992.
11. Texas Department of Health (TDH): *Infection Control Manual for Public Health Clinics*, 2nd ed. Austin, TX, TDH, 1993.

thirteen

13

SAFETY AND FIRST AID

Chapter Objectives

Upon completion of Chapter 13, the learner is responsible for the following:

1. Explain the measures that should be taken for fire, electrical, radiation, mechanical, and chemical safety in a health care facility.

2. Describe the essential elements of a disaster emergency plan for a health care facility.

3. Explain the safety policies and procedures that must be followed in all phases of specimen collection and transportation.

4. Describe the safe use of equipment in health care facilities.

The goal of safety in the health care institution is to recognize and eliminate hazards and provide information on safety education so that employees can work in a healthy environment. Safe working conditions must be ensured by the employer and have been mandated by law under the **Occupational Safety and Health Administration (OSHA) standards** (1910.1030).[1] Knowledge of OSHA requirements and cooperation between the employer and employee concerning these requirements are necessary in all health care facilities, including home health care agencies (Fig. 13–1). The health care worker involved in blood collection needs to become aware of safety policies and procedures in his or her health care facility and to receive proper instruction on safety requirements.

1. Gloves must be worn during *all* phases of blood collection procedures (at inpatient and outpatient facilities). Health care workers should make every effort to avoid contact with blood, body fluids, nonintact skin, and mucous membranes.
2. Gloves must be changed between patient collections, and hands must be washed after gloves are removed.
3. A laboratory coat, a smock, or a gown must be worn during blood collection procedures and left at the laboratory or clinic when the health care worker leaves the work area. The laboratory coat must be cleaned at the health care facility.
4. A personal respirator should be used if exposure to aerosolized *Mycobacterium tuberculosis* is possible.
5. Facial protection must be provided at the health care facility and used by the health care worker if any possibility of body fluid or blood splashing exists.
6. Needles should *never* be recapped by hand.
7. All sharps, including needles and lancets, must be disposed of *carefully* in a rigid needle container.
8. Blood collection items must be disposed of according to the proper procedure for biohazardous waste disposal.
9. Blood collection devices and surfaces must be decontaminated after use.

Figure 13–1. Safety precautions for the health care worker.

SAFETY IN SPECIMEN HANDLING

Patients' specimens should be handled with caution to prevent the possibility of acquiring an infection such as hepatitis or one associated with acquired immunodeficiency syndrome (AIDS). Health care workers who are routinely exposed to blood and body fluids must take the simple precaution of wearing gloves to protect themselves from infection. Further discussion of precautionary measures for specimen handling can be found in Chapter 12, Infection Control.

PERSONAL HYGIENE

While on the job, nothing should be inserted into one's mouth (e.g., food, pencils). Hands should be washed frequently during the day; before and after contact with patients or patients' specimens; before and after eating, drinking, or smoking; and before and after using restrooms. Cosmetics should not be applied while on the job (Fig. 13–2). The health care worker should avoid biting his or her fingernails and rubbing the eyes. Eating, drinking, or smoking within the specimen control section and other laboratory sections must be avoided. No food should be placed in any laboratory refrigerator unless the refrigerator is designated "FOR FOOD ONLY." A laboratory coat should be worn completely buttoned while collecting specimens and removed prior to coffee breaks or lunch. Loose clothing such as scarves, which might become entangled in the centrifuge, should never be worn. Long hair must be tied so that it cannot come in contact with specimens or become entangled in the centrifuge. Open-toed shoes are usually prohibited in most clinical laboratories because of potential chemical and glassware hazards.

LABORATORY SAFETY

Laboratory safety includes a variety of policies. However, all health care workers should remember a few key safety rules at all times. First, the patients' specimens should be covered at all times during transportation and centrifugation. Second, centrifugation of specimens should be performed within a biohazard safety hood. Third, all wastes from specimen collections must be disposed of in the correct containers. Specific **Environmental Protection Agency (EPA)** and OSHA regulations, as well as state and local laws, regulate the disposal of wastes. Blood and body fluids may be poured down a sink into the sanitary sewer if permitted by local ordinances. Urine specimens are usually flushed down the drain with water or flushed down the toilet. These biological liquid wastes

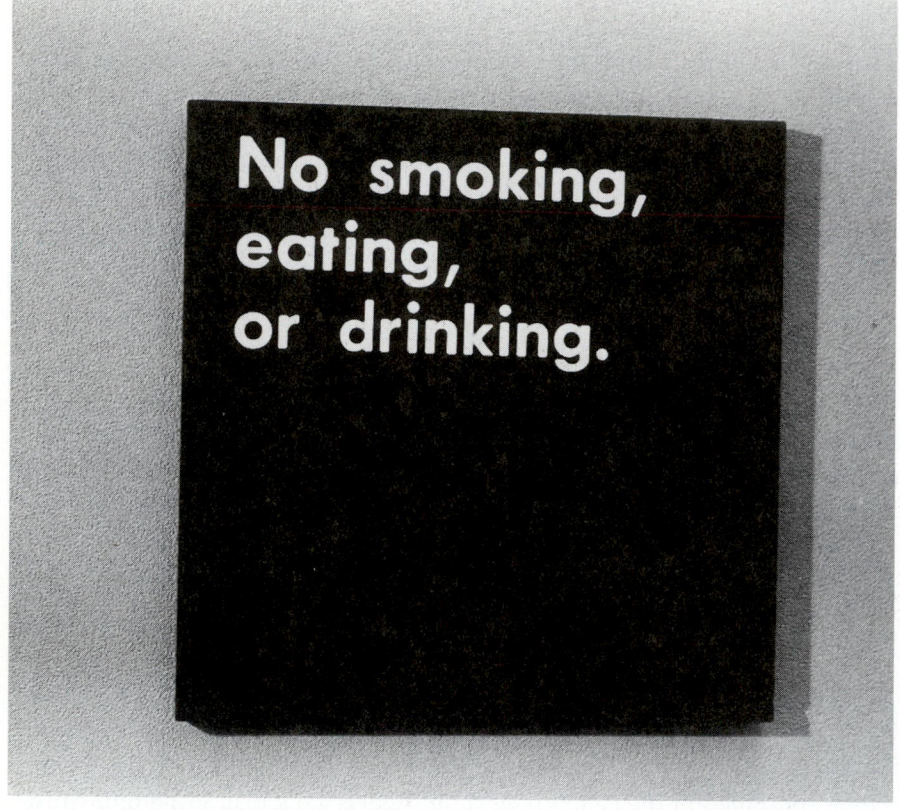

Figure 13–2. Required safety precautions during specimen collection.

should be disposed of gently so that they do not splash onto other objects, and hand washing should not occur in sinks used for disposal of these wastes. Needles *must not* be recapped before disposal (Fig. 13–3). Sharps such as needles and lancets should be disposed of in a special container that is spillproof, tamperproof, puncture resistant, and closable and that can be autoclaved. The sharps container must be labeled in red or orange, must be maintained upright, and must display the biohazard symbol (Fig. 13–4).

In addition, the specimen collection area should be decontaminated with a 1 : 10 bleach solution. Because a diluted bleach solution becomes unstable when exposed to oxygen, it must be prepared daily. Alternatively, a diluted bleach solution that is stable is available commercially. If blood or other body fluids are spilled, encapsulating powder, which is available from manufacturers of safety products (e.g.,

United Ad Label Direct, Brea, CA), should be used to gel the liquid for safe cleanup.

Colored biohazard labels must be affixed to all containers of regulated waste, refrigerators and freezers containing blood or other body fluids, and other containers used to store, transport, or ship these materials.

If an accident occurs, such as a needle stick, the injured health care worker should immediately cleanse the area with isopropyl alcohol and apply a Band-Aid. Then, he or she should notify the immediate supervisor, fill out the necessary incident and medical forms, undergo the appropriate laboratory tests [e.g., human immunodeficiency virus (HIV), hepatitis B], and receive a hepatitis B virus (HBV) vaccination. In addition, the health care worker should be counseled and evaluated for HIV infection at periodic intervals.

FIRE SAFETY

Fire safety is the responsibility of all employees in the health care institution. Health care workers should be familiar with not only the use and location of the fire extinguishers, but also the procedures to follow during a fire. They should also be knowledgeable of the exact locations of fire extinguishers and fire blankets. The blankets should be available to

Includes Blood and All Body Fluids

1. Wash hands BEFORE and AFTER patient care.

2. Wear gloves when likely to touch body substances, mucous membranes or non-intact skin.

3. Wear gown when clothing is likely to become soiled.

4. Wear mask and protective eyewear or a face shield when likely to be splashed with body fluids.

5. Place intact needle/syringe units and sharps in designated disposal container. DO NOT BREAK OR BEND NEEDLES.

UAL BHC

Figure 13–3. Universal precautions in patient care. *(Courtesy of United Ad Label (UAL) Co., Inc., Brea, CA.)*

Figure 13–4. Biohazard symbol.

smother burning clothes or to use as a fire shield if fire is blocking the exit. Health care institutions usually conduct periodic safety education programs in which the health care worker can participate and become skillful in and knowledgeable about the use of fire safety equipment.

Classification of Fires

The components of fire are fuel, oxygen, and heat, plus the necessary chain reaction. Four general classifications of fires have been adopted by the National Fire Protection Association (NFPA).[2] These classifications are as follows:

1. *Class A fires* occur with ordinary combustible material such as wood, rubbish, paper, cloth, and many plastics.
2. *Class B fires* occur in a vapor–air mixture over flammable solvents such as gasoline, oil, paint, lacquers, grease, and flammable gases.
3. *Class C fires* occur in or near electrical equipment.
4. *Class D fires* occur with combustible metals such as magnesium, sodium, and lithium. These fires are infrequently encountered in health care institutions.

Fire Extinguishers

Fire extinguishers are classified to correspond with each class of fire.

1. *Class A extinguishers* contain soda and acid or water and are used to cool the ordinary fire.

2. *Class B extinguishers* contain foam, dry chemicals, or carbon dioxide (CO_2) and are used to combat fires occurring in vapor–air mixtures over solvents.
3. *Class C extinguishers* contain dry chemicals, Halon (Allied Corporation, Morristown, NJ), or CO_2 (nonconducting extinguishing agents) and are used to combat electrical fires.
4. *Multipurpose (ABC) extinguishers* are frequently installed in health care institutions because they reduce the confusion associated with operating and maintaining different types of extinguishers.

As shown in Figure 13–5, the health care worker should learn how to use the various kinds of fire extinguishers in the workplace. Use of the wrong type of extinguisher may not only fail to put out the fire, but can actually spread it.

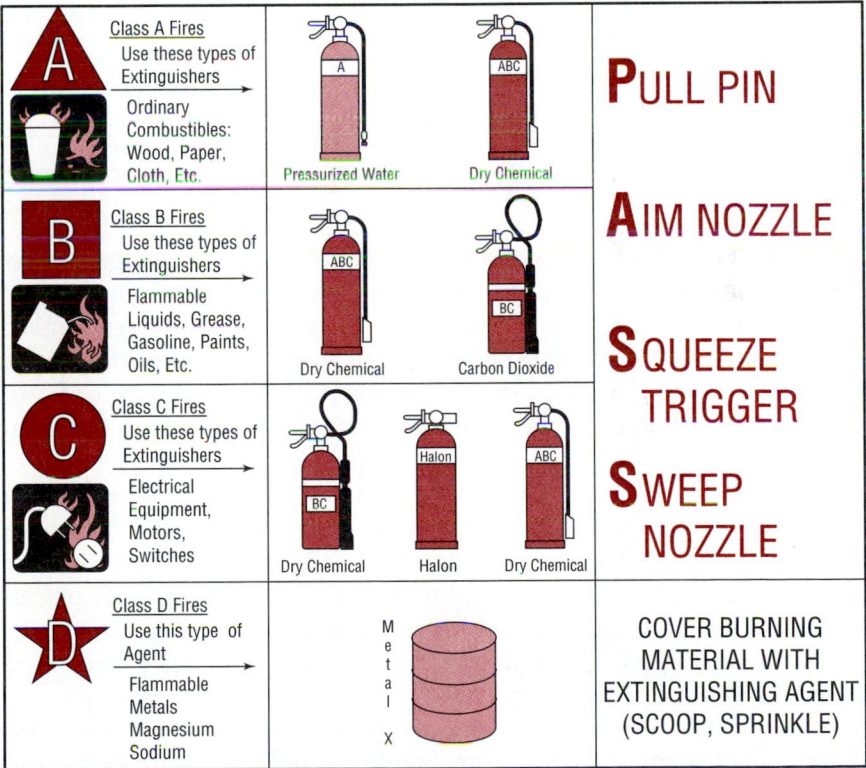

Figure 13–5. Proper use of fire extinguishers. *(Courtesy of Risk Analysis and Loss Control—Institutional Affairs, The University of Texas–Houston Health Science Center, Houston, TX.)*

In the event of a fire, the health care worker should *do* the following:

- Immediately pull the lever in the alarm box nearest the area he or she is in.
- Call the assigned fire number, which should be posted on or near each telephone.
- If the fire is small, attempt to extinguish it, using the proper extinguisher.
- If evacuation becomes necessary, use only the stairwells for exiting.
- Close all doors and windows before leaving the area.
- If clothing is on fire, drop to the ground and roll, preferably in a fire blanket.
- If caught in a fire, crawl to the exit. Because smoke rises, breathing is easier at floor level. Breathing through a wet towel is also helpful.

The health care worker should *not do* the following:

- Block entrances
- Reenter the building
- Panic
- Run

ELECTRICAL SAFETY

A major hazard in any area of a health care institution is the possibility of electrical current passing through a person. For example, in the clinical laboratory or physician office laboratory, the health care worker sometimes operates electrical equipment such as a centrifuge. He or she should be aware of the location of the circuit breaker boxes in order to assure a fast response in the event of an electrical fire or an electrical shock.

The health care worker should not use electrical equipment if power cords are frayed or if control switches and thermostats are not in good working order. The centrifuge or other electrical equipment must be unplugged before maintenance is performed. Any electrical instrument that has had liquid spilled on or in it or has had liquid come in contact with the wiring should be immediately unplugged and dried prior to further use.

If an electrical accident occurs involving electrical shock to an employee or a patient, the health care worker should be aware of the following two points:

1. The electrical power source must be shut off. If this is impossible, carefully remove the electrical contact from the

victim using something, such as asbestos gloves, that does not conduct electricity, or place your hand in a glass beaker and push the power supply away from the victim. The rescuer should not attempt to touch the victim without heeding these precautions.

2. Medical assistance should be called and **cardiopulmonary resuscitation (CPR)** started immediately. The victim should not be moved prior to the arrival of medical assistance. A fire blanket or other warm clothing should be put over the victim to keep him or her warm until medical help arrives.

RADIATION SAFETY

The three cardinal principles of self-protection from radiation exposure are time, shielding, and distance. Radiation exposure is cumulative; thus, limiting the length of exposure at any one time is a major factor in minimizing the hazard.

Areas where radioactive materials are in use and stored must have warning signs (Fig. 13–6) posted on the entrance doors. All radioactive specimens and reagents must also be properly labeled with the radioactive sign.

The health care worker will probably encounter potential hazards from radiation exposure only if he or she must collect specimens from

Figure 13–6. Sign for possible radiation hazard.

patients in the nuclear medicine or x-ray department or must take specimens to the radioimmunoassay section in the chemistry department. Thus, the health care worker should be cautious when entering an area posted with the radiation sign and should be knowledgeable of the institution's procedures pertaining to radiation safety. Health care workers who are pregnant should be aware of the potential hazard of radiation to the fetus.

MECHANICAL SAFETY

The centrifuge is a frequently used instrument for blood specimen preparation and testing. Thus, a health care provider who collects and prepares blood specimens for testing should learn how to maintain this instrument and become familiar with its parts. For example, he or she should know if the carriers are in the correct position prior to use. If the carriers are not in the correct position, they can swing out of the holding disks into the side of the centrifuge. Also, the wrong head, the wrong cups, or imbalanced tubes can lead to the same dangerous problem. If this particular type of accident occurs, tubes containing patients' specimens or spinning chemicals may be propelled onto the side of the centrifuge, and broken, and a dangerous, hazardous problem created. Thus, it is of utmost importance to abide by the preventive maintenance schedule and procedures for the centrifuge.

CHEMICAL SAFETY

Because a health care worker must sometimes pour preservatives such as hydrochloric acid (HCl) into containers for 24-hour urine collections and transport these specimens to the patients' floor, he or she should be knowledgeable of chemical safety. Labeling may be the single most important step in the proper handling of chemicals. Laboratorians should be able to ascertain from appropriate labels not only the contents of the container, but also the nature and the extent of hazards posed by the chemicals. Carefully read the label before using any reagents.

Chemical Identification

Various chemicals are needed in health care facilities, especially in the clinical laboratory department. Because chemicals may pose health or physical hazards, OSHA amended the *Hazard Communication Standard* (29 CFR 1910.1200, Right to Know/HCS Standard) to include health care facilities.[3,4] Thus, labels for hazardous chemicals must

(1) provide a warning (e.g., corrosive), (2) explain the nature of the hazard (e.g., flammable, combustible), (3) state special precautions to eliminate risks, and (4) explain first-aid treatment in the event of a chemical leak, a chemical spill, or other exposure to the chemical. In addition to mandating labels, the Right to Know law requires chemical manufacturers to supply material safety data sheets (MSDSs) for their chemicals. ✔ The MSDS is required for any chemical with a hazard warning label. An MSDS lists general information, precautionary measures, and emergency information.

The NFPA developed a labeling system for hazardous chemicals that is frequently used in health care facilities (Fig. 13–7). The system uses a diamond-shaped symbol, four colored quadrants, and a hazard rating scale of 0 to 4. The health hazard is shown in the blue quadrant, the flammability hazard is shown in the red quadrant, the instability hazard is indicated in the yellow quadrant, and the specific hazard is shown in the white quadrant.

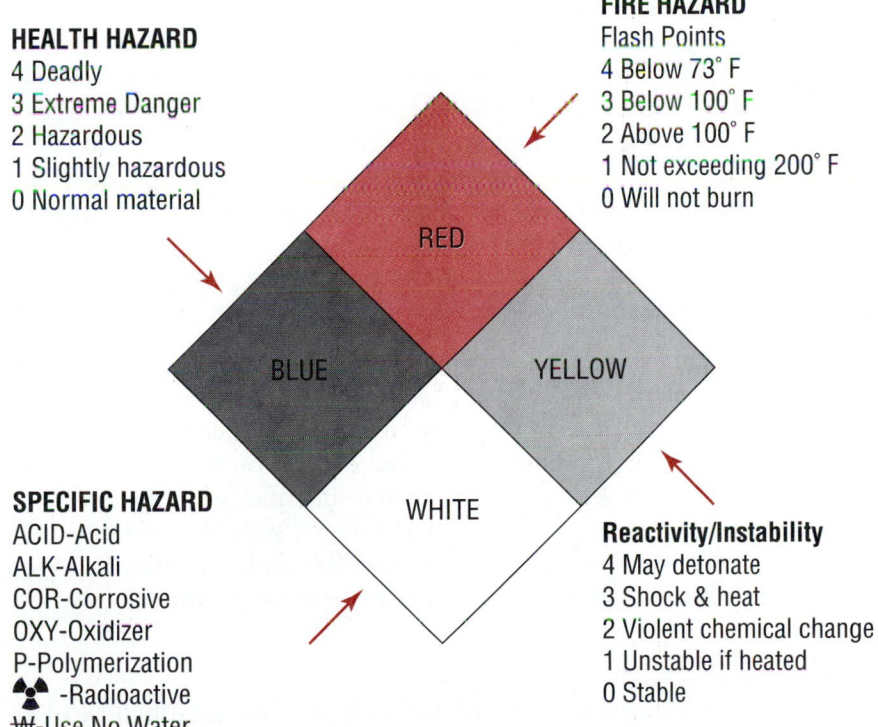

Figure 13–7. National Fire Protection Association (NFPA) 0 to 4 hazard rating system.

Protective Measures

The proper clothing must be worn when a health care worker is working with chemicals. A buttoned laboratory coat, safety glasses, and gloves provide protection and prevent skin contact. When transporting acids or alkalis, an *acid carrier,* should be used. It is a specially designed container for carrying large quantities of hazardous solutions.

The entrance of any room in which hazardous chemicals are in use or in storage must be posted with a caution sign specifying the types of chemicals present. No chemicals should be stored above eye level because of the danger of breakage or spillage involved in reaching. All explosives should be stored in an explosionproof or a fireproof room that is separate from the flammables.

Safety Showers and the Eyewash Station

Safety showers should be nearby for use if an accidental chemical spill occurs. Because permanent damage to the skin can result from chemical burns, the victim of a chemical accident must immediately rinse for at least 15 minutes after removing contaminated clothing.

In case of a chemical spill in the eye, the victim should rinse his or her eyes at the eyewash station for a minimum of 15 minutes. Contact lenses must be removed prior to the rinsing in order to thoroughly cleanse the eyes. The victim should not rub the eyes because doing so may cause further injury. If someone is hurt in a chemical spill, he or she should be taken to the emergency department for treatment after his or her eyes have been rinsed for 15 minutes.

Chemical Spill Cleanup

If a chemical spill occurs, the health care worker should obtain a spill cleanup kit from the clinical chemistry section. The kit includes absorbents and neutralizers to clean up acid, alkali, mercury, and other spills. The absorbent and neutralizer used depend on the type of chemical spill and have an indicator system that identifies when the spill has been neutralized and can be considered safe for sweepup and disposal. The health care worker should become familiar with the procedures for cleaning up chemical spills in his or her place of employment.

Disposal of Chemicals

Chemical wastes that are water soluble such as acids and alkalis, can be flushed down the sink with cold water; however, acids and alkalis should be poured into a large amount of water before flushing them down the sink. The acid *must* be added to the water and not vice versa to prevent a violent chemical reaction.

EQUIPMENT AND SAFETY IN PATIENTS' ROOMS

Each member of the health care team is responsible for the safety of the patient. All health care professionals are responsible for patient safety from the time the patient enters the health care setting until his or her departure. As a matter of general patient safety, the health care worker should do the following when in the patient's room:

1. Make certain that all specimen collection supplies, needles, and equipment are either properly disposed of or returned to the specimen collection tray after blood collection.
2. Check to see whether the bed rails are up or down. Always place bed rails up before leaving the patient if they were up when you entered the room.
3. Report unusual odors to the nursing station because a pipe may be broken and be leaking gas or liquid.
4. Check for food or liquid spilled on the floor, urine spills, or intravenous (IV) line leakage. Areas on which the patient and health care professionals walk must be dry. They should be free of obstacles and slipping hazards. Thus, in cases of spills, make certain that the area is cleaned and dried for the safety of the patient and hospital personnel.
5. During blood collection, be very cautious not to touch any electrical instrument located adjacent to the patient's bed because if the instrument malfunctions, the health care worker may ground the patient and, as a result, a microshock could pass through the health care worker and into the patient. A serious problem could result from such a shock if the patient has an electrolyte imbalance or is wet with perspiration or other fluid. Furthermore, the needle inserted in the patient's arm could produce ventricular fibrillation and death if the patient has a pacemaker or an unstable heart ailment.
6. Report the following problem immediately to the nursing station: If the patient has an IV line and the site is swollen and red, the IV needle is probably no longer in the vein and the IV solution is infiltrating into the surrounding tissues. Some chemicals in IV solutions are toxic to body tissue, so gangrene could result from such infiltration. Also, if blood is backing up the IV line from the needle insertion to the IV drip container, the IV solution container is empty. Report this problem immediately.
7. If the patient's alarm for the IV drip is sounding, report this problem to the nursing station immediately.
8. If the patient is in unusual pain or is unresponsive, notify the nursing station immediately.

PATIENT SAFETY OUTSIDE THE ROOM

Health care workers should be aware of possible hazards to patients outside the patients' rooms. As a matter of general safety practice, the following guidelines should be followed:

1. Because trays, carts, and ladders may be placed around a hallway corner, the health care worker should be careful not to travel too quickly from one room to another and around corners.
2. Items lying on the floor, such as flower petals, may cause someone to slip and should be reported for cleanup.
3. Avoid running in a health care facility because patients and visitors may become alarmed and begin to run as well. Also, someone may be hurt if the health care worker runs into him or her (e.g., a cardiac patient walking in the hall with an inserted IV stand or another health care worker carrying a specimen collection tray).

DISASTER EMERGENCY PLAN

Many health care institutions have developed procedures to be followed in case of a hurricane, flooding, earthquake, bomb threat, and other disasters. The health care worker should become familiar with these procedures because he or she must be prepared to take immediate action whenever conditions warrant such action.

EMERGENCY PROCEDURES

The health care worker should become knowledgeable of emergency care procedures because accidents do occur even though precautionary measures are in place. He or she must be able to detach him- or herself from the emergency situation to some degree in order to perform well and deliver the best possible health care. In an emergency situation, the following objectives must be met for the victim: prevent severe bleeding, maintain breathing, prevent shock and further injury, and send for medical assistance.

Bleeding Aid

Severe bleeding from an open wound can be controlled by applying pressure directly over the wound. A clean handkerchief or other clean cloth (compress) should be placed over the wound before applying pressure by the hand. In an emergency in which a clean cloth is not available, the bare hand should be used until a cloth compress can be located. Bleeding of a limb (i.e., an arm or a leg) can be decreased by elevation. The injured portion should be raised above the level of the victim's heart unless the injured portion is broken. However, even with elevation, pressure should be maintained on the wound until medical assistance arrives. A tourniquet should not be used to control bleeding except for an amputated, mangled, or crushed arm or leg, or for profuse bleeding that cannot be stopped otherwise.

Breathing Aid

When a victim's breathing movements stop or his or her lips, tongue, and fingernails become blue, immediate mouth-to-mouth resuscitation is needed. Any delay in using this technique may cost the victim's life. To perform mouth-to-mouth breathing, include the following:

1. See if the victim is conscious by *gently* shaking the victim and yelling, "ARE YOU OKAY?" If any possibility of a neck injury exists, do not shake the victim! If there is no response to the gentle shaking and yelling, call out for help and start aid immediately.
2. Place the victim on his or her back on a firm, flat surface. Caution must be exercised if the person has a spinal or neck injury. No twisting should occur to the victim's body.
3. Open the airway passage by checking for obstructions: tongue, chewing gum, vomitus, and so on.
4. Place one hand on the victim's forehead and, applying firm, backward pressure with the palm, tilt the head back (Fig. 13–8). Place the fingers of the other hand under the bony part of the victim's lower jaw, near the chin, and lift to bring

Figure 13–8. Head-tilt/chin-lift for emergency care.

the chin forward with the teeth almost to occlusion. The jaw should be supported as the head is tilted back. This position is called the *head-tilt/chin-lift.*

5. Listen and feel for return of air from the victim's mouth and nose for approximately 3 to 5 seconds. Also, simultaneously, look for the victim's chest to rise and fall.

6. If there is no breathing, maintain the head-tilt/chin-lift and pinch the victim's nose shut with the hand to prevent air from escaping. Open mouth widely, take a deep breath, and seal mouth over the victim's mouth (Fig. 13–9). Blow into victim's mouth. Watch for the victim's chest to rise. (If it does not, the airway is blocked and must be cleared.)

7. Give two full ventilations. If this still does not start an air exchange, reposition the head and try again. After two more ventilations, again look, listen, and feel for breathing. Improper chin and head positioning is the most common cause of difficulty with ventilation.

Circulation Aid

To maintain circulation in a victim, a health care provider must know the techniques of basic CPR. Thus, he or she should check with the supervisor about the availability of CPR classes at the health care institution because this emergency technique must be demonstrated so that the employee can learn the proper skills.

Figure 13–9. Breathing aid in emergency situation.

Shock Prevention

Shock usually accompanies severe injury. It may result from bleeding, extensive burns, an insufficient oxygen (O_2) supply, and other traumatic events. Early signs include pale, cold, clammy skin; weakness; a rapid pulse; an increased, shallow breathing rate; and, frequently, nausea and vomiting. The main objectives in treating a shock victim are to improve circulation, to provide sufficient O_2, and to maintain normal body temperature.

The following six actions are recommended if first aid is given to a shock victim:

1. Correct the cause of shock if possible (e.g., control bleeding).
2. Keep the victim lying down.
3. Keep the victim's airway open. If he or she vomits, turn head to the side so that the neck is arched.
4. In the absence of broken bones, elevate the victim's legs so that the head is lower than the trunk of the body.
5. Keep the victim warm.
6. Call for emergency assistance.

Actions that are *not* recommended include the following:

1. Giving fluids to a victim who has an abdominal injury (the person is likely to require surgery or a general anesthetic)
2. Giving fluids to an unconscious or a semiconscious person

✔ Key Terms

CARDIOPULMONARY RESUSCITATION
(CPR)

ENVIRONMENTAL PROTECTION
AGENCY (EPA)

MATERIAL SAFETY DATA SHEETS
(MSDSs)

OCCUPATIONAL SAFETY AND
HEALTH ADMINISTRATION (OSHA)
STANDARDS

Study Questions

The following may have one or more correct answers:

1. If a fire occurs in or near electrical equipment, which of the following fire extinguishers should be used?
   a. class A extinguisher
   b. class B extinguisher
   c. class C extinguisher
   d. ABC extinguisher

2. What are the major principles of self-protection from radiation exposure?
   a. distance
   b. time
   c. combustibility
   d. shielding

3. Which of the following safety rules should be maintained in patients' rooms?
   a. full ashtrays should be emptied into the trash can to prevent a fire hazard
   b. unusual odors in the patient's room should be reported to the nursing station
   c. health care providers should not touch electrical instruments located adjacent to the patient's bed
   d. if the patient has an IV line and the site is swollen and reddish, this problem should be reported to the nursing station

4. Which of the following precautions prevents infectious aerosol spray?

   a. popping the cap on a vacuum collection tube rather than twisting it

   b. inspecting vacuum tubes for cracks prior to centrifugation

   c. applying the centrifuge brake to save time during centrifugation of specimens

   d. pouring the specimens into the required aliquot tubes

5. The main objectives of treating a shock victim are to

   a. improve circulation

   b. provide sufficient drinking water

   c. provide sufficient oxygen

   d. maintain normal body temperature

6. In an emergency situation, which of the following is/are objective(s) that must be met for the victim?

   a. prevent severe bleeding   c. prevent shock

   b. maintain breathing   d. send for medical assistance

7. Which of the following should occur first if a fire breaks out in the health care facility?

   a. run from the floor where the fire is located

   b. call the assigned fire number

   c. use the fastest elevator to escape from the floor where the fire is located

   d. close all windows before leaving the area of the fire

8. The Right to Know law originated with the

   a. CDC   c. OSHA

   b. CAP   d. NFPA

9. The hazardous labeling system developed by the NFPA has the blue quadrant of the diamond to indicate:

   a. flammability hazard   c. instability hazard

   b. health hazard   d. specific hazard

10. If an electrical accident occurs involving electrical shock to an employee or a patient, the *first* thing that the health care worker should do is

   a. move the victim   c. start CPR

   b. shut off electrical power   d. place a blanket over the victim

REFERENCES

1. US Department of Labor, and Occupational Safety and Health Administration (OSHA): Occupational exposure to bloodborne pathogens; final rule (29 CFR 1910.1030). *Federal Register* Dec 6: 64004–64182, 1991.
2. National Fire Protection Association (NFPA): *National Fire Codes.* Quincy, MA, NFPA, Vol 1, 1990.
3. Occupational Safety and Health Administration (OSHA): *Hazard Communication Standard.* 29 CFR 1910.1200, Washington, DC, OSHA, 1986.
4. Occupational Safety and Health Administration (OSHA): *Toxic and Hazardous Substances.* 29 CFR 1910.1001-1047, Washington, DC, OSHA, 1989.

ADDITIONAL SOURCES FOR SAFETY INFORMATION

Centers for Disease Control and Prevention (CDC)
Division of Biosafety
1600 Clifton Rd, NE
Atlanta, GA 30333
(404) 639-3883

College of American Pathologists (CAP)
325 Waukegan Rd
Northfield, IL 60093
(703) 446-8800

Department of Transportation (DOT)
Materials, Transportation Bureau, Information Services Division
Washington, DC 20402
(202) 426-0656

Joint Commission for Accreditation of Healthcare Organizations (JCAHO)
875 N Michigan Ave
Chicago, IL 60611
(312) 642-6061

National Committee for Clinical Laboratory Standards (NCCLS)
771 E Lancaster Ave
Villanova, PA 19085
(215) 525-2435

National Fire Protection Association (NFPA)
One Battery March Park
Quincy, MA 02169
(617) 770-3000

Occupational Safety and Health Administration (OSHA)
US Department of Labor
200 Constitution Ave, NW
Washington, DC 20210
(202) 523-8148

fourteen

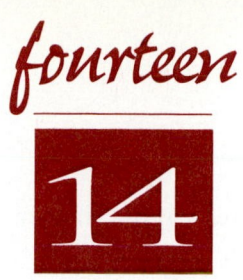

14

SPECIMEN DOCUMENTATION AND TRANSPORTATION

Chapter Outline

Chapter Objectives

Upon completion of Chapter 14, the learner is responsible for the following:

1. Describe the basic components of a clinical, or medical, record.

2. Identify six ways to enhance the intralaboratory communication network.

3. Describe essential elements of a requisition–report form.

4. Name three methods commonly used to transport specimens.

5. Name areas or departments that usually receive laboratory reports.

FUNDAMENTALS OF DOCUMENTATION

All health care organizations have methods of documenting information related to each patient and procedure that include some common elements. One document that can be found in all health care settings is the clinical (or medical) record for each patient. It is the definitive legal document that provides a chronological log of the patient's care. Figure 14–1 describes the components most likely to be found in a medical record. In addition, numerous other documents provide a record of actions and results of the numerous procedures that occur in the daily processes of providing health care services. Documentation in any health care setting is important for the following seven reasons:[1]

1. *Quality of care.* Documentation is used to describe what has been done and how the patient responds.
2. *Coordination of care.* Documentation is used to plan interventions, evaluate progress, and assist the health care team in making effective decisions.
3. *Accrediting and licensing.* The Joint Commission for Accreditation of Healthcare Organizations (JCAHO) and other such accrediting agencies require specific standards for documentation in each patient's clinical, or medical, record. They usually include some guidelines for containing an assessment, a plan of care, medical orders (e.g., laboratory, radiology, etc.), progress notes, and a discharge summary.
4. *Quality monitoring.* State and JCAHO regulations also mandate that ongoing quality assessment activities take place. For this purpose, the clinical record is used to collect objective, readily measurable indicators that allow these

Each health care facility has its own method for keeping track of information in the clinical record. The amount of data and degree of documentation required vary with the particular setting and the severity of each illness; thus, the clinical record in a physician's office is usually not as elaborate as one in a hospital. The following sections are commonly used in hospital clinical records:

FACE SHEET: Includes patient's name, birth date, social security number, address, and marital status; name of closest relative; list of allergies; admitting diagnosis; assigned diagnosis-related group; and physician's name

MEDICAL HISTORY AND PHYSICAL FORMS: Completed by the physician and the nurse; contain information about the initial assessment

ORDER SHEETS: Contain the physician's medical orders, including laboratory, radiology, pharmacy, and so forth

NURSING CARE PLAN: Covers the nurse's plans for the patient

GRAPHIC SHEETS: Flowcharts showing recordings of the patient's temperature, pulse rate, respiratory rate, blood pressure, weight, blood glucose levels, urinalysis results, and other assessments

MEDICATION ADMINISTRATION RECORDS: Contain information about medication dosage, route of administration, site, date, and time of administration

PROGRESS NOTES: Cover patient's progress, intervention, and treatment; provided by the physician and the nurse

DIAGNOSTIC TEST RESULTS: Include results from all tests performed on the patient, such as laboratory test results, radiology results, and so forth

HEALTH CARE TEAM RECORDS: Include notes from other departments such as physical therapy, respiratory, and the like

CONSULTATION SHEETS: Contain evaluations by clinical specialists (e.g., rheumatologists, infectious disease specialists, etc.) who have been called in for their treatment recommendations

DISCHARGE PLAN/SUMMARY: Reviews the patient's stay and plans for care after discharge from a hospital, including dietary, medication, and follow-up appointments

Figure 14–1. Components of a clinical record. *(From Clinical Skillbuilders:* Better Documentation. *Spring House, PA, Spring House Corporation, 1992, with permission.)*

agencies to assess the structure, process, and outcomes of patient care.

5. *Peer review.* Similar to quality monitoring, peer review organizations (PROs) also use documentation in the clinical records to evaluate the quality of care for specific indicators such as nosocomial infections, medical stability of patients, unnecessary procedures and tests, adequate discharge planning, and the occurrence of avoidable discomfort or death. PROs can impose fines, impose sanctions, or deny reimbursement for care if patient care is inappropriate.

6. *Legal protection.* Documentation in the clinical records can provide proof of the quality of care given. Documentation can serve as evidence in disability, personal injury, malpractice, and mental competency cases. Appropriate documentation is the key to winning or losing a case for individual members or employers of the health care facility.

7. *Research.* In teaching institutions, documentation can provide important data for clinical research on new therapies and procedures.

The general guidelines for documentation that should be adhered to involve accuracy, completion, and objectivity. Accuracy refers to recording the facts, not opinions or assumptions. Clinical records should *never* be falsified to cover a mistake. Complete documentation refers to making notes about each event, procedure, or problem that occurs. This includes writing down the information as soon as possible, making notations about the exact time of a procedure or an event, and identifying other sources of information about the process. For example, if a health care worker is unable to identify a patient because of a missing armband, the notation should include the time, the date, the name of the nurse who positively identified the patient, and the health care worker's name. Comments should avoid assigning blame (e.g., "blood was not collected from the patient because nurse Jones did not complete the proper requisition"). Also, unrelated information such as comments about staffing shortages or working overtime should not be recorded because it would be confusing in a courtroom in that it may or may not have a direct influence on the patient's condition. Each notation should be legibly written in blue or black ink, if possible, on the appropriate forms, and signed. Chapter 17 addresses other legal aspects of documentation.

PHYSICIAN–PATIENT–LABORATORY NETWORK

The major purpose of a clinical laboratory is the acquisition and determination of valid data by analytic procedures performed on patient specimens and the timely communication of those data to the physician. It is essential that a physician–patient–laboratory communication cycle be established to achieve this end. The number of persons and steps involved in this cycle varies greatly depending on the size of the institution and the type of laboratory involved. Clinical laboratories may be centralized or may be decentralized, with satellites, or minilaboratories, in various locations. With each additional location or person involved, another potential source of error or delay is introduced into the system. Therefore, the clinical laboratory must concern itself with all parts of the cycle rather than limit its attention solely to data acquisition. The individual who performs the phlebotomy is a vital link in this cycle and must communicate with the patient, the laboratory, the physician, and other members of the health care team.

Various illustrations conceptualize this cyclic pattern, ranging from a simplified version, as in Figure 14–2, to more complex representations such as those in Figure 14–3. Although these illustrations are quite different, they show that to deliver effective services, the clinical laboratory must be involved not only in activities of a central laboratory, but also

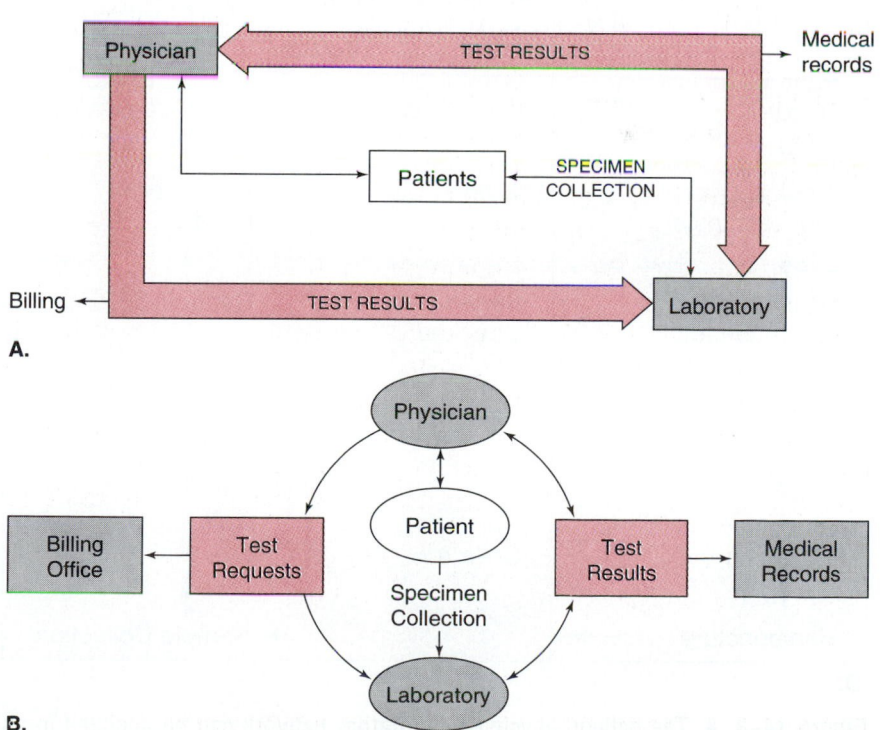

Figure 14–2. A. The patient–physician–laboratory network can be depicted simply. **B.** The network can be considered cyclic.

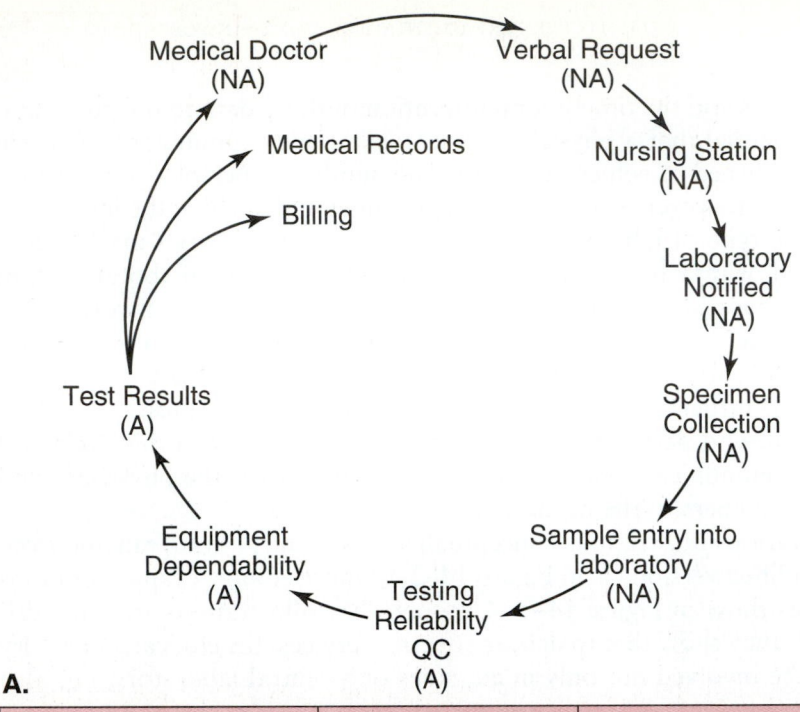

A.

PATIENT ORIENTED	OVERLAPPING FUNCTIONS	TEST ORIENTED
Patient Medical Records →	Compiled Recorded	Medical Doctor reviews/assesses
↓		↑
Medical Doctor requests tests →	Divided	Laboratory Record
↓		↑
Mechanism for test request →	Sorted Checked	Reporting
↓		↑
Health care worker receives orders →	Batched	Calculations Evaluations
↓		↑
Process of specimen collection →	Delivered Collated	Analysis
↓		↑
Venipuncture →		→ Sample Collection

B.

Figure 14–3. A. The patient–physician–laboratory network can be depicted in an analytic phase (A) and a nonanalytic phase (NA). QC, quality control. **B.** The network can also be divided into patient-oriented and test-oriented functions.

of the hospital unit, or of an outpatient clinic. There is a constant overlap and interaction between internal and external functions of the laboratory. This chapter addresses the importance of this network, both inside and outside the laboratory, as well as the various nonanalytic communication components of laboratory test request specifications, test requisitioning, patient and specimen identification, specimen transport, reporting of results, and distribution of results.

In a relatively small laboratory, as in the case of a physician's office laboratory, the communication processes, both within the laboratory (intralaboratory) and with all others outside the laboratory (extralaboratory), are essentially the same. As the size of the institution increases, however, the requirements for effective and efficient intralaboratory and extralaboratory communication are greatly expanded.

INTRALABORATORY COMMUNICATION NETWORK

Using well-written procedures in the clinical laboratory enhances the communication network by ensuring continuity of methods; avoiding shortcuts; minimizing the chances of errors, specimen re-collections, and reruns; preventing expensive substitutions of reagents; and enhancing quality control (QC), teaching, and safety. Overall, such procedures lead to more efficient data collection and reporting.

Policy Manual

Clinical laboratories have administrative or personnel policy manuals that can be consulted by all employees. The manual contains policies that are consistent with those of the larger organization (i.e., hospital, clinic). The manual is general in scope and particularly concerned with, but not limited to, such subjects as management authorizations, organizational charts, responsibilities, personnel practices (e.g., attendance and punctuality policies, dress codes, and rules about coffee breaks), and professional protocol. The policies are generally approved and signed by the laboratory director. Because many changes occur in the clinical laboratory, the policies must be reviewed by the supervisory staff and updated at least annually with a signature and a date to document the review. A staff technologist, technician, or other health care worker who accepts a position in a clinical laboratory section should become acquainted with the laboratory policies.

Procedure Manuals

Written procedures about a specific situation, event, technique, or protocol to be followed should be available to employees who will be performing the procedures or who need to know about safety procedures. An example is depicted in Figure 14–4).

Technical Procedures. Technical procedures describe in detail the steps to be followed in the performance of specimen collection and each laboratory test. Technical procedures are approved and signed by the supervisor, the medical director, or both individuals from the section responsible for the performance of the particular laboratory test. The College of American Pathologists (CAP) requires technical procedures to be made available, on-site at all times, to technical personnel who perform specimen collection procedures and laboratory assays.[2] The technical procedure format includes the name and title of the procedure, a description of the method, specimen requirements, procedural steps, a discussion of reagents and preparation, **reference ranges,** the clinical significance of the results, quality control instructions, calculations, reporting requirements, approval signatures, dates, and references. Not all these sections apply to phlebotomy procedures, but they would be found when reviewing specific laboratory testing procedures.

Laboratory Administrative Procedures. The following topics are generally covered in an administrative procedure manual:

- Technical procedure format
- Assignment of test code numbers to laboratory procedures
- Communication with physicians and other health care professionals
- Time cards and attendance records
- Laboratory equipment identification and centralization of specification files
- Handling of samples for reference laboratory work
- Acceptable symbols, abbreviations, and units of measure
- Handling of laboratory charges
- Purchase and maintenance requisitions
- Performance evaluation procedure and disciplinary policies
- Employee folders, color-blindness records, certification records
- Distribution of laboratory documents
- Quality assurance procedures
- Quality control procedures
- Safety procedures, including fire, chemical, and radiation safety procedures and a disaster plan
- Loan of laboratory equipment
- Compensatory time off, annual leave, and overtime policies
- Employee accidents
- Laboratory library resources
- Inventory lists of capital equipment

Collection Logbook Verification

1. Requests on computer-generated labels that serve as requests for phlebotomy are checked against the logbook prior to the drawing of blood. Any discrepancy should be brought to the attention of the unit secretary or nurse for resolution of orders. Any test deleted from the log by request of a unit will be circled and an explanation of the deletion, along with requester's name, will be written in the log. Any tests added to requests also should be added to the logbook. If any tests are added but not requested on computer labels, a stamped request must be made by the nursing unit personnel.
2. After the appropriate specimens have been collected, each patient's collection that is complete will be initialed by the health care worker collecting the blood and time of draw will be entered in the appropriate box in the logbook. At the bottom of the list of patients, a line is drawn and "EOR," or End of Run, is written to signify that all is complete.

Inability to Draw Specimen

1. A maximum of two laboratory employees will attempt to obtain blood from a patient.
2. Any unsuccessful attempt to obtain blood *must* be documented in the logbook and on the request slip.

Patient Unavailable

1. If you are unable to obtain blood when requested because a patient is unavailable (gone to x-ray or surgery, out of room), hold these slips until you have completed all other patients on that nursing unit. Check the patient's room again before leaving unit.
2. If the patient is still unavailable, notify the primary nurse, if available, or unit clerk. Leave the slip(s) at the desk, circle the orders, and write the following in the logbook:

Reason patient is unavailable
Time and intials of collector
Name of nurse notified
The patient's blood will then be drawn on the next scheduled run.

Patient Refused

If the patient refuses to have blood drawn, notify his or her primary nurse. Often, the nurse can convince the patient to cooperate. If not,

Figure 14–4. Sample procedures for documenting specific phlebotomy situations.

leave slips at the unit desk, with the following information written in the logbook:

Patient refused
Time and initials of collector
Name of nurse notified

Patient Missed

If at any time the person collecting blood is unable to obtain the blood, he or she should check to see whether another collector is available to help. If no other health care worker is available, notify the patient's nurse that the patient was missed and that another person from the laboratory will try on the next run unless the nurse requests that the attempt be made sooner. Leave the slips at the desk, with the following information written in the logbook:

Unable to collect specimen
Time and initials of collector
Name of nurse notified

Upon returning to the laboratory, notify the supervisor. If the second person is unable to obtain the specimen, a nurse is again notified and the previous information is again documented on the requisition form and in the logbook. At this time, request that a physician draw the blood.

Combative Patient

In cases when an adult patient is combative or verbally abusive of laboratory personnel, and nursing staff is unavailable, the health care worker should notify the supervisor. If the health care worker is instructed by the supervisor to refuse to draw blood, the primary nurse should be notified of the refusal and it must be documented in the logbook, noting:

Reason for refusal
Name of the nurse notified

Unidentified Test Requested

If a test is requested that cannot be found in the specimen requirement book, the nurse should be asked to consult the doctor to clarify the request. Meanwhile, the health care worker can call the laboratory for a more familiar name for the test and test requirements. If no

Figure 14–4. (*continued*)

other name can be found and no clarification is offered, he or she *must* refuse to draw a specimen for the test. The logbook should be marked "no such test," the primary nurse notified, and his or her name recorded in the logbook. The supervisor of the laboratory also should be notified.

Figure 14–4. (*continued*)

- Consent to donate blood and urine specimens
- In-service records
- Clinical laboratory samples referred from outside sources
- Hepatitis testing of laboratory personnel
- Dress code

Safety and Infection Control Procedures. Safety procedures should be distributed to all management staff and made known to all personnel. One book of safety procedures should be available in each laboratory section, including the specimen collection areas. Safety manuals should include fire safety, internal and external disaster plan, radiation safety, and biological hazard, as well as a **hazard communication manual** and infection control manuals. The infection control manual usually includes procedures for handling specimens, isolation procedures, handling precautions, disposal policies, decontamination procedures, and hand-washing procedures. Chapter 12 of the textbook provides more detailed information on these procedures. If phlebotomy personnel are decentralized, these policies should be accessible to them at their workstations.

Hazard Communication Manual. The Occupational Safety and Health Administration (OSHA) Hazard Communication Standard enacted in 1986 requires that employers maintain documentation related to any hazardous substances. This act is known as the **Right to Know Law.** Employers must have a written communication program, training for employees, sophisticated tracking and documentation of hazardous substances, and material safety data sheets (MSDSs). The manual must include copies of the federal act as well as any state laws and regulations. All employees must be trained to read and understand MSDSs and biohazard labels and must know the appropriate ways to react to accidents in the laboratory. These topics are covered in greater detail in Chapter 13 of the text.

QC Procedures. QC procedures pertain to the conduct of diagnostic laboratory testing. These procedures should be available in each laboratory section, including the specimen collection area, or they can be indicated in each technical procedure. QC records include information about hazards; proper use, storage, and handling; stability; expiration dates; and indications for measuring the precision and accuracy of analytic processes.

Instrument and Maintenance Manual. Other manuals or procedures that might be used in the clinical laboratory are instrument and equipment maintenance manuals or procedures. These include records of maintenance adjustments, malfunctions, and service calls regarding instruments.

Continuing Education

In addition to procedure manuals, ongoing laboratory in-service education programs help increase communication, safety, and efficiency in patient care. With the increasing complexity of patient care services and responsibilities, it is essential for health care workers to attend in-service education sessions within the institution and elsewhere. Certain types of continuing education, such as training about universal precautions, fire safety, and radiation safety, may be required periodically.

Staff Meetings

Intralaboratory communication is improved when regularly scheduled staff meetings are held within each laboratory section, such as the specimen collection area. They are useful for discussing problems, new policies, and procedures, and for planning. Decisions made in such meetings are usually conferred to all members of the laboratory by written memoranda, by minutes of meetings, or by telephone contact in some cases. Minutes of these meetings should be reviewed by employees who were absent from the meeting. Employees in remote off-site locations can participate by using conference calls. This saves the time and travel expense of leaving a work site to come to "headquarters" for meetings. If the health care worker works as a hospital unit–based employee rather than a laboratory-based employee, there is a greater emphasis on meeting the needs of the patients and medical staff on that particular unit.

Other Modes of Intralaboratory Communication

Bulletin boards, posters, checklists, memoranda, and clipboards are noncomputerized suggestions for disseminating current information.

One person from each laboratory should be responsible for periodically checking and changing poster information. Computer software and hardware are also available for networking within the laboratory. **E-mail** (electronic mail), voice mail, electronic bulletin boards, product recall notices, and facsimiles (faxes) are all effective ways of communicating. Sometimes off-site laboratory facilities also have a speed-dialing telephone exchange. All individuals who practice phlebotomy must be familiar with the communications technology in their facilities.

EXTRALABORATORY COMMUNICATION NETWORK
Provision of Information

Communication with other health care workers working outside the laboratory can be enhanced by the use of an information bulletin or a *floor book* of laboratory services, made available at least in every patient unit, both inpatient and outpatient. This book contains a directory of the laboratory sections with listings of the key staff members, the location of the laboratory, telephone numbers, operating hours, reference ranges, instructions, and pertinent standard procedures of the laboratory. The methods used for collection of all specimens, as well as the proper identification, storage, preservation, and transportation mechanisms to be used, are clearly specified. In addition, an alphabetical listing of all laboratory determinations, specimen requirements, special instructions, and normal values for each measurement are included. (Refer to Figure 14–5.) A health care worker involved in specimen collection should be familiar with the floor book in order to answer questions related to the clinical laboratory specimen collections and procedures. In some hospitals, this information can be reproduced as a pocket-sized resource. This is particularly helpful to medical students, residents, fellows, and trainees.

Periodic hospital and departmental newsletters or bulletins, circulated to all departments and medical staff, are another method of communicating information about new institutional and departmental services or policies.

Use of the Telephone

The telephone is the most frequently used method of two-way communication in any setting. Health care workers must be aware of the procedures for operating it, such as how to transfer calls, how to put someone on hold, how to use an intercom system or voice mail, and how to use conference call and speaker phone functions, and should be able to

TEST #	PROCEDURE	SPECIMEN	AVERAGE TURNAROUND TIME	REQUEST FORM	COLLECTED BY	INSTRUCTIONS
517	Herpes simplex, virus culture	Must specify source	2 weeks	Special test	Physician/nurse	Contact Serology Laboratory (Ext. 3515). Performed by Reference Laboratory.
550	Heterophile anti-body (Monospot)	Blood 7 cc—RT	24 hours	Serology	Laboratory	
586	HI titer—St. Louis Encephalitis	Blood 7 cc—RT	2 weeks	Special test	Laboratory	Performed by Reference Laboratory.
861	Histamine 10 cc—GT	Blood	5 days	Special test	Laboratory	Collect on ice. Do not spin. Performed by Reference Laboratory.
526	Histoplasmosis, complement fixation (fungal serology)	Blood 10 cc—RT	2 weeks	Serology	Laboratory	Performed by Reference Library.

3	HLA typing (microcytotoxicity)	Blood 10 cc—GT		Special test	Laboratory	*Do not* refrigerate or freeze.
707	Homovanillic acid (HVA)	Urine 24-hour	6 days	Chem urine II	Nurse	72-hour dietary restrictions: coffee, tea, vanilla ice cream, anti-hypertensive drugs. Obtain specimen container with 25 mL 6N HCl from Room C3.007. Performed by Reference Laboratory.
761	Human chorionic gonadotropin (HCG) (Immuno-assay—beta)	Blood 10 cc—RGT	24 hours	Chemistry III	Laboratory	Available Mon–Fri only.
762	Human chorionic gonadotropin (HCG)	Urine 24-hour	6 days	Chem urine II	Nurse	Performed by Reference Laboratory.

Figure 14–5. Sample of a hospital unit's *floor book* of laboratory information listing pertinent requirements for collection and testing. In some settings, this information may also be available by computer.

write legible messages. In addition, conversational techniques and manners should be reviewed. Figure 14–6 provides suggestions that may help the health care worker communicate effectively and politely on the telephone.

Confidentiality

Each state has statutes related to privileges between physicians and patients. Communications between a physician and a patient are generally considered privileged and must not be shared with other people without written consent of the patient. Verbal communications and clinical documents must be kept confidential. Clinical documents include the results of testing (e.g., laboratory and radiology) and monitoring. Exceptions to this are matters for legal consultation. Health care workers who have access to patient information must be careful not to disclose results or other patient information in a casual, unnecessary fashion. Discussion

---

- Always speak in a polite and professional tone.
- State the department, clinic, or unit name.
- To establish a cooperative relationship, always use phrases such as the following:

  May I help you?
  Please spell your name.
  I am sorry that I cannot assist you with that matter, let me refer you to someone who can.
  Thank you.

- If speaking to patients and family members, try to use words that are easy to pronounce, concise, direct, and uncomplicated.
- Spelling a term may help you or the receiver understand or recognize what is being said.
- Restate sentences to make sure that you understand the message or instructions.
- Remain neutral in a controversy.
- Reflecting on a response before answering will help clarify your answer; however, pauses that are too long may indicate a lack of interest.
- Ask pertinent questions and have the ability to say that you do not know the answer.

Figure 14–6. Telephone tips.

that does not directly relate to the health care worker's role in caring for the patient should be avoided.

Electronic Transmission (Facsimile) of Printed Materials

Each laboratory or health care institution should have clear policies related to the use of test requests or patient information that has been sent by facsimile, or fax. Most laboratories find the use of a **fax machine** efficient, timely, and cost effective, especially when off-site services are offered. However, precautionary measures should be detailed in procedure manuals that relate to receiving an official laboratory order from the requesting physician. In addition, older fax paper copies have been known to fade with time. In cases when the paper fades, a reproduction (photocopy) of the fax is necessary to provide a more permanent version.

COMPUTERIZED COMMUNICATIONS

Personal, mini-, and mainframe computers have become essential instruments in the clinical laboratory and health care setting; thus, the health care worker needs to become acquainted with information systems. For example, in the clinical laboratory, the functions of a laboratory computer system include (1) entering lists of test requisitions for a patient; (2) printing patients' labels, specimen collection lists, and schedules; (3) updating the laboratory specimen accession records; (4) printing lists that identify which test procedures need to be performed on patients' specimens; (5) entering test results into the computer manually or through clinical laboratory instrumentation; (6) storing test results; (7) sending laboratory test results to the nursing stations; and (8) sending patient charges to the accounting office.

Computers are composed of the same basic units that can transmit information, store information, and perform various types of calculations. The computer system has three main components: (1) central processing unit (CPU), which performs the arithmetic operations and regulates the functions and sequence of events in the system; (2) main memory, which stores data and programs for immediate use; and (3) peripheral devices such as printers.

Computerization of the collection process can significantly decrease errors. Without a computer, collection and specimen information must pass through several people before the sample is actually processed in the laboratory. With a computer, data are continually being checked against the computer files, and authorized individuals can add to and receive information from the accumulated data.

REQUISITION FORMS

Requested patient laboratory tests occur by means of the laboratory ✔ **requisition form** or a computer-generated order. Therefore, the information or instructions must be explicit and the design and format of the request forms or computer screens to be used must be carefully considered in order to minimize handwriting, permit convenient handling, generate inexpensive and legible copies, and obtain all necessary information for laboratory testing.

Multiple-part forms, which serve as both request and report forms, represent one of the most widely used traditional formats for a manual health care facility's laboratory system. The forms are usually of a convenient size to be easily attached to 8½ × 11-in. paper as is customarily used for patients' medical records. Also, these forms are easy to transport, handle, sort, and store, and they are cost effective. For example, the manual requisition forms designed for use at The University of Texas M.D. Anderson Cancer Center, Houston, TX, are 3¼-in. wide by 7⅜-in. long and are usually positioned horizontally, as seen in Figure 14–7A. Each form is divided into sections, one for request information and the other for results. The information in the request section (e.g., physician's name, collection time and date, clinic section) is arranged so that it always appears in the same order. This consistency allows standardization between departments and facilitates correct use. The request information must designate time specifications, or the promptness with which the test results are needed (STAT, routine, and so on); patient condition specifications or the circumstances at the time of specimen collection (preop, admission); and patient category specifications such as inpatient or outpatient. The request side also allows room for all patient identification information, whether added by means of an Addressograph machine (Addressograph Company, Chicago, IL) or handwritten. Each form is identified by name (e.g., hematology, coagulation, chemistry) and is divided into test categories usually coinciding with the different sections of the laboratory. The forms are manufactured to provide clear copies and easy detachment (perforated edges). Color coding can be used for different request forms for ease of identification, both in the ordering of tests and in the charting of results. The name of the institution is usually included on each request form.

Certain additional specifications may be included on request slips that are to be used with a laboratory computer system or with instrumentation that generates printed results. Some request forms are used with a computerized reporting system but are designed to serve also as temporary report forms on a backup basis (Fig. 14–7A). Exact spacing

Figure 14–7. A. Multiple-part requisition forms that also serve as report forms can be stamped with Addressograph machines. These forms can be used with a computerized reporting system but are designed to serve as temporary report forms on a manual backup basis. **B.** If needed, bar-coded labels can be printed with the same information. *(Courtesy of The University of Texas M.D. Anderson Cancer Center, Division of Laboratory Medicine, Houston, TX, with permission.)*

specifications must be met when the request form is to be used as a printout report for certain test results.

Other variations of computerized requisitions may also be used, such as those with bar-coded identification numbers. The use of bar-coded labels (Fig. 14–7B) on patients' samples is becoming more commonplace to reduce transcription errors and speed up sample processing.

Bar codes represent a series of light and dark bands of varying widths. The configuration of these bands relates to specific alphanumeric symbols (i.e., numbers and letters). In other words, each letter of

Figure 14–7. (*continued*)

the alphabet and each number has a specific code (black and white bars of varying widths). When these bands are placed together in a series, they can correspond to a name (patient or test) or a number (identification or test code). When the bar is scanned with a sensitive light, or laser scanner, the series of numbers and letters is read into a computer in a precise manner. This technology has been shown to be very accurate and fast. It saves time and personnel from entering or typing information, and it reduces clerical errors substantially. Bar codes not only represent patients' names and identification numbers, but also the test codes, billing codes, and inventory records. Many instruments used in the clinical laboratory are functioning with automatic scanners to read a barcoded label directly from the patient's simple tube as it is run through the analyzer. In addition, many laboratory supplies are packaged with bar-coded inventory labels. Figure 14–8 shows some of the many uses for bar codes in a health care facility.

TRANSMITTAL OF THE TEST REQUEST TO THE LABORATORY

The test request mechanism formally initiates the cyclic procedure of the physician–patient–laboratory communication network. Two systems are commonly used for this activity. Orders for test requests can be transmitted directly to the clinical laboratory from the requesting authority through an on-line interactive computer system. In many institutions, however, manual requesting systems are still in use, sometimes using bar codes, which are then entered into the computer, other times involving a totally manual system in which the request form also serves as the final report.

On-line computer input of request information is the most error-free means of making requests. Because a computer system can perform automatic checks on the input, it does not accept a request for any test that is not in its test-information database. Likewise, it does not accept a sample of plasma or urine for a test restricted to serum. It also allows the person entering the test request to obtain accurate and up-to-date information about specific determinations, such as revised specimen collection requirements, delivery instructions, assay techniques, reference ranges, and fees.

In a manual system, the multipart request forms are commonly completed at each patient unit or nursing station by a nurse or a ward clerk and delivered to the laboratory. This type of system is more subject to human error. The requisition slips could be lost by the nursing service or the ward clerk prior to arriving in the clinical laboratory or by the laboratory personnel after the slips reach the laboratory. Another

A.

Figure 14–8. The use of bar codes can facilitate the following: **A.** Printing labels and requisition forms. **B.** Labeling specimens. **C.** Labeling blood smears. **D.** Identifying serum aliquot tubes. **E.** Processing blood samples. *(Courtesy of TimeMed Labeling Systems, Burr Ridge, IL, with permission.)*

B.

C. **D.**

E.

Figure 14–8. (*continued*)

common source of error comes from requests that are prepared in duplicate or not at all as a result of lack of communication in the nursing unit. These problems can be minimized by instituting a few organizational procedures. Providing a central location in the laboratory where all requisition forms are to be delivered or scheduling laboratory personnel to make designated pickups of all request slips usually alleviates the problem of misplaced or lost forms. A sorting system is maintained once the requisition slips reach the laboratory. The problem of determining whether a particular request has been made can be solved by removing one copy of the multipart form that can be kept in the patient unit as a record of the test requested. A blood collection log sheet at the nurses' station can also be used for this purpose. The request slips are kept with the blood collection log and compared by the health care worker when the blood is drawn. This system provides the added advantage of allowing the health care worker to make comments on the log sheet regarding problems in obtaining the blood specimens and provides a means of communicating this to the nursing personnel.

Some health care worker's have decentralized the phlebotomy functions to the patients' areas such that personnel are trained by the hospital clinical laboratory but stationed at the various nursing units. This approach is designed with several purposes in mind: (1) to maintain accurate and efficient communication with the physicians, nursing service, ward clerks, patients, and family members regarding laboratory services; (2) to speed up the cycle (turnaround time) from specimen collection to receipt of test results; and (3) to provide cost-effective cross-training capabilities for a more productive staff. These individuals are usually responsible for the collection of all blood work requested in their assigned unit, for delivery of these specimens to the laboratory, and for the collection and/or transportation of all other specimens requested in the unit. Additional duties may include performing clerical functions in the unit, conducting bedside testing such as glucose screening, assisting with other simple laboratory tests, maintaining a log of all specimens collected (Fig. 14–9), reviewing charts to ensure that the laboratory test requests have been accurately transcribed to the request slips, and charting results. It is easy to see how these responsibilities could alleviate problems encountered in request transcription, request delivery, specimen collection, and so forth.

Verbal test requests are occasionally used in cases of emergency. The request should be documented on a standardized form in the laboratory prior to the specimen collection (Fig. 14–10). After the blood is collected, the formal laboratory request slip can be filled out and accompany the specimen to the laboratory in the routine manner.

Figure 14–9. Daily log sheet documenting all specimens collected and delivered by the specialized phlebotomy personnel called *laboratory liaison technicians (LLTs). (Courtesy of The University of Texas M.D. Anderson Cancer Center, Division of Laboratory Medicine, Houston, TX, with permission.)*

STAT REQUESTS

Nurse:

Requesting Physician:

Location: ICU_____ ER _____ Other_____
              Room:_____

Patient:

Pick up orders on unit:

Tests Ordered:_____
_____
_____
_____
_____

Requested by: _____

Order taken by:_____
Date _____ Time _____ AM_____ PM _____

Figure 14–10. Sample of a documentation form used by the laboratory in cases of verbal test requests. ICU, intensive care unit; ER, emergency room. (*Adapted from a form used at The University of Texas M.D. Anderson Cancer Center, Houston, TX, with permission.*)

SPECIMEN LABELS AND BLOOD DRAWING LISTS

Clear and accurate specimen identification is essential and must begin immediately upon collection and continue through disposal of the specimen. Identification methods vary from manually copying all patient identification information onto the container to using prenumbered barcoded labels. Manually labeling specimens can be time consuming and is prone to transcription errors. These problems can be prevented by using preprinted labels, which are available from many commercial sources. Some labels are gummed hospital labels that can be attached to specimens. Other labeling systems include those that can imprint a patient identification card or electronically print patient identification information onto the specimen label.

Among the most sophisticated, accurate, and efficient labels are those generated by a hospital computer system. Requisition slips for the morning draw can be sent to the laboratory in the afternoon of the previous day or entered into the computer at any time. On the basis of the laboratory orders, the computer can generate enough labels containing all the appropriate patient identification criteria for each tube required to be drawn. The labels also list the specific tests requested, the types of specimen collection tubes required for the requested tests, and unique accession numbers or sample numbers to be used for that particular collection time. Bar codes can be used for any alphanumeric symbols. Smaller transfer labels may also be printed to label special aliquot tubes, collection tubes, cuvettes, and microscope slides. This type of system eliminates the manually written entry log used at many hospitals for recording the tests and accession number requested for each patient. Additional test requests ordered later in the day are entered into the computer, which assigns a specific time to the tests so that they can be easily separated from those requested in the morning. Labels for later collection can be computer printed or made with an Addressograph machine. Blood-drawing lists are also printed by the computer to provide a list of patients on each floor requiring blood work for the morning draw and the tests ordered, and to identify the assigned sample accession number. The health care worker initials this list after the patient's blood has been drawn, and a copy is left at the nursing unit so that caregivers attending the patient can see which specimens have already been collected. Any additional specimens collected later in the day are documented in the logbook on the floor (see Figure 14–9). In this way, the personnel in the hospital unit have a complete list of the specimen collections taken from each patient throughout the day.

SPECIMEN TRANSPORTATION AND DELIVERY

Both the communication network and the quality of laboratory test results depend on the time that specimens are received for processing. Blood and other specimens must be delivered expeditiously.

Basic Handling Guidelines

Every hospital or clinic has a specific protocol for specimen transportation and processing. Many institutions require the use of a leakproof plastic bag for insertion of the specimen container. This bag protects the health care worker from pathogenic (disease-producing) organisms during specimen transportation. Usually, this special transport bag has a pouch on the outside for the laboratory request slip. Thus, the potential for contamination of the request slip is eliminated with the use of this outer pouch. If possible, the blood in evacuated tubes and microcollection tubes should be maintained in a vertical position to promote complete clot formation, if required, and to reduce the possibility of hemolysis. It is also imperative to handle and transport blood specimens in a gentle manner to prevent hemolyzing the specimens.

Glycolytic action from the blood cells interferes in the analysis of various chemicals (e.g., glucose, calcitonin, aldosterone, phosphorus, enzymes). Because of this, the blood samples should be transported to the clinical laboratory within 45 minutes from the time of collection so that the serum or plasma can be separated from the blood cells. The serum or plasma that is separated from the cells must be handled according to the laboratory procedure. The National Committee for Clinical Laboratory Standards (NCCLS) suggests a maximum time of 2 hours from the time of collection to separation of sera from plasma. Once separated, sera may remain at room temperature, be refrigerated, be stored in a dark place, or be frozen, depending on the prescribed laboratory method.[3]

Chilled Specimens

For special types of specimens, chilling is required. If a health care worker is requested to transport an arterial specimen for blood gas analysis, he or she should be aware that the specimen must be transported in an airtight heparinized syringe and placed in a mixture of ice and water. The airtight container and the ice water decrease the loss of gases from the specimen. It is important to use ice water rather than solid chunks of ice; otherwise, parts of the specimen may freeze and hemolysis will result. Speed in specimen transportation is essential to prevent the loss of blood gases. Other specimens that may require chilling are those for gastrin, ammonia, lactic acid, renin, catecholamine, parathyroid hormone, prothrombin time (PT), partial thromboplastin time (PTT), and glucagon determinations.[4]

Protection of Specimens from Light

Some chemical constituents in blood such as bilirubin are light sensitive and decrease in value if exposed to light. Thus, blood collected for chemical analysis should be protected from bright light with an aluminum foil wrapping around the tube. Other tests, which are light-sensitive, are Vitamin B_{12}, carotene, and folate, and urine specimens for detection of porphyrins.

Microbiological Specimens

Blood and urine specimens for microbiological culture need to be transported to the laboratory as quickly as possible so that the blood can be transferred to culture media and the urine analyzed. This enhances the likelihood of detecting pathogenic bacteria. Specimens for blood cultures can also be collected directly into culture media, which minimizes possible contamination and speeds the contact with the culture media. (Refer to Chapter 4 for additional information about blood culture tubes.)

Warmed Specimens

Specimens that require warming (to body temperature, 37°C) include those for testing cold agglutinins and cryofibrinogen. These special cases require a heat block for transportation and handling purposes.

Laboratory Processing of Specimens

Processing specimens may occur in one location of the clinical laboratory or in each laboratory section (e.g., hematology, clinical chemistry, clinical immunology, blood bank, coagulation), depending on the organization of the laboratory. Specimen processing can also occur in satellite laboratories. Wherever the site, it is important to know the processing requirements of the clinical laboratory so that specimens are transported and processed as quickly as possible. As discussed in Chapters 12 and 13, safety devices should be used to gain access to the blood to prevent splashing and aerosol spray from the blood sample. Efficient and safe processing of the specimens leads to better clinical laboratory test results and thus better patient care.

In many laboratories, the specimen collection area has a medical technologist (clinical laboratory scientist) or a medical laboratory technician who centrifuges the specimens and makes the appropriate aliquots for each section. These aliquots are then distributed to the clinical laboratory sections for testing. Some specimens must be prepared for shipping to referral laboratories. This preparation sometimes involves special packaging requirements such as freezing the specimen to maintain stability and packaging it in a Styrofoam mailing container.

Hand Delivery

Many systems for specimen delivery involve hand-carried specimens and require standards for ensuring promptness. The laboratory is most often the department responsible for the collection and delivery of blood specimens. The laboratory may also be responsible for the delivery of all other patient specimens as well. Health care workers may make scheduled pickups as well as deliveries of stat specimens. The specimens should be placed in an assigned area in each hospital unit after being documented in the log book. The patient's name, hospital number, and room number; the specimens delivered; the date; the time; and the initials of the person transporting the specimen should be included on the log sheet, as shown in Figure 14–11. Specimen transportation can be more easily monitored when all personnel involved use the appropriate documentation procedures and communicate openly with one another.

Most health care workers organize blood collection trays or carts to accommodate patient specimens that need to be taken to the laboratory. A test-tube rack, slide rack, plastic holder, or cup is sufficient to hold the collected specimens. Some specimens require ice for transport, so it is wise to carry a small container with a slurry of ice water that will not leak and will fit conveniently on the tray.

Transportation Department

Specimen delivery may also be performed by a transportation department within the hospital. Typically, the transportation escort or order-

Patient Name	Location	Specimens						Date	Time	Escort Name
		CSF	Blood	Urine	Sputum	Other	Test Ordered			

SPECIMEN DELIVERY

Figure 14–11. Sample of a log sheet used by the laboratory to document delivery of patient specimens by the institution's transport service.

lies are responsible for moving patients from their nursing units to service areas such as diagnostic radiology, physical therapy, and so forth. When a specimen and a requisition form are to be delivered to the laboratory by the transportation department, the following information is usually required: type of specimen, name and hospital identification number of the patient, date and time of specimen collection, and destination of the specimen. After obtaining this information, the escort takes the specimen to the laboratory. The test request slip accompanying the specimen can also be clocked in at this time so that the actual delivery time can always be obtained. If any complications arise with the specimen, the escort notifies the nursing staff. Occasionally, specimens, especially stat or timed requests, may be collected and delivered to the laboratory by a nurse or a physician. Again, the requisition should be clocked in.

Pneumatic Tube Systems

Some hospitals use **pneumatic tube systems** to transport patient records, messages, letters, bills, medications, x-rays, and laboratory test results. However, reports from health care institutions differ as to the effectiveness of using tube systems for transporting blood specimens. Considerations in the utilization of pneumatic tubes for transporting specimens are mechanical reliability, distance of transport, speed of carrier, control mechanisms, landing mechanism, radius of loops and bends, shock absorbency, sizes of carriers, and laboratory assessment of chemical and cellular components in transported specimens versus hand-carried specimens. It is generally recommended that blood collection tubes be placed in the pneumatic tube with shock-absorbent inserts padding the sides and separated from one another to prevent spillage or breakage. Plastic clear liners are also commercially available so that if leaks do occur, they are visible and are contained to prevent contamination of the tube system, the carrier, and the personnel handling the specimens.

Transportation by Vehicle

Some manufacturers provide transport systems that are automated, motorized, or computerized. Delivery of specimens can be by means of a small container car attached to a network of track that is routed to appropriate sites in the laboratory, the nursing stations, or other specimen collection areas. Again, a thorough evaluation of such automated delivery systems needs to include mechanical reliability, transportation distances, speed of the carriers, control mechanisms, soft-landing provisions, radius of loops and bends, shock absorbency, size of carriers, method of cleaning containers, and overall time- and cost-effectiveness. When plans are made to renovate a laboratory area so that it includes this type of transport system, extra space above the ceiling tiles should be considered because the transport vehicles require a sizable right-of-way.

Other Transport Equipment

Health care workers involved in specimen collection may also be required to order and use special transport containers. All should be evaluated for cost, protective ability, temperature control, sterilizing potential, appearance, labeling system, breakage, leakage, and tamper resistance.

Some hospitals send specimens to reference laboratories for special analysis. When packaging or receiving one of the specimens in a special transport container, care must be taken to pay attention to the following details:

1. Specimens such as human or animal feces, blood, body fluids, or tissue should be properly labeled and in containers that protect individuals from contamination.
2. Specimens containing viable microorganisms must be specially packaged so that they can withstand leakage of contents, pressure and temperature changes, and rough handling. It is recommended that the specimen be placed in a primary container surrounded by absorbent packing material. This container should be labeled with pertinent information and instructions about the specimen contents. It can then be placed in a secondary container. Thus, if the specimen contents are released, they are maintained in the primary container. Biohazard and mailing labels should be affixed to the outside container.[4]
3. Specimen requisition forms or special instructions should accompany the specimen.
4. Containers holding dry ice should be labeled—for example, "DRY ICE, FROZEN BIOHAZARDOUS MEDICAL SPECIMEN." Biohazard labels should be affixed so that they are easily visible to anyone handling the container.
5. It is recommended that, when shipping biohazardous material, the address and telephone number of the Centers for Disease Control and Prevention (CDC), Atlanta, GA, be affixed to the container. In the event of damage or leakage, individuals outside the health care professions may need advice on how to dispose of or clean up a biohazardous spill.
6. After receiving an intact specimen from an outside source,

the container must be identified by name, number, and source. This information should match that on the accompanying requisition and the specimen can then be processed accordingly.
7. If a leaky or broken specimen is received, it should be handled cautiously and according to safety procedures.

REPORTING MECHANISMS

Written Reports

The laboratory report is a feedback mechanism for transmitting vital data from the laboratory to the physician requesting the information. Both the JCAHO and the CAP state that the results should be confirmed, dated, and accompanied by permanent report copies that are kept in the laboratory as well as added to the patient's medical record. The CAP also states that each report should contain adequate patient identification, be stamped to record the date and hour when the procedures were completed, and be signed and initialed by the laboratory personnel performing the procedure. When computer-generated report forms are used, laboratory documentation on worksheets by personnel performing the procedures is sufficient. The CAP has suggested that health care personnel consider the following when designing a report form:[2]

1. Identification of patient, patient location, and physician
2. Date and time of specimen collection
3. Description, source of specimen, and labeled precautions
4. Compactness and ease of preparing the package for shipment
5. Consistency in format
6. Clear understandability of instructions or orders
7. Logical location in patient's chart for reference laboratory reports
8. Sequential order of multiple results on single specimens
9. Listing of normal ranges or normal and abnormal values
10. Assurance of accuracy of request transcription
11. Administrative and record-keeping value

Any unique institutional requirements for an acceptable report should be stated in the laboratory procedure manual and may include such criteria as QC limits, absolute limits, and delta checks. If these criteria cannot be met on the report form, a written policy including these requirements should be available when needed.

Results can be documented in one of the following three ways: manual recording of test results, laboratory instrument–printed reports, and computer-generated reports. As previously mentioned, in most manual systems, combination test requisition–report forms are used (see Figure 14–7A). These forms may include multiple copies. Most laboratory instruments in use today contain microprocessors that can generate digital outputs and printed reports.

Verbal Reports

The use of verbal and telephone reports has declined in recent years because computer access to laboratory data is prevalent in most health care environments. If laboratory personnel take an active role in educating clerical, nursing, and physician staff on the acquisition of computerized data, the number of phone requests will decrease.

Verbal reports, although useful for reporting stat results and "panic" values, may become a problem in laboratories. The possibility of error is so great that at a minimum, a laboratory should always require proper identification of the patient and the name of the person receiving the report. Written documentation of verbally issued reports is recommended and should include the following information: patient name and hospital number, name of person receiving the report, date, information given, and name of person issuing the report (Fig. 14–12).

Computerized Reports

Various computer-transmission devices can provide a rapid on-line report system, and are, in general, more reliable than verbal reports and faster than waiting for the written report. A hospital with an on-line laboratory computer system can have terminals located in each patient unit. After the tests have been completed and verified in the laboratory, the results can be immediately displayed in each patient unit. A printer can be attached to each terminal to generate a temporary hard-copy report. Another transmission method electronically transmits a handwritten report, which is generated in a similar form at the receiving end. A third transmission device transmits fax results. All these methods can provide a written report that is usually accurate, dependable, and consistent.

Interim Reports and Cumulative Summaries

Interim laboratory reports are typically sent to nursing units at specified times during the day (e.g., 10:00 AM and 2:00 PM). These reports may include test results completed or in progress. This type of reporting sys-

CULTURE RESULTS—TELEPHONE REQUEST

PATIENT NAME:_____

PATIENT ID NUMBER: _____

PHYSICIAN: _____

PERSON REQUESTING INFORMATION:_____

DATE   SOURCE   CULTURE #   INFO GIVEN

TIME OF INQUIRY: _____

DATE OF INQUIRY:_____

TECHNOLOGIST: _____

Figure 14–12. Sample form used by the microbiology laboratory to issue culture results for verbal requests.

tem is often used in facilities that are only partially computerized or as a backup process if the hospital computer system is malfunctioning or down.

Cumulative summaries are a compilation of laboratory reports on one patient over a designated period or after a certain number of tests have been performed on the patient. They are printed at designated times during the week and facilitate the medical record-charting process. They are helpful to nurses and physicians because groups of similar tests are reported together. Trends that reveal laboratory and physiological changes can be detected more easily than if each laboratory value were reported separately and charted in the medical record at random.

DISTRIBUTION OF RESULTS

The final communication involved in the physician–patient–laboratory network is the distribution of test results. Those who receive the laboratory data include nursing, phlebotomy, clerical, and medical record personnel (chart attachment); the hospital business office (patient billing); and the laboratory (department record).

Charting Reports

Manual Methods. So that a chronological type of reporting system is used on the patient's chart, the laboratory reports have traditionally been shingled one upon another. Color coding by the laboratory originating the results aids in coordinating them on a carrier page. The laboratory may also key chronological reports by having a master card prepared in the laboratory for each patient, beginning with the admitting laboratory test results. The results of each day are added to the card, which can be photocopied and sent to the physician.

Computerized Medical Records. A health care facility's computer system can easily provide daily printed reports and cumulative reports for the patient's medical record. All reports should be printed and delivered at times convenient for making clinical decisions by the medical staff. Some health care facilities send a second set of results directly to the physician in case errors or delays in chart attachments occur. This helps to ensure that the data are available to the physicians before they make their patient rounds.

The business office of the health care facility also receives laboratory test results. This office must be notified of all laboratory charges, according to data requested and procedural code for patient billing. It is financially advantageous to send reports promptly. Laboratory copies of test results from previous days, months, or years should be accessible because they are often requested to confirm charges for the hospital stay. A copy of the combined request–report form can be easily stored and used for information retrieval. In a manual reporting system, log books are often kept in the laboratory and usually serve as duplicate recording of patient results. They can be beneficial in permitting a more rapid retrieval of a patient's previous results and aid in providing a delta check procedure. However, computer systems are advantageous because they can store easily retrievable information for long periods, require no paperwork from laboratory personnel, be programmed to automatically display and flag delta checks, and generate management reports about workload, abnormal results, and the like.

Self Study

✔ Key Terms

BAR CODES

E-MAIL

FAX MACHINE

HAZARD COMMUNICATION
MANUAL

PNEUMATIC TUBE SYSTEMS

REFERENCE RANGES

REQUISITION FORM

RIGHT TO KNOW LAW

Study Questions

1. The key elements common to most medical records are
   a. face sheet
   b. medical history and physical evaluation
   c. physician's order sheet
   d. discharge plan

2. Medical records serve what purpose?
   a. allow coordination of care
   b. meet accrediting and licensing requirements
   c. provide legal protection
   d. provide research data

3. Why is the hazard communication manual required?
   a. to provide technical procedures on phlebotomy
   b. to provide personnel policies
   c. to inform employees about hazardous substances
   d. to describe a disaster plan

4. Which of the following data should be considered confidential?
   a. laboratory test results
   b. radiology reports
   c. patient's diagnosis
   d. universal precautions

5. Bar codes can be used for
   a. identification of patient names
   b. identification of patient numbers
   c. designation of test to be performed
   d. inventory of supplies

6. The most error-free method for requesting a laboratory test is the
   a. handwritten requisition   c. verbal method
   b. computerized method   d. verbal stat method

7. A specimen should be protected from light for which of the following determinations?
   a. bilirubin concentration   c. glucose level
   b. hemoglobin level   d. blood cultures

8. A specimen should be chilled for which of the following analyses?
   a. complete blood count (CBC)   c. blood gas
   b. bilirubin level   d. glucose level

REFERENCES

1. Clinical Skillbuilders: *Better Documentation*. Spring House, PA, Spring House Corporation, 1992.
2. College of American Pathologists (CAP): *Standards for Accreditation of Medical Laboratories*. Skokie, IL, CAP, 1990.
3. National Committee for Clinical Laboratory Standards (NCCLS): *Procedures for Handling and Processing of Blood Specimens*. NCCLS Document H18-A, Villanova, PA, NCCLS, 1990.
4. National Committee for Clinical Laboratory Standards (NCCLS): *Procedures for the Collection of Diagnostic Blood Specimens by Venipuncture*. NCCLS Document H3-A3, Villanova, PA, July 1991.

Phlebotomy Case Study

NEWBORN NURSERY COLLECTIONS

Two health care workers oversee blood collections in the newborn nursery on Saturday and Sunday of each week. On Sunday morning, the clinical laboratory scientist (CLS) overseeing the clinical chemistry section noticed that the bilirubin value for Baby McPherson was as follows:

DAY	TIME	BILIRUBIN VALUE (mg/dL)
Friday		15
Saturday	8:15 PM	12
Sunday	7:10 AM	2

Knowing that the ultraviolet light on newborn Baby McPherson could not make the bilirubin value decrease that dramatically from Saturday to Sunday, the CLS called in the health care worker who had collected the Sunday morning blood sample to ask him questions regarding the collection.

Questions:

1. What type of microcollection container should have been used to collect the bilirubin sample?

2. Does taking the blood immediately to the laboratory for testing make any difference?

3. Give two reasons why the Sunday bilirubin value for Baby McPherson was so different from the values of the previous 2 days.

QUALITY MANAGEMENT AND LEGAL ISSUES

V

*T*he final portion of the textbook covers professional issues such as assessment of the quality of services that are provided in phlebotomy practice, professional and ethical communication and management practices, and the sensitive issues of legal risk and regulatory matters.

Chapter 15, Total Quality Management, describes the role of quality-monitoring activities in improving the practice of phlebotomy and related procedures. Specific examples are provided that demonstrate how quality-improvement tools (e.g., flowcharts, Pareto charts, cause-and-effect diagrams) can enhance services to customers, who include patients, families, physicians, nurses, and other health care professionals.

Chapter 16, Communication, Professionalism, and Managerial Skills, covers the importance of professionalism in communicating with patients and other members of the health care team. Suggestions for improving verbal and nonverbal communication skills are included. Management issues such as organizing, budgeting, staffing, team building, and monitoring productivity are also addressed.

Chapter 17, Legal and Regulatory Issues, describes general legal principles such as statutory, administrative, and judicial law and provides definitions of legal terminology. Also covered are the following legal issues, which are particularly important to health care professionals who practice phlebotomy: confidentiality, human immunodeficiency virus (HIV) exposure, informed consent, implied consent, and legal claims. In addition, legal cases that are related to phlebotomy and laboratory practices are cited, and issues of how to manage legal risk, malpractice insurance, and protective equipment are highlighted.

fifteen

15

TOTAL QUALITY MANAGEMENT

Chapter Outline

Chapter Objectives

Upon completion of Chapter 15, the learner is responsible for the following:

1. Describe the importance of quality improvement and total quality management.

2. Describe the "5 Ds" in terms of negative patient outcomes.

3. Identify steps in monitoring and evaluating a specimen collection process.

4. Distinguish between quality control and quality improvement.

5. Give examples of improved patient outcomes for phlebotomy services.

Most of the credit for initiating the quality revolution in the United States goes to **Dr. W. Edwards Deming,** an American statistician who spent time in Japan and helped develop modern Japanese management theories. His work focused on minimizing variation in the manufacturing processes such as those in the automotive industry. This is similar to a laboratory's goal of minimizing the variations in laboratory testing. Other noted quality innovators are Drs. Joseph Juran, Avedis Donabedian, Philip Crosby, and Donald M. Berwick. Dr. Donabedian, a physician, pinpointed key aspects (structure, process, outcomes) of health care functions that needed to be monitored for quality improvement. The contribution of this framework has shaped the way health care providers view quality assessments.

The Joint Commission on the Accreditation of Healthcare Organizations (JCAHO) has been instrumental in bringing quality-improvement methodologies to health care. This commission based its guidelines on Juran's model of **total quality management (TQM)** and Deming's principles of **continuous quality improvement (CQI).**[1,2] The most widely used strategy for quality assessment of health care performance is the **JCAHO 10-step process** (Fig. 15–1). It provides a systematic process for improving health care processes and outcomes. Another commonly used strategy for quality improvement is the plan–do–check–act (PDCA) approach (Fig. 15–2). Both are examples of how health care organizations can use a common method to systematically assess the quality of their services.

Many terms are used to convey the idea of improving the quality of services. These include *total quality management, continuous quality improvement, quality assurance,* and *integrated quality assurance,* to name a few. The current JCAHO standards include wider accountability for performance improvement. The JCAHO describes a framework of performance as follows:

> Performance is what is done and how well it is done to provide health care. The level of performance in health care is
> —the degree to which what is done is efficacious and
>   appropriate for the individual patient; and
> —the degree to which it is available in a timely manner to
>   patients who need it, effective, continuous with other care
>   and care providers, safe, efficient, and caring and respectful
>   of the patient.

1. *Assign responsibility.* The director or chairperson is responsible for monitoring and evaluating service quality. A written plan should describe responsibilities, the laboratory setting, the populations served, and the quality assessment activities.
2. *Delineate the scope of care.* All major sections of the laboratory must be covered.
3. *Identify key aspects of care.* These include high-volume procedures, high-risk procedures, problematic procedures, and high-cost procedures.
4. *Construct indicators.* Indicators should specify which activities, events, or patient outcomes will be monitored.
5. *Define thresholds of evaluation.* Thresholds specify the lower limits of acceptable quality. Exceeding them should stimulate further evaluation and problem resolution.
6. *Collect and organize data.* Two basic types of monitors should be used: scanning monitors (to provide important statistics about the laboratory's operations) and focused monitors (to periodically collect data so that the causes, nature, or scope of a problem can be determined).
7. *Evaluate data.* This includes comparing performance to standards, analyzing patterns and trends, evaluating statistical significance and clinical relevance, and analyzing causes.
8. *Develop a corrective action plan.* The plan should detail who or what is to change and what specific actions will be taken and when; it should focus on improving the system or behavior.
9. *Assess actions and document improvement.* The corrective actions must be monitored until the problem is resolved.
10. *Communicate relevant information.* Complete reports (including objectives, findings, conclusions, corrective actions, and follow-up results) must be forwarded to the appropriate officials in a timely manner.

Figure 15–1. JCAHO 10-step process for quality assessment. *(From Martin BG (ed): The CLMA Guide to Managing a Clinical Laboratory. Malvern, PA, Clinical Laboratory Management Association, 1991, with permission.)*

These characteristics of what is done and how it is done are called "dimensions of performance."[1]

Figure 15–3 defines the JCAHO dimensions of performance. Key elements of the theorists' various approaches are briefly summarized in Table 15–1.

Plan a change.
Do the improvement, data collection, and analysis.
Check the results to see the effect of the change.
Act on what was learned by either rejecting the change, adjusting the change, or adopting the change as a standard part of the process.

Figure 15–2. Plan–do–check–act (PDCA) cycle.

TOTAL QUALITY MANAGEMENT

TQM is a process aimed at continuous quality improvement, not just meeting a minimum standard. The focus is on improving the entire process of health care so that patient outcomes are positive. It includes, but is not limited to, reducing outliers, variations, or errors in all types of health care settings. It involves all levels of the health care team, including the health care worker. And, perhaps most important, it focuses on meeting the needs of persons who are being served, or **customer satisfaction.** Customers include patients and other health care workers such as technologists, nurses, students, pathologists, and all physicians who use or are a part of the specimen collection and laboratory services. Examples of customers might include a patient care aide or clerk responsible for charting a result, a patient who needs blood drawn for surgery the next morning, an anesthesiologist waiting for a stat blood gas analysis result, and a pathologist who needs to review an abnormal blood smear (Fig. 15–4). Even the JCAHO current accreditation guidelines recognize the need for "customer input through patient feedback."[1]

The six major characteristics of hospitals with successful TQM are as follows:

1. The organized TQM approach permeates the hospital horizontally and vertically through the organizational chart.
2. The objective of TQM is continuous improvement in performance and outcomes instead of meeting fixed, predetermined standards.
3. Work groups, teams, or quality circles include multidisciplinary individuals, preferably experts from the major groups that contribute to the process being studied. Improvements are made across departments and units.
4. The groups or teams are accountable to customers (patients and other members of the health care team).
5. The professional standards improve with time.
6. There is a commitment to customer satisfaction.

I. Doing the Right Thing

The *efficacy* of the procedure or treatment in relation to the patient's condition
> The degree to which the care of the patient has been shown to accomplish the desired or projected outcome(s)

The *appropriateness* of a specific test, procedure, or service to meet the patient's needs
> The degree to which the care provided is relevant to the patient's clinical needs, given the current state of knowledge

II. Doing the Right Thing Well

The *availability* of a needed test, procedure, treatment, or service to the patient who needs it
> The degree to which appropriate care is available to meet the patient's needs

The *timeliness* with which a needed test, procedure, treatment, or service is provided to the patient
> The degree to which the care is provided to the patient at the most beneficial or necessary time

The *effectiveness* with which tests, procedures, treatments, and services are provided
> The degree to which the care is provided in the correct manner, given the current state of knowledge, to achieve the desired or projected outcome(s) for the patient

The *continuity* of the services provided to the patient with respect to other services, practitioners, and providers, and over time
> The degree to which the care for the patient is coordinated among practitioners, among organizations, and over time

The *safety* of the patient (and others) to whom the services are provided
> The degree to which the risk of an intervention and the risk in the care environment are reduced for the patient and others, including the health care worker

The *efficiency* with which services are provided
> The relationship between the outcomes (results of care) and the resources used to deliver patient care

The *respect and caring* with which services are provided
> The degree to which the patient or a designee is involved in his or her own care decisions and to which those providing services do so with sensitivity and respect for the patient's needs, expectations, and individual differences

Figure 15–3. Definitions of dimensions of performance. *(From Joint Commission on the Accreditation of Healthcare Organizations (JCAHO):* 1995 Comprehensive Accreditation Manual for Hospitals. *Oakbrook Terrace, IL, JCAHO, 1995, with permission.)*

TABLE 15–1. SUMMARY OF THEORETICAL APPROACHES TO QUALITY IMPROVEMENT

Theorist	Approach
Deming	Do not tolerate poor service. Constantly improve production and service. Institute training for all workers. Institute effective leadership. Drive out fear. Create a climate of trust and innovation. Break down barriers between departments. Eliminate slogans. Eliminate numerical quotas. Remove barriers to pride in job performance. Take action.
Juran	Promote customer satisfaction.
Donabedian	Structure. Process. Outcomes.
Crosby	Zero defects. Strive to be error free.
Berwick	*Kaisen*, the Japanese term for "continuous search for opportunities for all processes to get better." Shift away from a regulatory model or seeking out the "bad apples," and move to seeking opportunities for improvement through mistakes. Learn from the mistakes.

When these six characteristics are adopted, the success of the hospital, a team, a service, a private practice, a clinic, or an entire laboratory can then be measured by the rate of improvement, not just by compliance with preexisting standards.

TQM is an umbrella concept that encompasses assessment of structure, process, outcomes, prevention, and customer satisfaction. Traditionally, clinical laboratory services have focused primarily on **quality control (QC),** or monitoring the testing process, and secondarily on quality assurance, or outcomes assessment. Figure 15–5 compares traditional laboratory QC and CQI. When determining the quality of performance, the evaluator must look for evidence that the best strategy of care was selected and that it was implemented in a skillful manner. The type of information that health care workers collect fits into structure, process, or outcomes measures.[2,3]

Structure

Structure is defined as physical or organizational properties of the settings where care is provided. Assessments of structural components include the following:

- *Physical structure.* Facilities where services are provided, adequacy of supplies, safety measures, and availability and condition of equipment such as computers, sterilizers, refrigerators, thermometers, centrifuges, autoclaves, and glucose-monitoring devices.
- *Personnel structure.* Numbers of personnel and support staff for each service, ratios of staff to patients, qualifications of staff, and availability of the medical director or supervisors.
- *Management–administrative structure.* Updated, available procedure manuals; multidisciplinary composition of committees; adequacy of systems for record keeping; and open lines of communication throughout the organization.

Most assessments of structural issues are done by a multidisciplinary team who can determine the adequacy of environmental and physical conditions. Structural components in quality assessment may reveal potential problems that other assessments (process and outcome) cannot. For example, the use of outdated blood collection tubes may cause faulty laboratory test results, even though the blood collection, testing, and reporting (processes) are perfect and the treatment plan for the patient (outcome) is appropriate.

- Internal inpatients
- Outpatients
- Patients' families and friends
- Patients' support groups
- Blood donors
- Clinical laboratory scientists
- Clinical laboratory technicians
- Secretaries and clerks
- Pathologists
- Nurses
- Administrators
- Human resources personnel
- Attending physicians
- Students
- Research staff
- Research granters
- Anyone who provides financial support (e.g., insurance companies, taxpayers, foundations)

Figure 15–4. The customers.

Continuous Quality Improvement (CQI)

CQI is a theoretical framework and management commitment to improve health care structures, processes, outcomes, and customer satisfaction. It is ongoing and involves all levels of the administrative structure of an organization.

Quality Control (QC)

QC monitors a process. It adjusts the analytic process to meet specific standards. It includes activities such as developing technical policies and procedures, ensuring that supplies are functional and not outdated, calibrating and maintaining equipment, and performing function checks. QC involves running QC samples in parallel with patient samples and participating in proficiency-testing programs.

Figure 15–5. Continuous quality improvement and quality control—similarities and differences.

Process

✔ **Process** is defined as what is done to the patient or client. Process assessments are common throughout the specimen collection and clinical testing arenas. This is where traditional QC measures are applicable. However, in addition to the normal laboratory data collection routines, other methods are effective for monitoring process. These include evaluation of patient records for complications, correct technical skills, and correct documentation procedures; direct observation of practices; videotaping of health care interactions and practices; patient interviews; and questionnaires.

Outcomes

✔ **Outcomes** are what is accomplished for the patient. The ultimate goal of CQI is to improve patient outcomes. Most outcomes assessments rely on information in the patient's medical record. Chart reviews usually evaluate the health status after services are provided. Timing is usually an important component of these measures. Outcomes assessments are typically the most difficult to measure and often relate to recovery rates, cure rates, nosocomial infection rates, return to normal functions, and so on. Poor patient outcomes have been described as the "5 Ds":[4]

- Death
- Disease
- Disability

- Discomfort
- Dissatisfaction

Unfortunately, health care workers can have negative effects in each of these categories. For example, misidentification of a patient can result in an erroneous cross-match and blood transfusion, which could be fatal to a patient (death.) Inappropriate cleansing techniques or hand washing could result in transmitting nosocomial infections (disease). Poor venipuncture techniques such as improper needle insertion or excessive probing could result in nerve damage (disability) or severe pain (discomfort). And lengthy waiting times, rude behavior, or messy work sites can contribute to an overall feeling of patient dissatisfaction. Even though these examples are extreme, they do exist in reality and need to be improved.

Quality improvement efforts for phlebotomy services often involve evaluating the following: the health care worker's technique, complications such as hematomas, re-collection rates resulting from contamination, and multiple sticks on the same patient. All these issues have the potential to result in a negative outcome for the patient. Thus, continuous improvement in minimizing these problems would be most beneficial to the patient and the health care worker.

Satisfaction

The study of satisfaction among patients and health care workers is usually accomplished by using questionnaires, mail outs, and telephone or personal interviews. Although the information gathered by using these techniques may be subjective, knowing *why* customers are dissatisfied and *which* customers are unhappy is extremely valuable. This information can be used to improve targeted services or aspects of a service. Health care workers must remember that positive patient outcomes usually result in positively satisfied customers.

TOOLS AND TRENDS FOR CQI

In a laboratory, check sheets, run charts, and statistical tests can be used to review both the analytic and nonanalytic parts of the laboratory. In an analytic sense, clinical laboratory scientists and technicians use data collection to ensure test sensitivity, specificity, precision, and accuracy. In a nonanalytic sense, data can be used to assess the timeliness of responses to requests, turnaround time for reporting test results, and effective communication. Tools for implementing CQI include the following:[3]

- **Flowcharts.** Useful for breaking a process into its components so that people can understand how it works (Fig. 15–6).

- **Pareto charts.** Bar charts that show the frequency of problematic events; the Pareto principle suggests that "80 percent of the trouble comes from 20 percent of the problems" (Fig. 15–7).
- **Cause-and-effect (Ishikawa) diagrams.** Diagrams that identify interactions between equipment, methods, people, supplies, and reagents (Fig. 15–8).
- **Line graphs, histograms, scatter diagrams.** Pictorial images representing performance trends.
- **Brainstorming.** Method used to stimulate creative solutions in a group.

Westgard et al.[4] suggest a "5 Q" framework for clinical laboratories that focuses on the following:

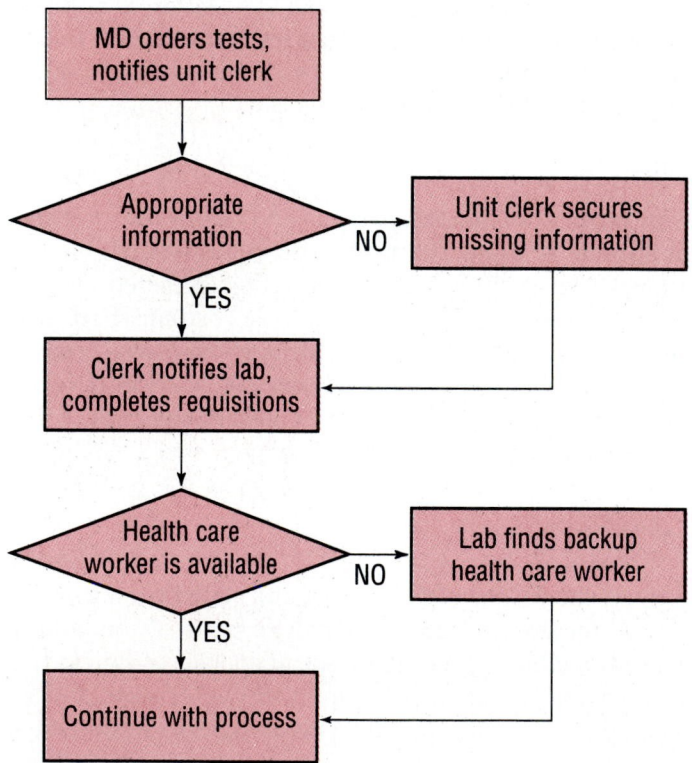

Figure 15–6. Flowchart. *(Adapted from Martin BG (ed): The CLMA Guide to Managing a Clinical Laboratory. Malvern, PA, Clinical Laboratory Management Association, 1991.)*

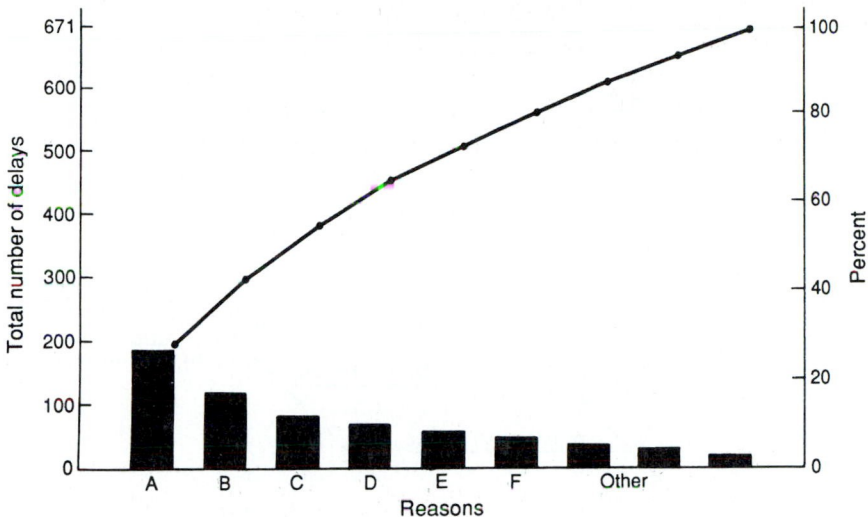

Figure 15–7. Pareto chart. *(From Martin BG (ed):* The CLMA Guide to Managing a Clinical Laboratory. *Malvern, PA, Clinical Laboratory Management Association, 1991, with permission.)*

- Quality planning (QP)
- Quality laboratory practices (QLP)
- Quality control (QC) of processes
- Monitoring performance, quality assessment
- Quality improvement (QI) when problems occur

This is a self-perpetuating, cyclic process that should become a way of life for all employees in the laboratory. However, each health care institution has different characteristics, and the laboratory's quality-management program will vary based on philosophy, mission, and tools selected for use.

CQI FOR SPECIMEN COLLECTION SERVICES

CQI studies for specimen collection services can be very revealing for laboratory employees, supervisors, and managers. A study by Howanitz et al.[5] indicated that 98.6 percent of patients in a study group from numerous hospitals were satisfied with many aspects of the phlebotomy services that they received. In this group, 97.3 percent of the patients had blood collected on the first phlebotomy attempt, and 16.1 percent of the punctures resulted in ecchymosis. In 25 percent of the cases, the

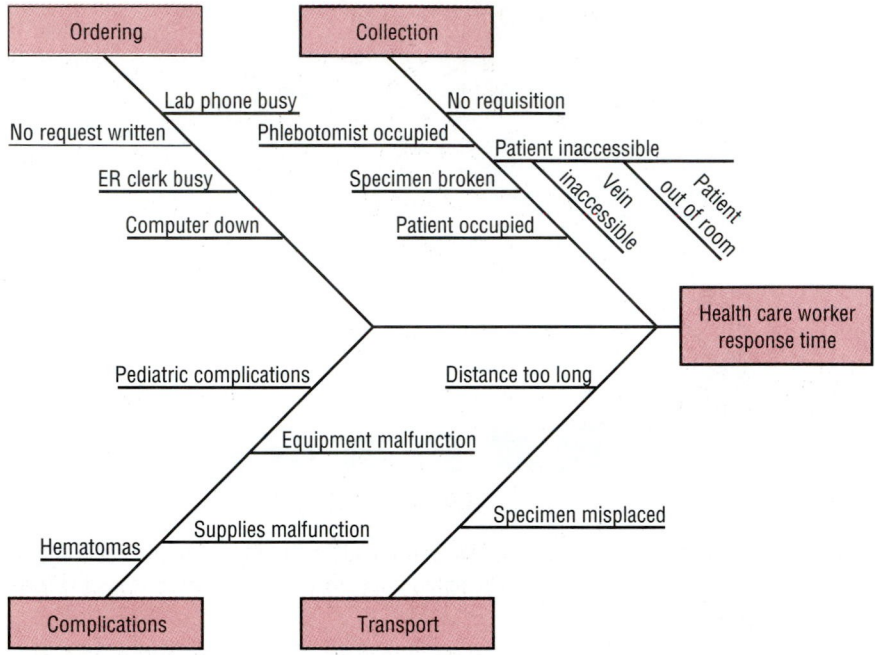

Figure 15–8. Ishikawa diagram. ER, emergency room.

time required for the phlebotomy procedure was 5 minutes or less. Each of these factors, in addition to numerous others, was analyzed, and areas for targeted improvement were identified. One of the general areas cited for suggested improvement was reduction of discomfort or pain caused by the puncture. Examples of CQI **monitors** that should be considered in specimen collection services are listed in Figure 15–9.

Monitors for quality assessment should fit specific criteria in order to be useful and valid. The **RUMBA model** is an easy check for determining the feasibility of a QI monitor.

- R—Relevant
- U—Understandable
- M—Measurable
- B—Behavioral
- A—Achievable

Before a study of a particular monitor (or problem) is begun, the RUMBA criteria should be applied. The following questions should be asked:

- Are the problems or variations in practices relevant to laboratory services or patient care?

- Are the items to be monitored understandable by those who will be collecting the data?
- Can measurable objective data be collected?
- Are there behavioral aspects that can be changed if necessary?
- Is the project realistic and achievable?

An important factor that can sometimes become a stumbling block for quality assessment is the data collection process. Most of the data can be collected from information already available in the patient care unit of the hospital or the laboratory, or by adding a brief tally or list to forms already in existence (Fig. 15–10). In addition, there are many other accessible sources of information (refer to Figure 15–4), although the use of some of these sources may require special permission.

COLLECTION PROCEDURES TO ENSURE QUALITY

Quality assurance in the clinical laboratory begins before the sample is collected from the patient. For perfect specimens, the patient and the specimen container must first be prepared. If the patient is inadequately prepared, the laboratory procedures and instrumentation cannot compensate for the shortcomings. Thus, the clinical laboratory must provide

---

- Health care worker response time (for inpatients)
- Patient waiting time (for outpatients)
- Time required for completion of the phlebotomy procedure
- Percentage of successful blood collections taken on the first attempt
- Number of phlebotomy attempts beyond the first attempt
- Number of phlebotomy attempts per patient by the medical service
- Number and size of hematomas
- Number of patients who faint
- Amount of time spent and number of telephone calls needed to acquire appropriate identification
- Number of redraws requested because of inadequate specimens
- Contribution of health care worker to turnaround times of designated laboratory tests
- Number of incomplete forms, documents, logs, and so forth
- Number of therapeutic drug monitoring tests that have incorrect documentation or timing
- Number of specimens received in incorrect tubes

Figure 15–9. Continuous quality improvement monitors for specimen collection services.

Medical records	Committee reports
Incident reports	Staff meetings
Accident reports	Marketing agents
Written complaints	Pathologists
Patient questionnaires	Attending physicians
Customer focus groups	Direct observation
Quality circles	Laboratory employees

Figure 15–10. Sources of information for quality assessment.

the nursing staff with a floor book that describes laboratory services, preparation of the patient, and special handling of patients' specimens. The health care worker should be aware of the protocol that is necessary to prepare patients and specimen containers for laboratory assays in order to instruct the nursing staff in this capacity and thereby lead to quality specimen collection. Thus, a monthly review of the laboratory's collection procedures and policies is recommended to reduce collection errors and, it is hoped, to lead to perfect specimen collection. Examples of the types of collection procedures and problems that the health care worker should review include the following:

1. Collection of blood specimens by skin puncture
2. Isolation techniques
3. Microcollection techniques on newborns
4. Collections for capillary blood gas analysis
5. Collection of blood specimens by finger stick
6. Intensive care blood collections
7. Pediatric blood collection techniques
8. Collection of specimens for intravenous glucose tolerance tests
9. Inability to collect blood specimen
10. Patient identification

Also, the health care worker should have access to a pocket-sized collection booklet that contains the same information as that in the floor book (e.g., laboratory test, laboratory section in which procedure is performed, required collection container, amount of required sample, preservatives for sample handling).

Anticoagulants and Preservatives: Quality Assurance

As discussed in Chapter 4, the health care worker uses various anticoagulants and preservatives in the collection of blood specimens. These tubes containing anticoagulants must be inverted promptly after blood is drawn to ensure mixture of the anticoagulant and the blood and thus to provide quality assurance of a perfectly collected specimen. As reviewed in Chapter 5, when several evacuated tubes of blood are collected from a patient, tubes containing anticoagulants should be filled in the appropriate order that proper inversion can occur and carryover of anticoagulants to clotted tubes will not occur.

For quality assurance, the anticoagulants and preservatives should meet the requirements established by the National Committee for Clinical Laboratory Standards (NCCLS). The manufacturer of the anticoagulants and preservatives must provide the shelf-life of these additives on the packages so that the user will know how long these additives are effective. When restocking the supply of collection tubes, health care personnel should place the tubes with a shelf-life (expiration date) nearest the current date at the front of the shelf so that these tubes are used first. In addition, for blood collection tubes, the manufacturers must test and verify draw and fill accuracy until the stated expiration date. The health care worker should be cognizant of expiration dates on any item used in specimen collection. Quality assurance accreditation standards require the health care institution to establish QC procedures for proper inspection of new lot numbers of evacuated blood collection tubes. In addition, quality can be obtained in specimen collection only with fresh specimens. If the blood specimen is not to be tested immediately, the health care worker must make certain that it is stored properly until the test is run.

Requirements for a Quality Specimen

The requirements for a quality specimen include the following:

1. Using universal precautions, the patient is prepared properly and medication interference is avoided, if possible.
2. The correct specimens are collected from the correct patients and are properly labeled. Because the policy of most clinical laboratories is to discard specimens that are unlabeled or labeled incorrectly, the health care worker must abide by the written laboratory policy describing acceptable identification of specimens to ensure perfect specimen collection. The potential errors in after-the-fact reidentification of a specimen by floor personnel can be extremely detrimental to the patient in question and must be avoided. (See Chapter 5 for identification and labeling procedures.)
3. The correct anicoagulants and preservatives are used with the sufficient amount collected (see Chapter 4).
4. The specimens are not hemolyzed.

5. The fasting specimens are collected in a timely fashion and are actually fasting samples.
6. Timed specimens are correctly timed and documented.
7. Specimens without anticoagulants are allowed to stand a minimum of 30 minutes so that clot formation can occur completely. (Gel separator tubes will shorten the time of clot formation, depending on the manufacturer's tubes.)
8. Specimens are transported to the clinical laboratory in a timely fashion to maintain freshness (within 45 minutes). If the laboratory does not have designated delivery times for specimens, the health care worker may suggest to his or her laboratory supervisor that such a system would ensure fresh specimens and, thus, high-quality laboratory test results. A list of the specimens that are delivered after the designated time limits should be maintained in a logbook. Such a list can usually help personnel detect the source of the problem so that quality assessments can be evaluated. The list reveals the number of specimens that were delivered after the allowable limits and how late they were. The supervisor of specimen control usually decides whether the late specimen should be discarded and a new one collected.

Number of Blood Collection Attempts

Another way to provide quality services to the patients is by monitoring and reducing the number of unsuccessful collection attempts. If the health care worker has had consecutively unsuccessful phlebotomy attempts on different patients, the supervisor and the health care worker will know that the problem in blood collection must be identified and solved to prevent future unsuccessful attempts. Most clinical laboratories have a written procedure on the inability to draw specimens that describes the steps that should be taken by the health care worker when (1) collection attempts are unsuccessful (usually no more than two sticks), (2) the patient is unavailable, or (3) the patient refuses to have blood drawn.

QC and Preventive Maintenance of Specimen Collection Instruments

The health care worker should be aware that QC checks and preventive maintenance of certain instruments and equipment most often occur in the specimen control section. Thermometers are one type of instrument that must be maintained by blood collection personnel. The sphygmomanometer is another instrument used in blood collection procedures that must be maintained and checked for quality assurance. Another instrument frequently used and maintained by health care workers is the centrifuge. In addition to undergoing preventive maintenance procedures, the centrifuge that is used to spin down the blood must be checked for accurate speed. The speed of the centrifuge can be checked with a tachometer, which indicates the speed in revolutions per minute (RPM). The relative centrifugal force, or g value, is then determined from a nomogram available in laboratories. The g value gives the efficiency of the instrument by determining the true force exerted by the centrifuge. A g force of approximately 1000 for 10 minutes is usually efficient for good separation of cells or clotted blood from plasma or serum. However, the health care worker must be sure to follow the manufacturer's directions when using gel separator devices to separate blood specimens. These collection tubes usually require a specified force higher than 1000 g for complete separation. The NCCLS publishes a manual entitled *Procedures for the Handling and Processing of Blood Specimens,* which provides more information on centrifugation of blood specimens.

✔ Key Terms

Cause-and-Effect (Ishikawa) Diagrams

Continuous Quality Improvement (CQI)

Customer Satisfaction

Dr. W. Edwards Deming

"5 Q" Framework

Flowcharts

Histograms

JCAHO 10-Step Process

Monitors

Outcomes

Pareto Charts

Process

Quality Control (QC)

RUMBA Model

Structure

Total Quality Management (TQM)

Study Questions

1. Of the following, which are examples of customers for phlebotomy services?
   a. outpatients
   b. patients' family members
   c. attending physicians
   d. nursing staff

2. Examples of poor patient outcomes include which of the following?
   a. excessive probing for a vein
   b. multiple sticks on the same patient
   c. nosocomial infections
   d. hematomas

3. Which of the following are examples of structural components of quality that should be periodically checked?
   a. expiration dates
   b. condition of supplies
   c. adequacy of supplies
   d. nosocomial infections

4. Which of the following are examples of process components of quality that should be checked?
   a. documentation procedures
   b. hematomas
   c. multiple sticks
   d. use of incorrect anticoagulants

5. Why is rapid delivery of specimens important?
   a. because cells should not remain in contact with sera for excessive periods
   b. so that the health care worker can hurry to the next patient
   c. to reduce turnaround time for results
   d. because laboratory test results are most accurate when fresh specimens are used

REFERENCES

1. Joint Commission on Accreditation of Healthcare Organizations (JCAHO): *1995 Comprehensive Accreditation Manual for Hospitals.* Oakbrook Terrace, IL, JCAHO, 1995.
2. Simpson KN, Kaluzny AD, McLaughlin CP: Total quality and the management of laboratories. *Clin Lab Manage Rev* November/December: 448–462, 1991.
3. Graham NO: *Quality in Health Care: Theory, Applications, and Evolution.* Gaithersburg, MD, Aspen Publishers, 1995.
4. Westgard JO, Barry PL, Tomar RH: Implementing TQM in health care laboratories. *Clin Lab Manage Rev* 5(5):354, 1991.
5. Howanitz PJ, Cembrowski GS, Bachner P: Laboratory phlebotomy—CAP Q-probe study of patient satisfaction and complications in 23,783 patients. *Arch Pathol Lab Med* 115:867–872, 1991.
6. Martin BG (ed): *The CLMA Guide to Managing a Clinical Laboratory.* Malvern, PA, Clinical Laboratory Management Association, 1991.

COMMUNICATION, PROFESSIONALISM, AND MANAGERIAL SKILLS

Chapter Outline

Chapter Objectives

Upon completion of Chapter 16, the learner is responsible for the following:

1. Describe the basic elements of effective communication in a patient care environment.

2. List examples of positive and negative body language.

3. Define helpful ways of communicating with patients.

4. List key management factors related to staffing for phlebotomy services.

5. Describe ways to be an active listener.

COMMUNICATION SKILLS IN THE PATIENT CARE ENVIRONMENT

As a vital member of the health care team, the health care worker provides the link between the patient and the analytic area. The quality of the blood specimens determines the quality of the diagnostic test results. However, the ease of collection of these specimens depends on the skills and abilities of the health care worker to perform the collection techniques and to interact successfully with the patient.

Bedside Manner

The climate established by the health care worker upon entering a patient's room begins before he or she leaves the laboratory area. The feeling of confidence that comes from the knowledge that the collection tray is clean and completely stocked is the first step in a good bedside manner. A pleasant face, a neat appearance, and a professional manner set the stage for a positive encounter with the patient. The first 30 seconds after the health care worker enters the patient's room determines how that patient perceives the clinical laboratory and, in some cases, the quality of patient care offered by that hospital. Most patients admit that the procedure they dread most is being "stuck" for blood collection.

As discussed in previous chapters, the health care worker should introduce him- or herself and then state that he or she is part of the hospital unit or laboratory staff. The patient should be informed that the specimen is being collected for a test ordered by the physician. A statement indicating that this is routine hospital protocol often reassures the patient. A lengthy discussion of why a certain test was ordered or what tests were ordered is inappropriate. These questions should be referred to the patient's physician. During all steps of the venipuncture, the health care worker should remain calm and professional. Before leaving the patient, he or she should make sure that the patient is no longer bleeding and thank him or her for cooperating.

Patient Interview

Hospitals and laboratories differ slightly in their guidelines for patient interviews. All agree that proper patient identification is essential, both by means of an armband and by verbal confirmation. If the patient does *not* have an armband, a positive confirmation must be made by a unit nurse who knows the patient. This process should be well documented by the health care worker. Special identification procedures should also be well documented for ambulatory patients. Armbands may not be routinely issued in ambulatory settings; however, an identification card usually is. It may include some demographic data. Again, this should be confirmed by the patient prior to collection of specimens. The patient should always be asked, "What is your name?" not "Are you Ms. Smith?" A patient on medication will often agree with anything that he or she is asked. Some institutions insist that the health care worker ask for the patient's complete address, whereas others require the mention of the patient's hometown, birth date, or street name to reinforce and confirm identity. Some prefer that patients spell an unusual last name. This portion of the specimen collection procedure ensures that the remainder of the diagnostic testing protocol provides information on the correct person.

It is important for the health care worker to remember that verbal and nonverbal cues (body language) play an important part in the communication of what the patient perceives and how he or she responds. In addition, listening skills are a valuable part of patient communication.

Teaching Patients

For most phlebotomy procedures to be successful, the patient must participate and cooperate. The health care worker must be willing and able to provide sufficient, understandable instruction to the patient for protocols to be accomplished. For example, in some clinical situations, patients with diabetes need to be instructed on the use of mechanical aids to perform finger sticks on themselves at home to check blood glucose levels.

Nursing staff or unit personnel may have instructed the inpatient that he or she will be fasting, or will have "nothing by mouth," until after the early morning blood collections. The health care worker should listen to patients' comments such as "I didn't have breakfast yet" and "they won't feed me." Even a question or a comment about food may inspire a response to confirm that the patient was truly fasting.

Even more critical are the timed tests such as the glucose tolerance test. In this test, patient understanding is essential. For the procedure to yield valid and reliable results, the patient must stay fasting, be in his or her room at the specified time, and drink enough water to provide the timed urine specimens. If the patient is a child, the parents or guardian must receive and understand the instructions. If the patient begins to feel ill or faint, the nursing personnel or the health care supervisor should be notified. If the patient is an outpatient, the health care worker and other laboratory personnel must monitor the patient's condition. A bed and bathroom must be convenient to the collection area to provide for the patient's comfort and safety.

Another timed specimen often used in laboratory medicine is the 24-hour urine specimen. For the test to fit into most laboratory schedules, the patient should void at 7:00 AM and discard the urine. The next urine and all urine voided for 24 hours is saved in the container provided. The patient should be cautioned that to have good results *all* the urine must be saved or the procedure will have to be started over.

For urine cultures, the patient must be instructed in proper specimen collection techniques to ensure valid results from microbiology. Occasionally, clinic patients require instruction in collection of stool specimens for culture, for examination for ova and parasites, or for occult blood tests. Also, the Scotch tape method for diagnosis of pinworms should be available in the procedure manual if needed for outpatient teaching. Although infrequent, the need to instruct the outpatient about the collection of a 24-hour stool specimen for fecal fat analysis may be necessary.

With therapeutic drug monitoring, the physician must know not only the time and date of collection, but also whether the blood was collected before or after medication was given. The length of infusion time is also a factor with some drug monitoring. Laboratory and/or hospital unit coordination necessitates a knowledgeable and readily available health care worker on the health care team as well as a positive working relationship with the nursing and pharmacy staff. Some hospitals designate only experienced health care workers as the collectors for drug-monitoring tests.

BARRIERS AND AIDS TO COMMUNICATION

Communication of information is essential not only for teaching and dealing with patients, but also for proper laboratory testing and interacting with hospital personnel. However, there are many barriers to good understanding and accurate communication. The following sections describe general concepts of communication.

Basic interpersonal communication can be depicted as a closed loop. The message must leave the sender and reach the receiver (Fig. 16–1). The receiver usually provides feedback to the sender. Without feedback, the sender has no way of knowing whether the message was accurately received or if the message was somehow blocked by extraneous factors. These factors can often filter out meaning from a message. Filters can be damaging to good communication. In the following sections, communication is broken down into its three more detailed components:

1. Verbal communication
2. Nonverbal communication
3. Active listening

Verbal Communication

A basic understanding of the language is needed for any health care worker to communicate with all patients, young and old. However, there are filters or barriers to simple verbal communication that can interfere greatly with the patient–health care worker relationship.

Basic Language Barriers. Many members of the health care team use jargon, or medical terminology, to explain things to the patient. This can often be confusing to laypeople. In addition, the meaning of words varies with the context and the age of the speaker. To promote understanding, a vocabulary that is easily understood should be used with patients whenever possible. This is particularly true with children. Also, children must *not* be told, "This won't hurt." Most blood collection procedures are slightly painful; therefore, it is important that the child be forewarned and prepared. It sometimes helps if the child is asked to hold something (e.g., a bandage) while the procedure is taking place.

Figure 16–1. Communication loop.

This allows the child to feel helpful and provides a distraction from the procedure.

Hearing Impairments. The more complex the directions, the greater the need to communicate. Thus, the health care worker should be more sensitive to patients who have impaired hearing. A question such as "How will you do this?" or "When will you begin to start this task?" yields better clues that the patient has heard and understood than "Do you understand?" If it is obvious that the patient did not hear, all efforts should be made to write down instructions for the patient. It is strongly recommended that writing tools be kept at the bedside of these patients and be accessible in an outpatient setting.

English as a Second Language. Patients often understand from nonverbal cues such as sign language, but the health care worker must know how to locate an interpreter, if available, when the patient does not speak or comprehend English. If a large segment of the patient population speaks another language, the hospital should provide interpreters who know the basic use of that language. In the southern and western United States, it is important to develop some skill in the Spanish language. (For basic requests in Spanish, refer to Appendix 1.) It is recommended that the health care worker practice the phrases with someone who can speak the language before attempting to communicate with a patient because mispronounced words may lead to more confusion. It might also be helpful to have printed cards in different languages that can be used to transmit information. Keep in mind that English language skills and understanding may vary greatly in the United States. The country's cultural diversity lends itself to language differences. The health care worker should always speak respectfully, in a highly professional manner, and with phrases that are clearly articulated. The dignity of the patient, whether he or she is English speaking or not, is of utmost importance. If a health care worker feels frustrated by an inability to communicate with a patient, the health care worker should seek assistance from a supervisor, a translator, a family member, or a physician. Each patient should be treated compassionately, fairly, and with the utmost of dignity, regardless of language abilities.

Age. The vocabulary of a teenager is different from that of someone 70 to 80 years old. The health care worker must be sensitive to word usage for each age group.

Tone of Voice. The tone of voice and the inflection used can change a positive sentence into a negative-sounding statement. Care must be taken to be *sure* that the pitch, or tone, of voice matches the words that the health care worker is attempting to communicate. Sarcasm is usually communicated just by tone of voice. Health care workers should make every attempt to avoid sending mixed messages to patients by practicing a calm, soothing, and confident tone of voice. Figure 16–2 is a practice exercise for health care professionals to use in observing their own facial expressions and voice tones.

Special Situations. The health care worker should realize that patients in the surgical suite, recovery room, or emergency room usually have the need for emergency (or stat) blood collection. This requires the health care worker to act with extra speed and accuracy without jeopardizing the "personal touch." Patients that are in the hospital or come in for chemotherapy often have veins that have been damaged or must be avoided and used only for treatment. Therefore, each patient must be considered in terms of his or her dignity and individual needs, not as the "burn case down the hall" or "the broken leg in 3C." As long as the

---

The following exercise is useful for improving verbal and nonverbal communication skills. Practice it in front of a mirror or with a co-worker.

1. Using a *nice tone of voice* (i.e., calm, compassionate, clear, professional tone), with a smile on your face, practice saying the following phrases:

   - "Please . . ."
   - "Good morning."
   - "How was your breakfast?"
   - "Have you had lunch?"
   - "May I check your identification bracelet?"
   - "Thank you."

2. Now, using a *degrading tone of voice* (i.e., sarcastic, whiny, angry tone), with a frustrated look on your face, repeat the phrases listed in step 1.
3. Contrast what you like about the first method with what you do not like about the second method.
4. Keep a mental impression of the positive aspects of your voice and expression.

Remember: A simple smile can often force a positive change in voice tone.

Figure 16–2. Practice exercise for observing the implications of facial expression and tone of voice.

health care worker is willing to provide care in a professional, respectful manner and to respond to each patient as an individual, the quality of care will improve.

Nonverbal Communication

It is often said that one of the most important parts of communication is the nonverbal component. Some educators believe that communication comprises 10 to 20 percent words and 80 to 90 percent nonverbal cues. These nonverbal cues, or body language, can be positive and helpful to understanding or can be negative and prevent communication. They are summarized next and in Figure 16–3.

Positive Body Language

Smiling. A simple, compassionate smile can set the stage for open lines of communication. It can make each patient feel that he or she is the most important person at that particular moment. In addition, most people look better with smiles on their faces than they do with frowns.

Positive Body Language

Maintaining erect posture
Having relaxed hands, arms, shoulders
Communicating face to face
Maintaining eye contact
Communicating at eye level when possible
Displaying good grooming habits
Maintaining zone of comfort
Smiling

Negative Body Language and Distracting Behaviors

Slouching, shrugging shoulders
Rolling eyes, wandering eyes
Looking at ceiling or window, staring blankly
Rubbing eyes, blinking excessively
Squirming
Tapping foot, fingers, pencil
Sighing deeply, moaning and groaning
Crossing arms, clenching fists
Wrinkling forehead
Thumbing through books or papers
Chewing gum
Repeatedly looking at clock or watch
Lining up objects on a desk
Stretching and yawning
Sitting backward on a chair (i.e., straddling it)
Peering over eyeglasses
Pointing a finger at someone

Figure 16–3. Nonverbal communication, or body language.

Health care workers should strive to be as compassionate as possible. Bedridden patients often feel intimidated because health care workers must repeatedly "look down" on them to provide care. Sometimes, these patients are depressed because of their condition or prognosis. This exercise will help you imagine yourself in the patient's condition and can make you a more compassionate member of the health care team. Practice the exercise with a co-worker.

1. Lie on a bed while your co-worker stands directly over you, looking down.
2. Have the co-worker go through the motions of a venipuncture procedure, including the greeting and identification process. Try to imagine the anticipation of the needle stick. Have the co-worker maintain eye contact with you while conversing.
3. Repeat step 2, without eye contact.
4. Mentally note the positive and negative aspects of this procedure.

Figure 16–4. Practice exercise for developing sensitivity to bedridden patients.

Eye Contact and Eye Level. The most expressive parts of the human face are the eyes. Therefore, eye contact is important in effective communication. Eye contact promotes a sense of trust and honesty between a patient and a health care worker. It can make the entire procedure less traumatic for the patient if he or she sees a sense of compassion and honesty in a health care worker's eyes.

In addition, eye level can be important. Unfortunately, bedridden patients must always look up to those in the room, including the caregivers and the health care worker. This can create a feeling of intimidation, being "looked down on," or weakness. Therefore, if a health care worker must explain a lengthy procedure to a patient, it should be done while seated at eye level with the patient. Other than this instance, it is rare that the health care worker would have a chance to be at eye level. However, health care workers must understand the concept so that they can feel what it would be like to be a bedridden patient. Figure 16–4 is a suggested exercise for understanding what it feels like to be bedridden.

Good Grooming. Physical appearance communicates a great deal about an individual. Neatly combed hair; clean fingernails; a clean, pressed laboratory coat; and an overall tidy appearance communicate a commitment to infection control, as well as overall cleanliness, and instill confidence in a person. This is particularly important in today's hospital environment, where patients and employees alike are deeply concerned about the spread of infectious diseases such as hepatitis and human immunodeficiency virus (HIV).

Erect Posture. Most of the time, health care workers perform their work while standing. However, there are occasions, particularly with ambulatory patients, when health care workers may sit while collecting blood. In these cases, erect posture conveys a sense of confidence and pride in job performance. Slouching conveys a sense of laziness and apathy.

Good posture is helpful for both the health care worker and the patient. Not only does it minimize the health care worker's back or neck strain and ease the patient's mind, but it also allows the patient to feel more confident in the health care worker. Relaxed hands, arms, and shoulders enable the health care worker to work more freely and to show the patient how to relax the arms and shoulders as well.

Face-to-Face Communication. When speaking, health care workers should face patients directly. Otherwise, the patients may feel that they are being avoided or neglected or that information is being withheld. However, if a patient turns away from a health care worker, it should be taken as a cue that the patient is either very frightened or angry, or in pain. The health care worker should try not to take it personally and to do everything to make the patient feel more comfortable during the phlebotomy procedure.

Zone of Comfort. Most individuals begin to feel uncomfortable when strangers get too close to them physically. A **zone of comfort** is the area of space around a patient that is private territory, so to speak. When a strange individual gets too close, it can cause the patient to feel nervous, fearful, or anxious. Health care workers must be understanding and approach nervous patients slowly and gently to avoid causing feelings of being threatened. This is particularly true with children, many of whom have a wide zone of comfort; that is, they do not like anyone to approach them except close relatives or friends. A skilled health care worker must be aware of his or her threat to a patient and approach the situation in a calm, professional, and confident manner.

In some cultures, the zone of comfort may be wide, and in others, people naturally speak more closely to each other. How much at ease a person feels with physical closeness can also vary with gender. Some women feel very uncomfortable having a male health care worker standing over them preparing to draw a blood specimen, and vice versa. It is particularly considerate if a health care worker recognizes this and responds accordingly. Again, respect for the patient's needs and dignity must be considered.

The health care worker can practice having the sensation that someone is "too close for comfort" by using role reversal. Figure 16–5 provides a brief exercise.

Negative Body Language and Distracting Behaviors

Wandering Eyes. In most cases, when people roll their eyes upward, they convey the sense of being bored, inattentive, or unwilling to perform a duty. Because this behavior is distracting, it should be avoided at all times when a health care worker is communicating with, listening to, or observing patients, co-workers, or supervisors.

Having respect for an individual's personal space, or zone of comfort, is part of being a compassionate health care worker. The comfort zone of each person varies with sex, culture, and situation. However, most people feel uneasy when strangers are touching them or are "too close for comfort." An example of this uncomfortable sensation is in a crowded elevator. People take great measures to move so that they are not touching strangers, and as people exit the elevator, the remaining people move and shift to provide more space around themselves. This same sense of uneasiness is felt by patients who are approached by unfamiliar health care workers.

To simulate a real patient–health care worker interaction, practice the following exercise with a co-worker who is not a close friend. Eye contact should be made during this exercise.

1. Lie on a bed as if you are a patient.
2. Have the co-worker slowly approach you. He or she should begin 10 feet away and pause between steps.
3. Note at what distance you begin to feel awkward or uncomfortable. (Usually, this distance is about 2 to 4 feet from the bed.) This distance is the boundary of your zone of comfort.
4. Repeat the exercise with the same co-worker. You will probably require a smaller zone of comfort because a person becomes a little more at ease after initial contact with an unfamiliar person.

Figure 16–5. Role reversal exercise for developing sensitivity to the zone of comfort.

The same can be said of gazing out the window or looking up at the ceiling. If a health care worker enters a patient's room and begins addressing the patient while looking out the window, the patient will feel neglected and the health care worker will appear unconcerned. If the window is too tempting to avoid a glance, the health care worker should include the patient in on the observations. The health care worker could make a friendly comment about the weather and so forth, then continue the specimen collection procedure when full attention can be given to the patient. The objective is to make the patient feel at ease through good communication techniques so that the procedure can be successful.

Nervous Behaviors. Some nervous behaviors such as squirming or tapping a pencil or a foot can be very distracting. These behaviors can make a patient feel nervous, hurried, or anxious about the venipuncture. It is important to present a calm and confident image for maximum patient comfort and trust. It is also important that health care workers recognize these nervous behaviors in patients, particularly children, so that a special effort can be made to relieve any fear. Allowing a few extra moments of conversation or preparation may help.

Deep Sighs. A deep sigh can convey a feeling of being bored or a reluctance to do the job. Health care workers must avoid this behavior, especially when communicating with an uncooperative or angry patient. Likewise, if a patient sighs deeply or moans at the mere sight of a health care worker, this behavior should be a cue that a little extra attention, conversation, or a smile might ease the reluctance for the procedure.

Other Distracting Behaviors. Many other actions can convey negative, distracting, or defensive types of emotions. Among these are crossed arms, a wrinkled forehead, frequent glances at a clock, rapid thumbing through papers or a book, chewing gum, smoking cigarettes, lining up objects on a table, or yawning and stretching. It is vital for health care workers to realize that these behaviors can detract from their professional image when they are communicating with patients, families, visitors, co-workers, and supervisors. It is also important to recognize what these cues mean if a patient exhibits them. Health care workers who are the most effective communicators can detect these signs immediately and deal with them in an honest, compassionate, and professional manner. It is strongly recommended that regular in-service or continuing education programs be directed at reminding health care workers to be aware of positive and negative body language, both in their own behavior and in that of patients.

Active Listening

Another key component of effective communication is the art of listening. **Active listening** helps close the communication loop (see Figure 16–1) by ensuring that the message that was sent can indeed be repeated and understood. Listening skills do not depend on intellect or educational background; they can be learned and practiced. Figure 16–6 provides tips for becoming an active listener.

FAMILY, VISITORS, AND SIGNIFICANT OTHERS

Sometimes, families and visitors are much more difficult to deal with than patients. Often, families and visitors make requests or demands that are beyond the scope of acceptable responsibilities for a health care worker. For example, a health care worker should not give hospitalized patients food without the physician's permission. It is safer to inform the nurse or the head of the care team of the patient's request.

If several visitors are in the room with the patient, they may be asked to step into the hall while the blood specimen is being drawn. If the health care worker believes that assistance is required, a family member may be asked to assist. This can make the family members feel helpful as well as provide reassurance to the patients, particularly children.

Physicians, priests, and chaplains have the right to visit privately with patients. Unless the blood specimen is timed, the health care worker should respect that privacy and return to the patient after completing the other draws in the unit or area. If the procedure is timed or stat, the health care worker can apologize for the interruption, explain the nature of the request, and ask permission to collect the specimen.

Families and visitors of patients should not be permitted in the clinical laboratory or provided with patient information, except by prior arrangement. Their safety and the confidentiality of patient records must be considered. Frequently, patients do not want their family members to know test results.

APPEARANCE, GROOMING, AND PHYSICAL FITNESS

In general, the white coat or smock is used to cover and protect clothing while the health care worker is in the technical or analytic area. However, some clinics, hospitals, and physicians' offices still follow the more traditional dress code. The following four rules generally apply to personnel who routinely interact with patients:

The following steps are presented as a starting point for the development of listening skills by health care workers. Because individuals can mentally process words faster than they can speak them, a good listener must concentrate and focus on the speaker to keep his or her mind from wandering. Development of these skills can help an individual in professional life as well as in personal life.

1. Concentrate on the speaker by "getting ready" to listen. Take a moment to clear your mind of distracting thoughts. Begin the interaction with an open, objective mind. Sometimes taking a deep breath can help clear your mind and prepare it to receive more information.
2. Use silent pauses in the conversation wisely by mentally summarizing what has been said.
3. Let the speaker know that someone is listening. Use simple phrases such as "I see," "Oh," "Very interesting," and "How about that" to reassure the speaker and communicate understanding and acceptance.
4. Keep personal judgments to yourself until the speaker finishes relaying his or her idea.
5. Verify the conversation with feedback. Make sure that everything was clarified. Ask for more explanation if necessary.
6. Mentally review the key words to summarize the overall idea being communicated.
7. Pay attention to body language and ask for clarification. Simple prompts such as "You look sad" and "You seem upset or nervous" can add more meaning to the conversation and encourage the speaker to verbalize feelings.
8. Listen for true meaning in the message, not just the literal words.
9. Maintain eye contact to communicate interest or concern.
10. Encourage the listener to expand his or her thoughts by using simple phrases such as "Let's discuss it further," "Tell me more about it," and "Really?"
11. Paraphrase the idea or conversation to ensure complete understanding.
12. Practice active listening at work and at home.

Figure 16–6. Steps for active listening.

1. *White uniform.* The complete white uniform should be worn with comfortable shoes (usually white shoes are preferred). Clogs, high heels, sandals, and other casual styles are not considered appropriate. The entire uniform and the shoes should be neat and clean.

2. *Jewelry, fingernails, makeup, and hair.* Jewelry should be limited to a few rings and a wristwatch, and fingernails should be filed short and kept clean. Hand lotion should be available because of drying due to frequent hand washing and prolonged use of gloves. Female personnel should remember to apply makeup sparingly because bright or dark colors look harsh with a white uniform. Hair should be kept neatly cut, styled, and clean. Long hair must be tied back because it may hide or contaminate the venipuncture site or get caught in laboratory equipment. Men who wear moustaches, beards, or both should keep them neat, trimmed, and clean. Many of these suggestions are also commonsense safety precautions.

3. *Smocks, tunics, or laboratory coats.* In some clinics and hospitals, health care workers wear white smocks, tunics, jackets, or laboratory coats with dark shoes and slacks. It is recommended that a light or white shirt or blouse be worn underneath. The sleeves of the smock or laboratory coat should be longer than the sleeves of the blouse.

4. *Protective clothing and equipment (laboratory coats, masks, etc.).* Protective clothing and equipment must be made available by employers. Most health care organizations launder and maintain a continuous supply of clean, pressed laboratory coats. This eliminates the need for employees to take their contaminated laboratory coats home to wash with other household clothing. This practice keeps laboratory workers safer, emphasizes a deep regard for cleanliness, and eases the patient's mind about the transmission of infectious diseases from dirty or soiled laboratory coats.

Supervisors should remember that the rules of dress must be applied impartially to men and women on the phlebotomy or health care team. In all cases, however, clothes should be clean and pressed.

A vital part of a nice appearance is careful attention to personal hygiene. A daily bath or shower followed by the use of deodorant is recommended. Perfume or aftershave lotion should be used sparingly because patients may be allergic or may find some scents overpowering and distasteful when they are sick. It is also important to maintain good health habits such as proper nutrition and exercise because the role of a health care worker requires physical stamina. Good health also improves the health care worker's appearance, attitude, and ability to cope with stress.

The proper uniform worn with the appropriate care, good grooming, and physical fitness all contribute to a professional appearance. With a pleasant smile, a positive attitude, and a neat appearance, the health care worker is more fully prepared to deal with patients, hospital visitors, family members, and other members of the health care team.

PATIENT RIGHTS

All members of the health care team must recognize that their first responsibility is to the patient's health, safety, and personal dignity. Many organizations such as the **American Hospital Association (AHA)** have recognized rights for patients in health care organizations. The AHA originally adopted a **Patient's Bill of Rights** in 1973 and has revised and reaffirmed it as needed. The key elements involve a patient's rights to the following:

- Respectful, considerate care
- Accurate information
- Informed consent
- Refusal of treatment
- Privacy
- Confidentiality
- Information about who his or her provider is
- Information about research procedures involved in his or her care
- Billing information

Issues in Specimen Collection

There are occasions during specimen collections when a patient's rights are particularly important. The patient may be rude, ill tempered, demanding, and/or uncooperative. However, it is important for members of the health care team to always deliver the best quality of care that they can give, being careful to show consideration, fairness, compassion, and respect for each patient.

Requests for certain laboratory tests and the results of clinical laboratory tests are part of the patient's treatment and are *strictly confidential*. This rule of confidentiality extends to all areas of a health care institution. A health care worker should *never* discuss patient information in a public place such as an elevator, a hallway, or the cafeteria. Family members or friends may overhear and be offended.

Health care workers are not to give patients (or their friends or family) information about why laboratory tests were ordered, the results, or the testing methodologies. Requests for this information can generally be handled correctly by saying to the patient, "your physician ordered blood to be drawn for testing; it would be best to discuss the tests with him or her." The remainder of the questions should be directed to the patient's physician. It is the physician's responsibility to communicate medical decisions to the patient. Sometimes, a talkative patient may want to share information of a personal and sensitive nature with the health care worker. It is appropriate to politely stop the patient from disclosure and continue with the collection procedure.

As part of the principle of informed consent, the health care worker should briefly explain to the patient the procedures used to collect the blood sample. The patient also has the right to know that the blood-drawing team member is part of the organization's staff and who he or she is. It is important for the health care worker to stress that the physician has ordered the tests. The patient also has the right to know if someone involved in his or her care is a student. It is helpful if the supervisor can reassure the patient of the student's competency to perform the procedure. Every effort should be made to have student–patient interactions be positive.

If a patient refuses to have a blood specimen drawn, the health care worker is responsible for reminding the patient that the physician ordered the clinical laboratory tests as part of the patient's medical care. If the patient still refuses, the health care worker should inform the nursing staff and, if possible, the physician. The health care worker should avoid any emotional confrontation or conflict with the patient. All the actions should be documented.

Clinical laboratory requisition slips contain demographic data that should not be exposed to the public, even if analytic results are not yet recorded. The hospital is responsible for the security of data in electronic information storage and retrieval systems and for making the information available only to those who specifically need it.

PROFESSIONAL BEHAVIOR

Accountability

Personal **accountability** cannot be calculated in a mathematical equation. Each health care worker has a personal responsibility for providing the best care possible. Personal integrity, or "doing what's right when no one is looking" (e.g., washing hands between patient collections, observing precautions to gown and scrub in isolation, and collecting timed tests at the proper time), reflects a health care worker's personal accountability or individual responsibility for actions.

Motivation and Social Behavior

Motivation has been defined as inducing people to act in a desired manner. People either perform of their own choice or are persuaded to perform. *Attitude,* however, is the personal feeling expressed in words or behaviors. Feelings that are expressed either verbally or in activities are a portrayal of attitudes. Ideally, the work setting should provide a climate that makes positive motivation and attitude development possible. Some people use the word *personality* to express what is meant about attitude. The right personality for the health care field can be defined as a caring personality coupled with a willingness to help and to do things for others. A cheerful disposition, an even temper, a methodical manner, and a reliable nature are valuable assets in any setting, but particularly in those involving patients. If the health care worker can be polite, tactful, efficient, and calm in emergencies, the interpersonal relationships between the health care worker and other members of the health care team can be pleasant.

Ethics

The principles of right and wrong conduct, as they apply to professional problems, are the ethics for that profession. Professions set standards of conduct for members, and members are expected to adhere to those standards of performance in their work. Standards of behavior are implied in the codes of ethics for each member of the health care team. The three major points common to most ethical standards are as follows:

1. Do no harm to anyone intentionally.
2. Perform according to sound technical ability and good judgment.
3. Respect the patients' rights (which include confidentiality, privacy, the right to know about their treatment, and the right of refusal).

As examples, the **American Society for Clinical Laboratory Scientists (ASCLS)** and the **National Phlebotomy Association (NPA)** developed codes of ethics for laboratory professionals and health care workers. The major themes of the codes are accuracy and reliability of laboratory test results, and confidentiality. Many hospitals across the country have also established codes of ethics. Often, these codes deal more specifically with specialty care for the hospital or with the specific mission of the hospital.

Health care workers, as in other areas of health care, must continue to upgrade and maintain the quality of their skills. They must know about new techniques, new tubes, changing time constraints on tests, computer data, and changes in scientific knowledge. Health care workers must accept the concept that patient safety and quality care come before saving time. They should also be willing to ask for assistance when dealing with a difficult patient or procedure. Health care workers should collect only the specimens ordered by the physician and those that they have been trained to collect.

When the implications of ethical behavior are considered, the concepts of *honesty, integrity,* and *regard for the dignity of other human beings* continue to be the personal foundations for professional codes. Only the health care worker dealing with patients on a one-to-one basis knows for sure whether the work that he or she performs each day is based on tenets for optimum behavior.

DEALING WITH STRESS

Stress is very prevalent in the workplace. Some people prefer to cope with the stress of illness by retreating from personal interaction. In a clinic or hospital setting, this is not possible. Thus, stress for health care professionals and patients can increase. Stress is usually defined by physiological changes such as the following:

- Elevated blood pressure
- Increased heart rate
- Increased respiration rate
- Increased body metabolism
- Increased blood flow to muscles

Stress may be caused by constant change with little escape from this change. Too often, the trauma associated with change is overlooked. For the health care worker, the change may involve a shift in work hours, the route covered, co-workers, the supervisor, new techniques and policies, or several or all of these.

A certain level of stress can push people to achieve, to win, and to compete. However, too much may incapacitate a person or make him or her ill. In fact, exposure to stress does not necessarily make withstanding greater stress easier. It may make the body even more vulnerable.

Rest can *almost* restore the body to the prior level of fitness. However, like a piece of elastic pulled too tight for too long, the body does not quite return to the original level of fitness after stress is relieved.

For these reasons, and so that the health care worker can maintain his or her professionalism, as well as communicate effectively with patients to ease *their* stress, the health care worker must be able to cope well with his or her own stress. Suggestions for lowering stress levels include the following:

- Take steps to mange time effectively.
- Associate with gentle people.
- Learn and practice the skill of relaxation.
- Exercise and eat nutritious foods to improve health.
- Engage in satisfying, meaningful work.
- Find time for privacy.
- Read interesting books and articles to get new ideas.

PROFESSIONAL ORGANIZATIONS

Three national organizations that recognize the health care worker as a definitive and vital part of the health care team are listed next. All are sponsors of certification examinations for health care workers.

1. *The American Society for Clinical Laboratory Scientists (ASCLS)* has recognized clinical laboratory personnel for more than 50 years. Several types of memberships are available depending on the education and experience of the individual. Currently, most health care workers are joining ASCLS as associate members as part of the phlebotomy section. The National Certifying Agency (NCA) offers a certification examination for health care workers and other laboratory professionals.
2. *The National Phlebotomy Association (NPA)* was established in 1978 to recognize the health care worker as a distinctive and identifiable part of the allied health team. This organization also offers a certification examination for health care workers.
3. *The American Society of Clinical Pathologists (ASCP)* allows nonphysician members to gain associate membership status. Through the society's Board of Registry, a Phlebotomy Technician Examination [Pbt (ASCP)] is offered annually. This is a criterion-referenced examination model. It covers the entry-level skills of a health care worker and uses taxonomy levels that assess recall (recognize facts), interpretive skills (use knowledge to interpret numeric data), and problem-solving skills (use applications of specific information to solve problems).

MANAGEMENT SKILLS IN THE PATIENT CARE ENVIRONMENT

The health care system is changing rapidly because of the dynamics of financial reimbursement through managed care arrangements, changing demographics and patient populations, and shifts away from specialization toward prevention and primary care. Health care professionals should be aware of the trends and how to make managerial and operational adjustments that do not compromise quality while being cost effective. Management is a dynamic process. When applied to phlebotomy services, it has both the technical responsibilities of providing services and the interpersonal components that deal with employees and customers.

Management can be described by functions that are performed by supervisors and administrators. These generally include planning, organizing, staffing, directing, and monitoring. In practice, these functions are performed simultaneously, but they are discussed separately for the sake of clarity. Issues affecting the management of phlebotomy services are given as examples.[1]

Planning

Planning occurs when managers project a vision for the future and a strategy for achieving that vision. At the senior levels of management, planning generally focuses on long-range planning, or **strategic planning,** which involves the organizational mission, goals, and objectives. The levels of management that are involved in day-to-day activities usually focus on operational planning rather than strategic planning. Supervisory personnel who are responsible for phlebotomy services are often involved in deciding when to offer a new testing methodology, deciding when to use new blood collection devices, planning the budget and expenses for the services, and preparing cost analyses for new services.

Organizing

Organizing consists of assigning activities to people so that tasks can be accomplished in an orderly and timely manner. Typically, an organizational chart depicts the network of authority, accountability, and communication. Some organizational charts promote a centralized authority, whereas others promote decentralization of the span of control. During changing times, many organizations redesign or restructure to match changing circumstances in the health care environment. Although it may be unsettling to some people, if organizations do not respond to changing market forces, they may go out of business.

Phlebotomy services are usually a part of a health care organization's redesign because basic venipuncture and skin puncture skills are conducive to cross-training among other health care workers. Likewise, health care workers have skills beyond the basics that are conducive to assisting with patient care services that are not a part of the traditional role. Examples might include expanded responsibilities in a hospital unit, such as assisting with clerical or charting functions, performing glucose monitoring or assisting with basic laboratory tests in a satellite laboratory, performing quality control on basic equipment, and checking inventories of supplies needed for patient services in the unit. The key to successfully managing a reorganization is the ability to be open minded and flexible about new opportunities to be an active member of the health care team.

Staffing

Staffing involves recruitment, selection, placement, training, development, compensation, scheduling, and evaluation of employees' productivity and performance. Larger organizations have Human Resources departments, which usually assist with some of these tasks such as recruitment, general training, compensation, and standardizing evaluations. However, for phlebotomy services, specialized training usually involves laboratory personnel; employee selection may involve hiring health care workers with specific skills such as drawing blood from donors, collecting blood for therapeutic drug monitoring, and so forth; scheduling involves having just enough staff on hand to provide essential services; and employee evaluations cover technical expertise, patient communication skills, the ability to work as a team member, and productivity assessments.

Directing

The management function of directing involves giving instructions, assignments, and directions in a professional, motivational manner. Many theories have been proposed about management styles, which include how a person directs others. It is often beneficial to managers and supervisors to reflect on their own style so that they may be cognizant about what works and what does not work with employees with varying personalities. Some employees need, and may want, closer supervision, whereas others prefer to work more independently. The most effective managers use a varying style of management according to each circumstance. For example, some health care workers may be able to perform venipunctures efficiently and rapidly, whereas others may prefer to spend more time talking to patients prior to a venipuncture, so they work more slowly. As long as the quality and efficiency of patient care is not compromised, supervisors should be sensitive and tolerant to the styles of these different employees.

Monitoring

Monitoring, another managerial function, involves ensuring that assignments are completed, that regulations and procedures are complied with, that problems have been handled appropriately, that the quality and quantity of services are continuously monitored and improved, and that services are performed in a cost-effective manner. These functions involve monitoring standards for time (such as turnaround times and productivity); measuring results or problems (such as redraws, hematomas, or incorrect documentation); comparing results to standards [such as Joint Commission on Accreditation of Healthcare Organizations (JCAHO) accreditation standards, National Committee for Clinical Laboratory Standards (NCCLS) recommendations, etc.]; monitoring technical performance (such as observation of the venipuncture procedure to ensure correct technique); checking inventory levels for supplies (such as amount, cost, and expiration dates of venipuncture tubes); and staying within the budgeted amount for the services provided (such as monitoring expenses on a monthly level and assessing cost-saving alternatives). Supervisors who collect, monitor, and undertand the revelant data will be in a position to constantly improve their services and thereby help make their organization more competitive in the health care market.

✔ Key Terms

ACCOUNTABILITY

ACTIVE LISTENING

AMERICAN HOSPITAL
ASSOCIATION (AHA)

AMERICAN SOCIETY FOR
CLINICAL LABORATORY
SCIENTISTS (ASCLS)

NATIONAL PHLEBOTOMY
ASSOCIATION (NPA)

PATIENT'S BILL OF RIGHTS

STRATEGIC PLANNING

ZONE OF COMFORT

Study Questions

1. After a venipuncture has been performed on an outpatient, what techniques should the health care worker follow before dismissing the patient?
   a. check the armband to verify identification
   b. check that the puncture site has stopped bleeding
   c. thank the patient
   d. help the patient sign the test requisition form

2. Which of the following can be barriers to communication?
   a. gender
   b. age
   c. cultural beliefs
   d. hearing ability

3. Identify the behaviors that exhibit positive body language.
   a. tapping a pencil or a pen
   b. making eye contact
   c. smiling
   d. having erect posture

4. Identify the topics in the Patient's Bill of Rights that are important for health care workers.
   a. properly notifying the patient of the charges for procedures
   b. maintaining confidentiality and privacy
   c. informing the patient of medical decisions
   d. respecting the patient's right to refuse a procedure

5. Identify the basic responsibilities of a health care manager or supervisor.
   a. evaluate technical performance
   b. schedule work hours
   c. monitor the budget and expenses
   d. measure turnaround times

REFERENCE

1. Taylor RJ, Taylor SB: *The AUPHA Manual of Health Services Management.* Association of University Programs in Health Administration, Gaithersburg, MD, Aspen Publishers, 1994.

seventeen

17

LEGAL AND REGULATORY ISSUES

Chapter Objectives

Upon completion of Chapter 17, the learner is responsible for the following:

1. Define major legal terms and explain how they relate to the health care setting.

2. Define risk and describe the major elements in a risk management program.

3. Describe the basic functions of the medical record.

4. Define *informed consent.*

5. Describe how to avoid litigation as it relates to specimen collection in a health care environment.

6. Describe CLIA '88 in perspective to blood collection and transportation responsibilities.

7. List the specimen collection requirements for toxicological analyses, including forensic specimens.

GENERAL LEGAL PRINCIPLES

The laws governing medicine and medical ethics complement and overlap one another. For many years, even centuries, the decision of the physician or health care professional was unquestioned. This has changed. Health care consumers and patients have become more aware, more critical, and much more willing to sue anyone that their lawyer believes has been at fault, including health care workers who are collecting blood specimens.

The legal system in the United States falls under legislative, regulatory, and judicial procedures at the federal, state, and local levels.

Statutory Law

Statutes are written laws enacted by state legislatures and the US Congress. Legislative activities performed by local government lead to written laws referred to as *ordinances.* Statutes and ordinances are **statutory laws** that are binding but in certain instances may require the courts (judicial law) to interpret how the statutory law applies to a given set of facts. For example, a statute may state that no sexual harassment will be allowed in the workplace. A court then may be called on to decide whether certain actions by a person are considered sexual harassment and therefore violate the law.

Administrative Law

Once enacted, statutes and ordinances must be implemented; this is **administrative law.** This process is performed by the executive branch, which has numerous departments and agencies. Administrative agencies (e.g., Health Care Financing Administration) write regulations that enforce the laws created through the legislative body. One department under the executive branch that has a major effect on administrative laws regarding health care workers is the US Department of Health and Human Services (DHHS). The DHHS is the main source of regulations affecting the health care industry.

Judicial Law

The function of the judicial branch of local, state, and federal governments is to resolve disputes in accordance with law. Most of the nation's **judicial law** actions occur at the state level. State and federal systems have trial courts, which are at the first level. The second level within the court system is intermediate courts (appeals courts), which review the decisions of the trial courts. The highest level within the judicial system is the supreme court of each state and of the federal system; these courts will hear only specific cases. Most of the written legal decisions occur from the appeals and supreme courts. However, more than 90 percent of all lawsuits are settled out of court, and many that are tried are settled before a final verdict is rendered.[1] Usually, phlebotomy cases are tried in state courts. However, if federal laws or regulations pertain to the case, the federal court system is used.

Legal Terminology

If a health care worker understands basic legal concepts, this understanding can help to define how personnel involved in the specimen collection process and area can be liable for activities that may occur in this field of health care. Such understanding can also reduce the conflicts between law and the health care workers. Liability for the lack of a proper standard of health care may be imposed on any health care worker, including health care institutions, physicians, nurses, laboratorians, patient care technicians, and phlebotomists. The number of substantial awards against health care workers as a result of improper care has grown in recent years as patients have become more sensitive to treatment complications.

Lawyers have become advisers to health care professionals and institutions in matters ranging from termination of treatment to approval of experimental protocols. Some lawyers specialize in hospital law or food and drug law; personal injury lawyers handle malpractice claims, and others are especially knowledgeable about Medicaid and workers' compensation benefits. No one lawyer can master all these areas. William J. Curran defined *health law* as a "specialty area of law and law practice related to the medical and other health fields—such as dentistry, nursing, hospital administration, and environmental law."[2]

To grasp the legal implication of health care, the health care provider must have some knowledge of basic legal terminology. The avoidance of legal conflicts through education and planning is called **preventive law.** Thus, there is a need to understand basic legal definitions and, it is hoped, to develop a preventive law approach in the procedures and techniques of blood collection. A few major definitions with health care examples follow:

- **Assault.** The unjustifiable attempt to touch another person or the threat to do so in such circumstances as to cause the other to believe that it will be carried out, or to cause fear. An assault may be permissible if proper consent has been given (e.g., consent to obtain a blood specimen).
- **Battery.** The intentional touching of another person without consent; also, the unlawful beating of another or carrying out of threatened physical harm. Because battery always includes an assault, the two are commonly combined in the phrase *assault and battery*. The receiver of the battery does not have to be aware that a battery has been committed (e.g., a patient who is unconscious and has surgery performed on him or her without his or her approval, either expressed or implied). The law provides a remedy to the individual when consent to a touching has not been obtained or if the act goes beyond the consent given. Thus, the injured person may initiate a lawsuit against the wrongdoer for the damages suffered. Liability of hospitals, physicians, and other health care workers for acts of battery is most common in situations involving lack of or improper consent to medical procedures, such as blood collecting. For example, a small boy who refused to have his blood drawn was locked in the blood collection room by the health care worker and was forced to have his blood drawn by the health care worker. The patient's parents sued and won. As another example, a patient is feeling stressed because of pain and not knowing what medical procedures will be occurring. If a health care professional displays behavior in a threatening manner, this can lead to legal intervention. The health care worker must obviously avoid directing threatening language to a patient (e.g., "If you don't let me collect your blood, your illness will probably become critical"). If the patient feels threatened by these words, he or she can "claim intentional infliction of emotional distress." The stress of collecting blood from numerous patients in a short period can lead some health care workers to think about

threatening difficult patients, but, of course, this could be detrimental to all involved.

- **Breach of duty.** An infraction, violation, or failure to perform.
- **Civil law.** Not a criminal action; the plaintiff sues for monetary damages.
- **Criminal actions.** Legal recourse for acts or offenses against the public welfare; these actions can lead to imprisonment of the offender.
- **Defendant.** The health care worker or institution against whom the action or lawsuit is filed.
- **False imprisonment.** The unjustifiable detention of a person without a legal warrant.
- **Felony.** Varies by state but generally is defined as public offenses, if the defendant is convicted, he or she will spend time in jail.
- **Invasion of privacy.** Physical intrusion upon a person; the publishing of confidential information, although true, but of such an objectionable or personal nature as to be offensive.
- **Liable.** Under legal obligation, as far as damages are concerned.
- **Litigation process.** The process of legal action to determine a decision in court. Many malpractice cases are negotiated and settled out of court.
- **Malpractice.** Improper or unskillful care of a patient by a member of the health care team, or any professional misconduct, unreasonable lack of skill, or infidelity in professional or judiciary duties. Malpractice may be described as *professional negligence*.
- **Misdemeanors.** The general term for all sorts of criminal offenses not serious enough to be classified as felonies.
- **Negligence.** Failure to act or to perform duties according to the standards of the profession.
- **Plaintiff.** The claimant who brings a lawsuit or an action.
- **Respondeat superior.** The concept whereby actions of one individual may be imputed to another person having control. This suggests that a technician's negligent act can be imputed to a laboratory corporation. Under this concept, supervisors and directors may be held liable for the negligent actions of their employees. This concept is also referred to as **vicarious liability.**
- **Tort.** A legal wrong in which the person who commits it is liable for damages in civil action. The tort system is a substructure of the judicial system. It is basically concerned with resolving two-party disputes over whether some harm to one party, or his or her property, was caused by the actions or inactions of another party. A tort is a harm or an injury that is civil, not criminal, in nature and does not constitute a breach of contract. Civil law does not deal with crimes. Torts and other civil wrongs must be proved by a *preponderance of the evidence. Preponderance* is taken to mean a majority; 51 percent or more implies that the defendant more likely than not committed the act.

Negligence. In the past decade, the number of legal cases in which the laboratory has been directly or indirectly involved has increased noticeably. Negligence is "a violation of a duty to exercise reasonable skill and care in performing a task."[3] Four factors, or key points, must be considered in alleged negligence cases.[3]

1. *Duty*—relates to what duties or responsibilities the hospital or health care worker had toward the patient; it also includes all the individuals who had a duty toward the patient to use the appropriate standard of care.
2. *Breach of duty*—relates to whether the duty was breached and if it was avoidable. The plaintiff must be able to show what actually happened and that the defendant acted unreasonably.
3. *Proximate causation*—relates to whether the breach of duty actually contributed to or caused injury; also concerns all the parties involved in contributing to the alleged injury. There must be a direct line from the conduct to the injury.
4. *Damages*—relates to whether the plaintiff was actually injured and when these injuries were discovered. Once negligence and causation are established, plaintiffs must be able to show that they were actually damaged by the negligent act.

Many circumstances could be considered negligence if health care workers are not extremely careful. For example, there have been legal cases in which confusion of patient samples led to a patient's death.[4]

Patient Confidentiality. Negligence cases can also arise out of violation of the right to privacy or of **patient confidentiality.** "No one except the patient may release patient results without a clinical need to know." Patient or employee laboratory test results must be considered *strictly* confidential. Negligence can be claimed if employees' or patients' drug abuse test results are released to anyone other than the attending physician or other authorized individuals. This is particularly true regarding employee or athlete drug or alcohol abuse screening and human immunodeficiency virus (HIV) testing. Confidential materials include communications between the physician and the patient, the patient's verbal statements, and nonverbal communications such as laboratory test results.

CONFIDENTIALITY AND HIV EXPOSURE

An increasing concern for health care workers collecting blood from patients who are homebound is the health care worker's rights in relation to accidental exposure to blood or body fluids, whether by a needle stick or some other means. In some states, laws allow health care workers to know the identity of a patient who has acquired immunodeficiency syndrome (AIDS) or who is HIV positive. However, many states do not provide for the easy acquisition of this sensitive patient information. A home health care worker who routinely collects blood specimens from homebound patients should obtain information on the state's law regarding confidentiality and HIV status.[5] It can be obtained from the health care worker's employer, from legal counsel, or from a national or state health professional organization.

It is important to use the proper blood collection techniques with safety precautions and required infection control procedures for homebound patients. If exposure to the blood occurs through a needle stick, a lancet, or another means, the home health care worker needs to be certain of obtaining the patient's HIV status to ensure that the proper immediate and long-term self-protective procedural steps can be taken. Even if the report from the HIV test is negative for the health care worker, continued negative status is not guaranteed. However, just because a patient's status is HIV positive, the health care worker exposed to the blood may not become HIV positive.

If employed by a health care facility, the health care worker should follow the guidelines established by the facility. If he or she is self-employed, it is important to monitor his or her own HIV status. Also, counseling should be sought to obtain emotional support during this stressful time.

If employed by a health care facility, the exposed health care worker must file an incident report concerning the accidental exposure. If the health care worker is self-employed and working for various agencies, he or she must report the incident to these agencies. The health care institutions and agencies must report accidental exposure incidents to the **Centers for Disease Control and Prevention (CDC).** The CDC maintains national surveillance of health care workers' accidental exposures. These statistics assist in developing better safeguards (e.g., new blood collection equipment) against accidental exposure.

MALPRACTICE

Malpractice, or professional negligence, is defined as improper or unskillful care of a patient by a member of the health care team, or any professional misconduct or unreasonable lack of skill.

The relationship between doctor and patient is, in the legal sense, a contractual one. The basic elements involved are common with those of other contracts. The elements of contracts are as follows:

- **Offer.** The physician offers to provide a service, either by opening an office or being on a hospital staff or both. Thus, he or she has made him- or herself available to patients who seek care.

- **Acceptance.** The patient visits the physician for treatment of a disease or a disorder and may agree to accept medical care.
- **Consideration.** The patient accepts treatment and pays for the care provided by the physician.

By completing these steps, the physician and the patient engage in a contract that implies obligations on both their parts. The physician is obligated to provide medical care to the patient if he or she follows directions and pays for the service. There is even a question about the length of grace period in terms of payment. Also, the patient generally must refuse treatment before the physician is legally freed from his or her obligation. By agreeing to provide service, the physician is required to provide a standard of care.

If the physician is the medical director overseeing clinical laboratory testing, in most cases he or she is responsible under the law for the standard of care and the performance of all aspects of laboratory testing. Therefore, a breach of standard on the part of the health care worker collecting blood for laboratory assays could place both the physician and the health care worker at risk.

STANDARD OF CARE

If a patient has suffered injury due to blood collection for laboratory testing, the patient must show that the health care worker who collected the blood failed to meet the prevailing **standard of care.** All health care workers must conform to a specific standard of care to protect patients. In legal cases, the standard of care is determined by what a reasonably prudent person would do under similar circumstances. It is a measuring stick representing the conduct of the average health care worker in the community. The community has been expanded to be a national community as a result of national laboratory standards and requirements. Examples of setting the standard of care include statutes, licensing requirements, rules and regulations of regulatory or professional organizations (e.g., American Hospital Association, Joint Commission for Accreditation of Healthcare Organizations (JCAHO), Health Care Financing Administration, etc.), internal health care facility rules, and regulations and professional publications.

INFORMED CONSENT

Informed consent is voluntary permission by a patient to allow touching, examination, and/or treatment by health care providers. It allows patients to determine what will be performed on or to their bodies. Without informed consent, intentional touching can be considered a criminal offense. This type of consent can be obtained through word or action. Thus, the consent may be given orally, expressed by nonverbal behavior, or expressed in writing. Following is an example of nonverbal consent. The physician orders laboratory tests for diagnosis and the patient comes to the laboratory with a rolled-up sleeve. The patient is giving consent for the health care worker to take the blood samples. Integral to consent is the patient's belief that the person to whom consent is given has the knowledge, skills, and technical ability to perform such tasks. Consequently, the patient can expect the blood collector to know the proper venipuncture, arterial puncture, and/or skin puncture technique. For the blood collection, the health care worker should briefly explain to the patient the procedure used to collect the blood specimen. It is important for the health care worker collecting the blood to stress that the physician ordered the test. Health care workers are becoming more cognizant of the informed consent principle because this is the largest area of litigation. Minors must have the consent of their parents or legal guardians for medical care, including blood collections. With the increased amount of immigration to this country, language can be a barrier to informed consent. An interpreter may be necessary so that information for consent may be given in the native tongue.

Most states have enacted legislation requiring that informed consent be obtained before most HIV testing is performed. The statutes indicate the type of information that must be given for the patient to be considered informed. These laws usually require that the patient be counseled on the following: (1) an explanation of the test, including its purpose; (2) potential uses of the HIV test; and (3) testing limitations and the meaning of its results. The American Medical Records Association has a pamphlet entitled *Guidelines for Handling Health Data on Individuals Tested for HIV Virus,* which includes forms for request and consent for testing and a suggested procedure for conducting a confidential screening program. (More information may be obtained by writing the American Medical Records Association, 875 N Michigan Ave, Suite 1850, Chicago, IL 60611.)

IMPLIED CONSENT

Implied consent exists when immediate action is required to save a patient's life or to prevent permanent impairment of the patient's health. In other words, an emergency removes the need for consent. Implied consent differs in legalities from one state to another. Health care providers need to know the legal boundaries of implied consent because they may become involved in an emergency situation (e.g., giving cardiopulmonary resuscitation).

SPECIMENS FOR TOXICOLOGICAL ANALYSIS AND FORENSIC SPECIMENS

In toxicological analysis, very small amounts of analytes are usually found in the blood, urine, or other specimens obtained for analysis. Thus, the type of specimen (e.g., venous blood, arterial blood), materials, and equipment used for collecting specimens for toxicological analysis can greatly affect analytic results. The type of glass or plastic composing the collection tube, cover, or both may contain materials that will react with the analytes or absorb the analytes. Thus, for toxicological specimens, the health care worker must strictly adhere to the facility's laboratory guidelines for collection of these types of specimens.

Many states have provisions under which drivers suspected of being intoxicated by the arresting police officer must voluntarily give implied consent to the performance of certain laboratory assays to determine the level of blood alcohol. In some states, this statute applies only to the testing of urine and breath samples. Thus, as a health care worker working in emergency care centers, it is advisable to determine the medically acceptable manner for obtaining blood specimens from patients for alcohol analysis.[6] If blood alcohol specimens are collected in the facility, the blood collector must cleanse the patient's skin with a *nonalcohol* disinfectant, and all tubes of blood must be clearly labeled.

When a specimen is collected for toxicological studies involving drug abuse testing, or for another medical application related to civil or criminal law, these specimens are referred to as **forensic specimens.** They require a **chain-of-custody form** (Fig. 17–1) that must be completed showing specific identification, who obtained and processed the specimen, the date, the location, and the signature of the subject documenting that the specimen in the container is the one that was obtained from the person identified on the label. The specimen must be placed in a specimen transfer bag that permanently seals the specimen bag until it is cut open for analysis. The seal ensures a tamper-evident transfer of contents until it reaches its destination for analysis.[7]

Many sports associations, major companies, and industrial complexes are requiring urine drug screens for athletes and employees. Usually, the screening is done without prior notice; therefore, the procedures for specimen collection, processing, analysis, and reporting results can be very strict and well defined. The **National Institute on Drug**

Name of subject: _____

Subject's SS#: _____ – ___ – _____

Specimen type: Blood ___ (Specify if venous, arterial, or capillary and if any additives
in container)

Urine ____

Other (Specify) _____

Amount of specimen in mL: _____ mL

Collected by (please print name here): _____

Signature of collector: _____

Date, time, and location of collection: _____

_____

Witness(es) _____

_____

- -

Signature of courier: _____ Date and time: _____

> Received in lab by (please print) _____
>
> Date & time: _____ (signature) _____
>
> Condition of seals:
>
> 1. Outside container sealed: _____ Yes _____ No
> 2. Specimen sealed: _____ Yes _____ No
>
> Seals broken and tested by: _____
>
> Date: _____ Time _____
>
> Additional transfers
>
> From: _____ Date: _____ Time: _____
>
> Reason: _____
>
> To: _____ Date: _____ Time: _____

Figure 17–1. Chain-of-custody form.

Abuse (NIDA) defines requirements for collection, processing, and testing. The following five precautions are usually involved:

1. Sterile, airtight specimen containers that can be sealed are strongly recommended. Special preservatives may be required for the analyses.
2. A proctor should be present during the urine collection process to ensure that the specimen was obtained from the appropriate person. Specialized facilities should be maintained for specimen collection, particularly urine collections.
3. The specimen must be properly labeled to establish a chain of

custody. A split sample may be required for parallel testing, confirmation, or both.

4. Specimens should be sealed and locked in a transport container during transfer from the collection site to the testing site to prevent tampering.
5. Careful documentation of who received the specimen must be maintained.

STATUTE OF LIMITATIONS

✔ The **statute of limitations** is a law that defines how soon after an injury (e.g., malpractice) a plaintiff must file the lawsuit or be forever barred from doing so. The purpose of this law is to prevent the threat of a lawsuit from hanging over a possible defendant's (e.g., health care worker's) head forever and to force legal action before memories and records are not available and witnesses die. The statute of limitations for professional negligence in most states is 2 years. A complete and accurate medical record with laboratory testing results is the best defense in these cases because the attending physician and health care workers for the patient may have little recollection of the events in question.

LEGAL CLAIMS AND DEFENSE

In a malpractice lawsuit, the first pleading filed in a negligence action is the complaint. It is the first statement of a case by the plaintiff(s) against the defendant(s) and states a cause of action, notifying the defendant(s) as to the basis for suit.

✔ Several steps follow, and if the case is not dismissed before trial, the parties to a lawsuit have the right to **discovery**—to examine the witnesses before the trial. Examination before trial is a method used to enable the plaintiff(s) and defendant(s) to learn more regarding the nature and substance of each other's case. This discovery process consists of oral testimony under oath and includes cross-examination by the
✔ lawyers. The **deposition** is the testimony of a witness that has been recorded in a written legal format. Either party in the lawsuit—plaintiff or defendant—may obtain a court order permitting examination and copying of laboratory reports, incident reports from personnel files, medical records, phlebotomy and laboratory policies and procedures, training manuals, and so forth, and other facts and information that may help in the discovery.

In addition to the deposition, the parties may undergo cross-examination at the time of the trial. They will provide testimony that will be recorded and filed with the court regarding the cause for the case.

If a health care worker receives a summons to provide a deposition before a trial and/or testimony during a trial for a lawsuit, some helpful guidelines include the following:

- Answer only the questions asked.
- Be organized in your recollection of the facts regarding the incident.
- Do not be antagonistic in answering the questions.
- Explain the laboratory and/or blood collection procedures and policies in simple terminology for the jury.
- Do not overdramatize the facts that you are presenting.
- Dress neatly and be groomed appropriately.
- Be polite, sincere, and courteous.
- Be sure to ask for clarification of questions that you did not clearly hear and questions that you did not understand.
- If you are not sure of an answer, indicate that you do not know the answer or that you are not sure.

Expert Witness

Expert testimony, as well as scientific or medical data, is sometimes used to assist in establishing the standard of care required in any given situation. An **expert witness** may be used to assist a plaintiff in proving the wrongful act of a defendant or to assist a defendant in refuting such evidence. At the time of testifying, each expert's training, experience, and special qualifications will be explained during the deposition and later to the jury during the trial.

Evidence

Evidence during the trial is used to prove or disprove the lawsuit. Evidence must be competent, relevant, and material. It may include such items as vacuum tube holders and tubes, needles, safety apparatuses such as biohazardous waste containers, infection control logs and reports, JCAHO standards, board certification standards for health care workers, and laboratory policies and procedures.

Advice to Avoid Lawsuits

Justice is expensive in the United States. Lawyers' fees typically range from $100 to $500 per hour, and associated costs can lead to thousands of dollars in legal fees. Also, legal proceedings are time consuming, expensive, and, most of all, emotionally devastating to both the plaintiff(s) and the defendant(s). Thus, to avoid a malpractice lawsuit, the health care provider should heed the following tips:

- Provide the patient with proper blood collection techniques comparable to national standards [e.g., National Committee for Clinical Laboratory Standards (NCCLS) guidelines, JCAHO regulations, etc.].
- Obtain consent for collection of specimens.
- Regularly participate in continuing education programs.
- Properly handle all confidential communications (e.g., HIV testing) without violation.
- Maintain all required blood collection equipment on trays and/or in collection areas for proper collection, including safety apparatuses such as gloves and disposal containers.
- Be a good listener and let the patient identify his or her anxieties.
- Report incidents immediately and document them.

Respondeat Superior

✔ **Respondeat superior** (Latin term meaning "let the master answer") is the concept whereby actions of one individual may be imputed to another person having control. It is a legal doctrine that holds employers responsible for acts of their employees within the scope of the employment relationship. Liability predicated on respondeat superior may be imposed on an employer only if a master–servant relationship exists between the employer and the employee and the wrongful act of the employee occurs within the scope of employment. Because the law holds negligent persons responsible for their negligent acts, employees are not released from liability when the health care institution is held liable through the application of respondeat superior. Not only may the injured party sue the employee directly, but the employer, if sued, may also seek indemnification from the employee. Indemnification is compensation for the financial loss suffered by the employee's act.

MEDICAL RECORDS

✔ **Medical records** are vital. A health care worker cannot be expected to remember a patient from whom blood was drawn 3 to 4 years ago. The medical records must be neat, legible, and accurate. They are extremely important if a medical malpractice case goes to court. Medical records have four basic purposes:

1. Allow for continuity of the patient's care plan
2. Provide documentation of the patient's illness and treatment
3. Document communication between the physician and the health care team

4. Provide a legal document that can be used by patients and
   hospital or health care workers to protect their legal interests.

Medical records are also used for nonmedical reasons that are not directly tied to medical services, such as billing, utilization review, quality improvement, and so on.

Health care workers and their supervisors have a legal duty to keep records, documentation, and laboratory test results confidential. This duty may be waived only if a patient has given express permission for the information to be released, if the patient has sued the institution or its health care personnel, or if the health care worker is specifically obligated to release patient information (e.g., to the CDC). But even in these situations, the confidentiality of patient records and reports cannot be breached while they are communicated or in transit. It is important to remember that many cases are not cited in the literature because often health care institutions or health care workers negotiate, arbitrate, and settle out of court.

LEGAL CASES RELATED TO CLINICAL LABORATORY ACTIVITIES

Most phlebotomy cases are settled after a lawsuit is filed but before the court renders a judgment. The following sections discuss cases that are of interest to health care workers involved in blood collection.

Schmerber v. State of California

Nurses, technologists and health care workers are concerned about drawing a blood sample from an unconscious patient or lacking the patient's consent when requested by police. The US Supreme Court ruled in *Schmerber v. State of California* that tests performed on a blood sample drawn by a hospital physician from a person arrested by the police were admissible in a court action. This may vary by state.

Lazernick v. General Hospital of Monroe County (PA 1977)

A patient who was pregnant for the first time had her blood typed in January 1971. The report sent to her physician indicated that her blood type was A-positive. The patient gave birth to her second child on June 1977. The child was brain damaged and paralyzed on the right side of the body as a result of hemolytic blood disease. The laboratory records in 1971 and 1977 showed that the mother's blood type was O-negative. In a malpractice suit, the parents charged that the physician's and his employees' negligence caused the child's injuries. The physician, who was chief of the laboratory when the blood test was performed, was found liable, as was the health care worker.

Walton v. Providence Hospital

A patient was admitted to Providence Hospital for treatment of pneumonia. On the second day, the patient complained of coldness and numbness in his right hand. On the fourth day, a vascular surgeon examined the hand and ordered 4000 U of heparin in hopes of restoring blood flow. The hand had to be amputated. In court, the expert witness testified that a blood pressure cuff had been left on for an extended period. The patient was awarded $40,000.

Helmann v. Sacred Heart Hospital

Failure to follow proper isolation techniques, such as proper hand washing and prevention of cross-contamination, is a major area of concern for hospitals. The patient in *Helmann v. Sacred Heart Hospital* [62 Wash. 2d 136, 381 P. 2d 605 (1963)] had multiple fractures in the area of the left hip socket. After surgery on his hip, he was returned to a semiprivate room. His roommate complained of a boil under the right arm. Eight days later, a culture was taken of the roommate's wound drainage. Three days later, the laboratory identified the wound infection as *Staphylococcus aureus*. The infected roommate was immediately placed in isolation for the wound. However, for the preceding 11 days, the hospital attendants administered care to both patients without washing their hands between patient care.

The patient with the hip injury developed a *S. aureus* infection at the site of his hip incision. The infection penetrated into the hip socket, destroying tissue and leading to additional surgery and a hip fused in a nearly immovable position. Negligence on the part of the hospital personnel was identified as the cause of the injury as a result of deviation from the accepted standard of care.

Stepp v. Review Board of the Indiana Employment Security Division

Another type of legal case involved a laboratory technician in *Stepp v. Review Board of the Indiana Employment Security Division* [521 N.E. 2d 350 (Ind. Ct. App. 1988)]. She was found to have been properly dismissed from her position in the laboratory because of her refusal to perform laboratory tests on patients' specimens with AIDS warnings attached.

Paros v. Hoemako Hospital

The chief x-ray technician in *Paros v. Hoemako Hospital* [681 P. 2d 918 (Ariz. Ct. App. 1984)] was found to have been properly dismissed because of a chronic hostile and argumentative attitude inconsistent with managerial supervisory responsibilities. The ruling was appealed, and the appeals court upheld the lower court's decision.

Cases Resulting from Improper Technique and Negligence

Health care workers who collect blood by venipuncture must be thoroughly trained and skilled in proper technique, safety, and the use of collection equipment. Problems that can arise include hematoma and abscess at the puncture site, and the patient may faint, fall, and injure him- or herself during or after the blood collection process. In one of two separate cases settled out of court, a health care worker had not received proper blood collection training. She performed a venipuncture by inserting the needle approximately 2 inches above the antecubital fold. The needle went through the vein, through muscle, and into the nerve, severely injuring the patient's arm, which remained permanently damaged even after three surgeries to repair the damage from the resultant hematoma and nerve injury. The other case involved a medical technologist under pressure to collect specimens as quickly as possible. One of the patients in this pressure mill stated prior to blood collection that she had fainted during the blood collection at a previous time. However, the technologist took no precautions and collected her blood and allowed her to leave immediately. She fainted at the elevator and suffered permanent loss of smell and has a permanent "ringing sound" in her ears. In another case, a health care worker collecting and performing bedside glucose results misread the glucometer and caused the deaths of three patients with diabetes.

DiMarco v. Lynch Homes–Chester County, Inc.

In *DiMarco v. Lynch Homes–Chester County, Inc.* [Pennsylvania Superior Court, April 14, 1989, 559 A. 2d 530 (PA Super 1989)], a blood collector suffered a needle puncture wound when a nursing home patient from whom she was collecting blood kicked her. The blood collector received follow-up treatment from her physician, who advised her that she may contract hepatitis up to 6 weeks after the incident. Thus, she was told, she should avoid sexual relations during this time to prevent the possibility of infecting her boyfriend. After 8 weeks, the blood collector resumed her relationship with her boyfriend. However, after this length of time, the blood collector contracted hepatitis and her boyfriend also was diagnosed with the disease. The boyfriend sued the physician and the nursing home. Through the appeals process within the state, the boyfriend won the case. The Pennsylvania Superior Court concluded that someone who renders services to another should recognize the need to protect the third party (the boyfriend) and is liable to the third party who is injured.

Booker v. Duke Medical Center

A similar case was *Booker v. Duke Medical Center* [2565.E. 2d 189 (N.C. 1979)], in which compensation was awarded to the wife of a laboratory technician who died after being exposed to viral hepatitis. The court ruled that the technician's employment exposed him to a greater risk of contracting the disease than members of the public or employees in general.

Veronica Prego v. The City of New York

In *Veronica Prego v. The City of New York* (Kings County Hospital, New York City Health and Hospital Corporation, Kings County, New York Supreme Court, Index No. 14974/88), in January 1983 a health care worker at Kings County Hospital pricked her finger on a needle used to collect blood from a patient dying of AIDS. The plaintiff tested positive for AIDS in March 1985. The health care worker stated that the hospital failed to dispose of used needles properly, claiming that needle boxes should have been provided in each room. The health care worker won the lawsuit and more than $1 million in damages.

HIV-RELATED ISSUES

If a health care worker becomes infected with HIV during employment at a health care facility, coverage by workers' compensation benefits are usually available. However, the health care worker must demonstrate a causal connection between his or her HIV infection and his or her employment. This causal connection includes having a documented incident report at the health care facility involving a needle-stick injury, a puncture wound, or other exposure to HIV-contaminated blood or body fluids. In addition, the health care worker's lifestyle will be investigated to determine whether the exposure occurred elsewhere. Preemployment health evaluations may prove useful later should the health care worker allege contraction of infection during the time of employment.

If a health care worker resigns because of contracting AIDS, unemployment benefits may be available if the worker can show that he or she believed in good faith that continued employment would jeopardize his or her health.

In a letter to the *New England Journal of Medicine*,[8] a resident physician who acquired HIV from a patient stated the following: "Workers' compensation works well to cover medical expenses and income lost because of occupational injuries that result in temporary or minor disabilities such as muscle tears or bone fractures. But these are not the accidents that a physician (health care provider) is likely to suffer at work. The main threats today are catastrophic, and workers' compensation is grossly inadequate for catastrophic illness."

LEGAL CASE PROTECTION

If an incident occurs (e.g., a patient develops a hematoma), the blood collector must write an incident report and provide it to the supervisor. The incident report can be helpful in a lawsuit to identify the real cause, the time, and other details of the incident. It may be of great assistance to the health care worker who is the defendant in the case in recalling the reason for the patient's (plaintiff's) alleged suffering and truth. However, the health care worker must not tamper with evidence in a lawsuit by writing an incident report after being sued by a patient for malpractice. In one case in which a health care worker was sued for damaging a patient's median nerve as a result of probing with a needle to find the vein, the health care worker "after the alleged fact" wrote an incident report for the incident that occurred prior to the filed suit. Eventually, through court proceedings, it was discovered that the health care worker had not actually filed an incident report at the time of the patient's needle-stick injury. The falsification of documentation immensely affected the plaintiff's award for damages.

LAWS ON MEDICAL DEVICES AND PROTECTIVE EQUIPMENT

Blood collection involves the use of many types of equipment and supplies. Blood collectors and patients have been injured as a result of malfunctioning equipment. In 1990, the federal government issued the Safe Medical Devices Act, which states that any malfunctioning devices (e.g., in vitro diagnostics, reagent kits, clinical analyzers, blood collection equipment) must be immediately reported to the federal government with a description of the malfunctioning incident (e.g., breakage of needle in arm). After an investigation of the incident, a nationwide alert is generally provided to health care institutions regarding the failure(s) of the health care device. This law was enacted to protect health care workers and patients from injuries due to health care devices.

✔   To avoid the possibility of malfunctioning equipment, the **Food and Drug Administration (FDA)** evaluates the safety, clinical efficacy, and medical efficacy of the equipment and supplies used in blood collection.

✔   Another federal agency, the **Environmental Protection Agency (EPA)** monitors and enforces environmental requirements for the safe disposal of chemical and biological hazards.

Another federal rule affecting health care workers who collect blood is the Occupational Safety and Health Administration (OSHA) rule for personal protective equipment (PPE) that became effective on July 5, 1994. The rule describes the following:

- PPE must be of a safe design and construction for the work to be performed.
- PPE must be provided, used, and maintained in a sanitary and workable condition.
- PPE must be selected for employees based on an assessment of the hazards of the work environment (e.g., safety shields over needle apparatus).
- Employees must be trained in the proper use of PPE.

MALPRACTICE INSURANCE

Because hospitals are places where seriously ill patients are admitted and treated with highly sophisticated medical technology, the likelihood for problems is greater there than in other health care settings. Often, the health care staff in the hospital or clinical laboratory are part of a blanket malpractice insurance policy. However, if the health care worker is employed by a pathologist who has a contract with an institution or owns a clinic, the staff may be protected by the pathologist's malpractice insurance policy.

Malpractice insurance rates for pathologists are generally the lowest premiums charged because of their low risk level. At the bench and administrative levels, laboratories have rarely been named in malpractice suits. Part of the reason for so few cases is that under the legal concept of respondeat superior, responsibility for wrongful acts of the employee (agent–servant) rests on the employer (principal–master). Also, another reason for not being named in a suit is the *deep pocket concept.* The health care worker, with less money or no insurance, in the past has not been a target for suit. However, the advances in technology and increased complexity of health care have increased legal exposure for allied health professionals. Often, laboratorians feel safe from legal responsibilities because of limited interaction with patients. However, the health care worker and any other staff member that routinely deals with the public in patient–health care worker relationships are indeed liable. Therefore, each individual should examine the possibility of malpractice suits and the need for malpractice insurance from a personal standpoint.[9]

If the health care worker decides to purchase malpractice insurance, four factors should be carefully considered:

1. Is adequate dollar value coverage provided? In recent lawsuits, total damages of $1 million or more have been awarded against physicians.
2. What are the coverage limitations?
3. What are the procedures that must be followed for the policy to provide coverage? Some policies state that divulging the amount of coverage or the fact of coverage voids the policy.
4. The health care worker should not assume that the lawyers representing the hospital, laboratory, or clinic will have his or her best interests at heart. The attorney's first obligation is to serve those who have hired him or her. There have been cases in which the hospital was cleared of all charges but the allied health professional was held liable for damages. For the health care worker, if an adult patient seems alert and does not object to the blood specimen collection, consent is implied. Proceeding without consent may give rise to assault and battery charges, as well as civil suits.

With the purpose of malpractice professional liability insurance, the attorney's fee and court costs are usually covered. Some professional organizations offer professional liability insurance at a reasonable or reduced rate. With the advent of organ transplantations, renal dialysis, and hyperbaric care, the avenues of liability are widened. A genuine concern for others and careful attention to technique are good investments of the health care worker's time. A record of continuing education courses, seminars, workshops, and academic credits should be a part of each health care worker's personal file.

MANAGEMENT OF RISK

Concepts of Risk

Risk can be described as "exposure to the chance of injury or loss."[10] Health care workers face many risks daily. It is important for health care workers, supervisors, and managers to reflect on their personal risk and that of their employers. Active steps should be taken to understand risk factors and to minimize areas of risk for the benefit of patients and the protection of employees and employers. Risk can be managed by using carefully planned objectives that can be categorized as preloss (to reduce or prevent losses) and postloss (how the facility can recover from a loss). The goals and objectives of the institution or department can guide the risk management program. A generic model of **risk management** might involve the following levels:

- *Risk identification and analysis*—analysis and measurement of identified risks
- *Risk treatment*—use of tools (e.g., safety manuals, policies and procedures, public relations tactics) to prevent harm or losses
- *Education*—of patients, employees, and visitors
- *Risk transfer or postponement*—shifting risk to other parties (e.g., liability insurance, contract services, and employees)
- *Risk evaluation*—assessment of what should be done

One way to identify risk is to review *incident, accident,* or *occurrence* reports that involve laboratory or phlebotomy services. Employees must be continually encouraged to use these tools because without an effective reporting system, proper investigations and risk assessments cannot be made. An incident or occurrence does not have to result in injury. The older term *accident report* is rarely used anymore because it implies that an error occurred, which may not always be the case. Trends of events that deviate from normal, but fortunately do not harm any patients, are most revealing and controllable.

Risk treatment has two elements: loss or risk control, and risk financing.[10] Loss or risk control means that the department should attempt to reduce the frequency of errors or events that can potentially cause financial loss. Similar to quality-improvement programs, the aim would be to reduce adverse outcomes such as excessive venipunctures on the same patient, reducing the number of hematomas, and so on. *Risk financing* refers to how to pay for losses once they occur (liability insurance or other means). If a patient faints during venipuncture and injures him- or herself, care should be taken to assist and provide free services for the person to recover. Documentation should clearly indicate the details of the accident and each step of the follow-up.

Education and communication are also vital to the risk management process. If employees do not know about new procedures, they cannot be expected to follow them.

Risk transfer through the use of liability insurance is also an important part of the risk management process. Contracting for services has also traditionally shifted some of the liability to other parties. However, federal and state laws are changing to include contract personnel and contract services (e.g., reference laboratories, diagnostic radiology services) under the respondeat superior concept. This trend suggests that health care facilities might be held liable for services performed by those with whom they have contracts.

Evaluation of all the elements of risk management just discussed may show a need for changes in procedures, employee counseling, or educational programs. Table 17–1 indicates some common sense tips for minimizing risk in a phlebotomy setting.[10,11]

Clinical Laboratory Improvement Amendments

In October 1988, the US Congress passed Public Law 100-578, **Clinical Laboratory Improvement Amendments (CLIA).** This public law is administered by the **Health Care Financing Administration (HCFA).** CLIA '88 regulations became effective on September 1, 1992, as a means to ensure the quality and accuracy of laboratory testing by creating a uniform set of provisions governing all laboratories that examine human specimens either for the diagnosis, prevention, or treatment of disease or for the impairment of, or the assessment of the health of, human beings.[12] CLIA '88 essentially applies to every clinical laboratory testing facility in the United States and requires that the facility be certified by the federal government. The certification requires an inspection by federal and/or state agencies to determine whether the laboratory testing facility uses methods to test patients' specimens that lead to accurate, reliable, and quality test results. Only laboratories that perform "waived" laboratory tests (e.g., simple tests such as dipstick urinalysis) are not required to undergo an inspection. If the laboratory test is not categorized as waived by the CLIA '88 federal regulations, it falls into the category of "moderately complex" or "highly complex," depending on the difficulty of conducting the test and the risk of harm to the patient if the test is not performed correctly. For the moderately complex or highly complex testing, the inspection considers all procedural steps in laboratory testing—preanalytic, analytic, and postanalytic. Thus, the blood collection procedures area is a major part of CLIA inspections. The HCFA states that a laboratory with moderately complex or highly complex testing must have available and follow written policies and procedures for the following:

- Protocols for the preparation of patients
- Specimen collection
- Specimen labeling

TABLE 17–1. LAWSUIT PREVENTION TIPS FOR MINIMIZING RISKS

Common Issues in Lawsuits Against Health Care Providers	Prevention Tips for Phlebotomists, Nurses, and Others Involved in Blood Collection
Documentation	Always document the time, date, and blood collector's initials on the blood collection containers.
Reporting of incidents	Document the information legibly and spell correctly.
	If an adverse incident occurs to the patient and/or the blood collector before, during, or after blood collection, report the incident to your immediate supervisor and complete the appropriate documentation in a legible manner.
Failure to follow hospital procedure	Be knowledgeable of the health care facility's and clinical laboratory's policies and procedures.
	If you must deviate from a policy or a procedure, discuss the incident with your immediate supervisor and decide on the appropriate action.
Failure to ensure patient's safety	Monitor the patient in an appropriate, timely manner during and after blood collection.
	Return bed rails to the raised position if the bed rails were raised prior to blood collection.
	Lock the patient in the blood collection chair for the blood collection procedure.
	If an outpatient says that he or she faints during blood collection, place the patient in a supine position to collect blood, and monitor the patient for at least 20 minutes after collection before allowing him or her to stand up and leave the facility.
Improper treatment and performance of treatment	Use proper technique and equipment (e.g., gloves) when performing procedures
	Follow the health care facility's and clinical laboratory's procedures when performing treatments.
	Update your collection skills and techniques through continuing education classes.
Failure to monitor and to report	Report any significant changes in a patient's condition (e.g., patient continues to bleed from puncture site after blood collection).
Equipment use	Learn how to use blood collection equipment as designed.
	Use biohazardous waste containers as indicated in procedures.
	If involved in off-site blood collections, carry biohazardous waste containers.
Patients with HIV	Be conscious of actions that could result in a lawsuit: Discrimination in treatment Nosocomial transmission of the virus Breach of confidentiality
	Follow health care facility's procedures for blood collection and disposal of biohazardous waste.

- Specimen preservation
- Conditions for specimen transportation

Written instructions may be supplemented by oral explanation of the instructions to patients for proper preparation and specimen collection (Sections 493.1101 and 493.1103 of the February 28, 1992, CLIA rule).

From the test requisition section of the CLIA (Section 493.1105), the HCFA has defined test requisition requirements for laboratories performing moderately or highly complex testing that include the following:

- The laboratory must perform tests only at the written or electronic request of an authorized person.
- Oral requests for laboratory tests are permitted only if the laboratory subsequently obtains written authorization for testing within 30 days.
- Records of test requisitions or test authorizations must be retained for a minimum of 2 years.
- The patient's chart, or medical record, if used as the test requisition form, must be retained for a minimum of 2 years and must be available to the laboratory at the time of testing and available to the DHHS upon request.
- The patient's name or other unique identifier must be on the laboratory requisition or test authorization form.
- The laboratory requisition or test authorization form must include the name and address of the authorized person requesting the test, and, if appropriate, that of the individual responsible for utilizing the test results or the name and address of the laboratory submitting the specimen, including a contact person to enable the reporting of imminent life-threatening laboratory test results or panic values.
- The test(s) to be performed and the date of specimen collection must be on the laboratory requisition or test authorization form.

For the moderately or highly complex testing laboratories, the test record system (Section 493.1107) must provide documentation as listed under the test requisition section and including the following:

- Patient's identification number, accession number, or other unique identification of the specimen
- The date and time of specimen receipt into the laboratory
- The condition and supposition of specimens that do not meet the laboratory's criteria for specimen acceptability
- Records and dates of all specimen testing, including the identity of the personnel who performed the test(s), which are necessary to ensure proper identification and accurate reporting of patient test results

Other sections of the CLIA that are relevant to blood collection include subpart K and subpart M.

Subpart K: Quality Control

Section 493.1201 General Quality Control. The laboratory must establish and follow written quality control procedures for monitoring and evaluating the quality of the analytic testing process of each method to ensure the accuracy and reliability of patient test results and reports.

Section 493.1204 Standard: Facilities. The laboratory must provide the space and environmental conditions necessary for conducting the services offered (including space, ventilation, utilities, and safety precautions for protection against physical hazards and biohazardous materials).

Section 493.1205 Standard: Test Methods. The laboratory must utilize test methods, equipment, instrumentation, reagents, materials, and supplies that provide accurate and reliable test results and test reports.

Section 493.1211 Standard: Procedure Manual. (1) A written procedure manual for the performance of all analytic methods used by the laboratory must be readily available and followed by all laboratory personnel. (2) The procedure manual must include, when applicable to the test procedure, requirements for specimen collection and processing, and criteria for specimen rejection.

Section 493.1215 Standard: Equipment Maintenance and Function Checks. The laboratory must perform equipment maintenance and function checks that include electronic, mechanical, and operational checks of equipment, instruments, and test systems to ensure accurate and reliable test results and reports.

Section 493.1221 Standard: Quality Control Records. The laboratory must document and maintain records of all quality control activities. (See Chapter 15, Total Quality Management, for methodology to comply with CLIA '88.)

Subpart M: Personnel

Section 493.1423 Standard: Testing Personnel Qualifications. Personnel must possess a current license issued by the state in which the laboratory is located, if such licensing is required; must have earned a high school diploma or its equivalent; and must have documentation of training that ensures that the individual has the skills required for proper specimen collection, including preparation, if applicable; labeling; handling; preservation or fixation; processing or preparation; transportation; and storage of specimens.[12]

✓ Key Terms

ADMINISTRATIVE LAW

ASSAULT

BATTERY

BREACH OF DUTY

CENTERS FOR DISEASE CONTROL AND PREVENTION (CDC)

CHAIN-OF-CUSTODY FORM

CIVIL LAW

CLINICAL LABORATORY IMPROVEMENT AMENDMENTS (CLIA)

CRIMINAL ACTIONS

DEFENDANT

DEPOSITION

DISCOVERY

ENVIRONMENTAL PROTECTION AGENCY (EPA)

EVIDENCE

EXPERT WITNESS

FALSE IMPRISONMENT

FELONY

FOOD AND DRUG ADMINISTRATION (FDA)

FORENSIC SPECIMENS

HEALTH CARE FINANCING ADMINISTRATION (HCFA)

IMPLIED CONSENT

INFORMED CONSENT

INVASION OF PRIVACY

JUDICIAL LAW

LIABLE

LITIGATION PROCESS

MALPRACTICE

MEDICAL RECORDS

MISDEMEANOR

NATIONAL INSTITUTE ON DRUG ABUSE

NEGLIGENCE

PATIENT CONFIDENTIALITY

PLAINTIFF

PREVENTIVE LAW

RESPONDEAT SUPERIOR

RISK MANAGEMENT

STANDARD OF CARE

STATUTE OF LIMITATIONS

STATUTORY LAW

TORT

VICARIOUS LIABILITY

Study Questions

For the following, choose the ONE best answer:

1. The legal term for improper or unskillful care of a patient by a member of the health care team, or any professional misconduct, unreasonable lack of skill, or infidelity in professional or judiciary duties is

    a. a misdemeanor
    b. malpractice
    c. litigation
    d. liability

2. What are the factors, or key points, that must be considered in alleged negligence cases?
    1. duty
    2. breach of duty
    3. proximate causation
    4. damages

    a. 1, 2, and 3 are correct
    b. 1 and 3 are correct
    c. 2 and 4 are correct
    d. only 4 is correct
    e. all are correct

3. One agency affecting regulations on blood collection is the HCFA, which stands for

    a. Home Care Financing Administration
    b. Health Care Financing Administration
    c. Health Care Financial Agency
    d. Health Care Funding Agency

4. Which of the following legal branches writes regulations that enforce the laws?

    a. administrative branch
    b. judicial branch
    c. US Supreme Court
    d. executive branch

5. The avoidance of legal conflicts in blood collection through education and planning is called

    a. administrative law
    b. executive law
    c. preventive law
    d. preparatory law

6. A child who refused to have his blood drawn was locked in a room by a phlebotomist and was forced to have his blood collected. This scenario is an example of

    a. invasion of privacy
    b. informed consent
    c. a misdemeanor
    d. assault and battery

7. The standard of care currently used in malpractice legal cases involving health care providers is based on the conduct of the average health care provider in the

   a. state
   b. city
   c. national community
   d. local community

8. The voluntary permission by a patient to allow touching, examination, and/or treatment by health care providers is

   a. implied consent
   b. assault and battery
   c. battery
   d. informed consent

9. Which of the following evaluates the safety, clinical efficacy, and medical efficacy of the equipment and supplies used in blood collection?

   a. EPA
   b. OSHA
   c. CDC
   d. FDA

10. When a specimen is collected for toxicological studies involving drug abuse testing, it is what type of specimen?

   a. FDA specimen
   b. forensic specimen
   c. CDC specimen
   d. fulgurate specimen

REFERENCES

1. Richards EP, Rathburn KC: *Law and the Physician*. Boston, Little, Brown and Company, 1993.
2. Curran WJ, Hall MA, Kaye DH: *Health Care Law, Forensic Science, and Public Policy*. Boston, Little, Brown and Company, 1990.
3. Rakich JS, Longest BB, Darr K: *Managing Health Services Organizations*. Baltimore, Health Professions Press, 1992.
4. *Parker v. Port Huron Hospital*, 105, N.W. 2d 854 (1981).
5. Brent NJ: Confidentiality and HIV status: The nurse's right to know. *Home Healthcare Nurse* 8(3):6–8, 1990.
6. Jones AW, Jonsson K-A, Korfeldt L: Differences between capillary and venous blood alcohol concentrations as a function of time after drinking, with emphasis on sampling variations in left vs. right arm. *Clin Chem* 35:400, 1989.
7. Bittikofer J: Toxicology, in Bishop M, Duben-Engelkirk J, Fody E (eds): *Clinical Chemistry: Principles, Procedures, Correlations*. Philadelphia, J.B. Lippincott, 1992, pp 599–613.
8. Aoun H: When a house officer gets AIDS. *N Engl J Med* 321(10):695, 1989.
9. Pozgar GD: *Legal Aspects of Health Care Administration*. Gaithersburg, MD, Aspen Publishers, 1993.
10. Troyer GT, Salman SL: *Handbook of Health Care Risk Management*. Rockville, MD, Aspen Publishers, 1986.

11. Bunting RF: Risk management and prevention in the clinical laboratory. *Clin Lab Sci* 5 (Jan/Feb):1, 35–37, 1992.
12. Department of Health and Human Services (DHHS), Health Care Financing Administration (HCFA), Public Health Service: 42 CFR 405 *et seq,* 57 FR 7002-7186, Feb 28, 1992.

Phlebotomy Case Study

COMMUNICATION

Ms. Nancy Garcia, a 78-year-old Hispanic female, was admitted to River Bend Hospital as a result of complications from diabetes mellitus. When the health care worker arrived to her hospital room to collect blood for laboratory tests, he introduced himself and asked her name. She did not respond and looked perplexed.

Questions:

1. What should the health care worker do next?
2. What could a health care facility provide to assist in this situation?

appendix

BASIC REQUESTS IN ENGLISH AND SPANISH

The following translations are designed to present the health care worker with a *very basic* means of communicating with patients who speak Spanish. Before speaking with patients, the health care worker should practice using these phrases with someone who knows the correct pronunciation. Otherwise, the patient may become even more confused. Another alternative is to have the key phrases printed on cards that the health care worker may point to or use as a reference when he or she is communicating with the patient.

English	Spanish
one	uno
two	dos
three	tres
four	cuatro
five	cinco
six	seis
seven	siete
eight	ocho
nine	nueve
ten	diez
twenty	veinte
thirty	treinta
forty	cuarenta
fifty	cincuenta
sixty	sesenta
seventy	setenta
eighty	ochenta
ninety	noventa
one hundred	ciento

Hello.	Hola.
Good day.	Buenos dias.
Good morning.	Buenos dias.
Good afternoon.	Buenas tardes.
Good evening.	Buenas noches.
Mother	Madre/mama
Father	Padre/papa
Sister	Hermana
Brother	Hermano
Son	Hijo
Daughter	Hija
Husband	Esposo/marido
Wife	Esposa
Infant/baby	Niño/niña
Grandfather	Abuelo
Grandmother	Abuela
Friend	Amigo/Amiga
Mister	Señor
Mrs.	Señora
Miss	Señorita
Doctor	Doctor
Nurse	Enfermera
My name is . . .	Me llamo . . .
I work in the laboratory.	Trabejo en el laboratorio.
I speak . . .	Hablo . . .
We are going to analyze	Vamos analizar
. . . your blood.	. . . su sangre.
. . . your urine.	. . . su orina.
. . . your sputum.	. . . su esputo
Do you understand?	Entiende Usted (ud.)?
I do not understand.	No entiendo.
Please (pls.)	Por favor (p.f.)
Thank you.	Gracias.
You are welcome.	De nada.
Speak slower, pls.	Hable mas despacio, p.f.
Repeat, pls.	Haga me el/favor de repetir.
Relax.	Relajese.
What is your name?	Como se llama?
What is your address?	Su domicilio?
What is your birth date?	En que fecha nacio?
How old are you?	Cuantos años tiene ud.?
Have you been here before?	Ha estado ud. aquí antes?
Who is your doctor?	Quien es su doctor?

Your doctor wrote the order.	El doctor/la doctora escribio la orden.
Here is the bathroom.	Aquí esta el baño.
Here is the call light.	Aquí esta la luz de emergencia.
You may not eat/drink anything except water.	No debe de comer/beber nada solamente agua.
You may not smoke.	No puede fumar.
Have you had breakfast?	Ya tomo el desayuno?
We need a blood/urine/stool sample.	Necesitamos una muestra de su sangre/orina/del excremento.
Please	Haga me el favor de (or Por favor . . .)
. . . make a fist.	. . . cerrar el puño.
. . . bend your arm.	. . . doblar el brazo.
. . . roll up your sleeve.	. . . levantarse la manga.
. . . open your hand.	. . . abrir la mano.
. . . sit down here.	. . . sientese aquí.
. . . change your position.	. . . cambiarse de posición.
. . . turn over.	. . . voltearse.
. . . change to the left.	. . . cambiarse a la izquierda.
. . . change to the right.	. . . cambiarse a la derecha.
I need to	Necesito
. . . take a blood sample.	. . . sacar sangre.
. . . stick/prick your finger.	. . . picarle su dedo.
It will hurt a little	Le va a doler un poquito.
The needle will stay in your arm while I am collecting the blood sample.	La aguja se quedara en su brazo durante el tiempo necessario para obtener la muestra.
I am finished.	Ya termine.
Press this gauze on your arm/finger until I can make sure that the bleeding has stopped.	Comprese esta banda en su brazo su dedo hasta que pare la sangre.
Are you lightheaded?	Esta usted mareado?
Do you feel as if you are going to faint?	Se siente como si se va a desmayar?
You must lie down.	Necesita acostarse.
Collect the midstream portion of the urine in the container or bottle.	Coleccione la porción del medio de la orina en el vaso.

2

UNITS OF MEASUREMENT AND SYMBOLS

α	alpha
Å	angstrom
amp	ampere (unit of electric current)
c	centi- (10^{-2})
°C	degrees Centigrade or Celsius (unit of temperature; convert to Fahrenheit by multiplying by 1.8 and adding 32)
cc	cubic centimeter (same as mL, 1/1000 L)
cd	candela (unit of luminous intensity)
cm	centimeter
cu mm	cubic millimeter
d	deci- (10^{-1})
da	deca- (10^{1})
dL	deciliter (1/10 of a liter)
°F	degrees Fahrenheit (unit of temperature; convert to Centigrade by subtracting 32 and multiplying by 0.555)
g or gm	gram (1/1000 of a kilogram, unit of mass)
G%	grams in 100 mL
h	hecto- (10^{2})
hpf	high-power field on microscope
IU	international unit
k	kilo- (10^{3})
°K	degrees Kelvin (thermodynamic temperature; convert to Centigrade by subtracting 273.15)
kg	kilogram (1000 g, or 2.2 lb)
L	liter (1000 mL or 1000 cc, unit of volume)
lpf	low-power field on microscope
μ	micro- (10^{-6})
μci	microcurie (1/1000 mCi)
μg or mcg	microgram (1/1000 mg)
μm	micron

m	meter (unit of length)
m	milli- (10^{-3})
mCi	millicurie
mEq or meq	milliequivalent
mg or mgm	milligram ($\frac{1}{1000}$ g)
mg%	milligrams in 100 mL (same as dL)
min	minutes
mIU	milli–international unit ($\frac{1}{1000}$ IU)
mL	milliliter ($\frac{1}{1000}$ L, same as cc)
mm	millimeter ($\frac{1}{10}$ cm)
mm^3	cubic millimeter
mm Hg	millimeters of mercury
mmole	millimole
mol, M	mole (unit of substance)
mOsm	milliosmol
N	normality
n	nano- (10^{-9})
ng	nanogram ($\frac{1}{1000}$ mg)
p	pico- (10^{-12})
pg	picogram ($\frac{1}{1000}$ ng)
QNS	quantity not sufficient
sec or s	second (unit of time)
SI	international system
sp *g*	specific gravity
U	international enzyme unit
WNL	within normal limits
WNR	within normal range
wt	weight
w/v	weight/volume
$\cong$	approximately
$\leq$	less than or equal to
$\geq$	greater than or equal to
+ or (+)	positive
− or (−)	negative
$\sum$	summation

3

METRIC CONVERSION CHART

LENGTH

1 inch (in.) = 2.54 centimeters (cm)
1 foot (ft) = 30.48 centimeters (cm)
39.37 inches (in.) = 1 meter (m)
1 mile (mi) = 1.61 kilometers (km)

MASS

1 ounce (oz) = 28.35 grams (g)
1 pound (lb) = 453.6 grams (g)
2.205 pounds (lb) = 1 kilogram (kg)

VOLUME

1 fluid ounce (fl oz) = 29.57 milliliters (mL)
1.057 quarts (qt) = 1 liter (liter or L)
1 gallon (gal) = 3.78 liters (liter or L)

appendix

4

FORMULAS AND CALCULATIONS

Area | square meter (sq m or m^2)
Clearance | liter/second (L/s)
Concentration and conversions |
   Mass | kilogram/liter (kg/L)
   Substrate | mole/liter (mol/L)

% w/v to M or vice versa:

$$M = \frac{\% \text{ w/v} \times 10}{\text{molecular wt (mol wt)}}$$

% w/v to N or vice versa:

$$N = \frac{\% \text{ w/v} \times 10}{\text{eq wt}}$$

mg/dL to mEq/L or vice versa:

$$\text{mEq/L} = \frac{\text{mg/dL} \times 10}{\text{eq wt}}$$

M to N:

$$N = M \times \text{valence}$$

N to M:

$$M = \frac{N}{\text{valence}}$$

Density | kilogram/liter (kg/L)
Dilutions | Final concentration = Original concentration $\times$ dilution 1 $\times$ dilution 2, and so forth
Electrical potential | volt (V) = kg m^2/s^3A

Energy	joule (J) = kg m^2/s^2
Force	Newton (N) = kg m^2/s^2
Frequency	hertz (Hz) = 1 cycle/s
Hematology math	Mean corpuscular volume (MCV) = average volume of red blood cells (RBCs); expressed in cubic microns (μm^3) or femtoliters (fL)

$$MCV = \frac{Hct \times 10}{RBC \text{ count (in millions)}}$$

Hct = hematocrit value

Mean corpuscular hemoglobin (MCH) = Average weight of hemoglobin in RBC; expressed in picograms (pg)

$$MCH = \frac{hgb \text{ (g)} \times 10}{RBC \text{ count (in millions)}}$$

hgb = hemoglobin value

Mean corpuscular hemoglobin concentration = Hemoglobin concentration of average RBC

$$MCHC = \frac{hgb \text{ (g)}}{Hct} \times 100\%$$

RBC distribution width (RDW) = numerical expression of variation of RBC size, dispersion of RBC volumes about the mean

$$RDW = \frac{SD \text{ (standard deviation)} \text{ of RBC size}}{MCV}$$

Pressure	Pascal (Pa) = (kg/m)s^2
Quality control math	
Variance (s^2)	$s^2 = \dfrac{(x - \bar{x})^2}{n - 1}$
Standard deviation(s)	$s = \sqrt{s^2}$
% Coefficient of variation	$\%CV = \dfrac{s}{x} \times 100$
Relative centrifugal force (rcf)	Measures force of centrifugation acting on blood components and allowing them to separate. Can be used to calibrate centrifuges.

rcf = 1.118 × 10^{-5} × r × n^2
r = rotating radius (centimeters)
n = speed of rotation (revolutions per minute)

Solutions	Specific gravity (sp g):

$$\text{sp } g = \frac{\text{wt of solid or liquid}}{\text{wt of equal volume of } H_2O \text{ at } 4°C}$$

Temperature

Celsius or Centigrade ($°C = K - 273.15$; $°C = °F - 32 \times 0.555$)

Kelvin $°K = °C + 273.15$ or $\frac{5}{9} (°F) + 255.35$

Fahrenheit $°F = (°C \times 1.8) + 32$

Volume
deciliter (dL) $= \frac{1}{10}$ of a liter
10 dL $= 1$ L
centiliter (cL) $= \frac{1}{100}$ of a liter
100 cL $= 10$ dL $= 1$ L
milliliter (mL) $= \frac{1}{1000}$ of a liter
1000 mL $= 100$ cL $= 10$ dL $= 1$ L

SELF STUDY AND CASE ANSWERS

CHAPTER 1

1. a
2. b
3. c
4. a
5. b
6. a, b
7. b, c, d
8. c
9. c
10. b

CHAPTER 2

1. a, b, c
2. c
3. b
4. a, b, c, d, e
5. a, b

6. a, b, d
7. b
8. c
9. d
10. b, c

CHAPTER 3

1. a, b, c
2. a
3. a, c
4. a
5. c, d, e
6. a, b, c, d
7. c
8. b
9. d
10. a, b, c, d

PHLEBOTOMY CASE STUDY: DORSAL HAND COLLECTION

1. *Dorsal* (proximal) refers to the back of the hand in this case. The anterior hand or wrist should not be used for venipuncture.

2. *Supine* means lying on the back, face upward.

3. An orthopedic floor is for patients with bone and joint disorders.

CHAPTER 4

1. a, b, c
2. d
3. a
4. b
5. c
6. b
7. a
8. a, b, c
9. c

CHAPTER 5

1. b, c
2. a, b, d
3. b
4. a, c, d
5. b, c
6. b, d
7. d
8. a
9. a, b, c, d
10. a, b

CHAPTER 6

1. a, b, c
2. b, d
3. c, d
4. a, b, c, d
5. b, c
6. b, c, d
7. b, c
8. b
9. a, b, c, d
10. c

CHAPTER 7

1. a, c, d
2. b, d
3. a, b, c, d
4. c
5. c
6. b
7. b
8. a
9. a
10. a, b, c

PHLEBOTOMY CASE STUDY: HOME CARE COLLECTIONS

1. | *Laboratory Assay* | *Color of Blood Collection Tube Top* |
   |---|---|
   | Calcium, ionized | green |
   | APTT | light blue |
   | CBC count | purple |
   | Protime | light blue |
   | Chemistry screen | red or red-speckled |
   | Digoxin | red or red-speckled |
   | Plasma potassium | green |

2. The order of draw was incorrect for blood vacuum tube collections. The correct order should have been red, light blue, green, and purple. The correct order prevents contamination of nonadditive tubes by additive tubes, as well as cross-contamination between the different anticoagulants.

3. The order of draw was incorrect for the syringe method. The green-topped tube should have been filled first so that the blood could immediately be mixed with the anticoagulant to prevent clotting. Then, the remaining blood should have been placed in the red or red-speckled tube to clot.

CHAPTER 8

1. a, b
2. b, d
3. a, b, d
4. c
5. a, d
6. d
7. b
8. a, b
9. a, b, d
10. c
11. b, c
12. b, d

CHAPTER 9

1. c
2. c
3. d
4. a
5. d
6. c
7. a
8. b
9. a
10. b

CHAPTER 10

1. c
2. d
3. b
4. c
5. d
6. b
7. b
8. a
9. a
10. c

CHAPTER 11

1. b
2. b
3. c
4. c
5. c
6. b
7. b
8. c
9. b
10. b

PHLEBOTOMY CASE STUDY: BEDSIDE GLUCOSE TESTING

1. The problem in this bedside glucose testing case is that the patient's meter was reading outside the control confidence limits. Thus, the glucose results are out of control and not considered accurate or reliable.

2. The phlebotomist, the nurse, and other health care providers involved in the bedside glucose testing for this patient should troubleshoot for

   a. Correct timing of the analytic procedure

   b. Reagents and controls stored at correct temperature and within appropriate expiration dates.

   c. Instrument blotting or wiping technique performed according to manufacturer's directions.

In this case, the control solution had expired March 2, 1995.

CHAPTER 12

1. d
2. b, c, d
3. b, c
4. a, b, c, d, e
5. b
6. b
7. c
8. c
9. b, c, d
10. b

CHAPTER 13

1. c, d
2. a, b, d
3. b, c, d
4. b
5. a, c, d
6. a, b, c, d
7. b
8. c
9. b
10. b

CHAPTER 14

1. a, b, c, d
2. a, b, c, d
3. c
4. a, b, c

5. a, b, c, d
6. b
7. a
8. c

PHLEBOTOMY CASE STUDY: NEWBORN NURSERY COLLECTIONS

1. Blood collected from a baby for a bilirubin determination should be collected in an amber microcollection tube or a tube covered with foil so that the microcollection tube is not exposed to light. Light breaks down bilirubin.

2. Because bilirubin breaks down in the presence of light, the longer a blood specimen is exposed to light, the more bilirubin is broken down. Thus, the bilirubin value will be falsely decreased.

3. Probably, the phlebotomist who collected Baby McPherson's blood on Sunday morning collected the blood in a clear microcollection tube and allowed it to remain in direct light for an extended period prior to delivering it to the clinical laboratory.

CHAPTER 15

1. a, b, c, d
2. a, b, c, d
3. a, b, c
4. a, b, c, d
5. a, c, d

CHAPTER 16

1. b, c
2. a, b, c, d
3. b, c, d
4. b, d
5. a, b, c, d

CHAPTER 17

1. b
2. e
3. b
4. d
5. c
6. d
7. c
8. d
9. d
10. b

PHLEBOTOMY CASE STUDY: COMMUNICATION

1. The phlebotomist should check with the floor nurse to determine whether Ms. Garcia speaks English and/or whether she has a hearing disability. If the patient speaks only Spanish, an interpreter or a written description of the phlebotomy procedure should be available in Spanish to assist in this situation. If the patient has a hearing disability, efforts should be made to write down instructions for the patient.

2. If a patient has a hearing disability, writing tools should be kept at the bedside of the patient. If a large segment of the patient population speaks another language, the hospital should provide interpreters who know the basic use of that language. Also, instruction sheets on phlebotomy steps should be made available in other languages for patients who do not speak English.

INDEX